TRENDS IN ANGIOGENESIS RESEARCH

TRENDS IN ANGIOGENESIS RESEARCH

Roberta V. Zubar
Editor

Nova Biomedical Books
New York

For permission to use material from this book please contact us:
Telephone 631-231-7269; Fax 631-231-8175
Web Site: http://www.novapublishers.com

LIBRARY OF CONGRESS CATALOGING-IN-PUBLICATION DATA:
Available Upon Request

ISBN: 1-59454-452-2

Published by Nova Science Publishers, Inc. ✦ New York

Contents

Preface		**vii**
Chapter I	Proteolytic Fragments of Extracellular Matrix Components as Angiogenic Regulators *A. R. Clamp and G. C. Jayson*	**1**
Chapter II	Studies of the Endothelial Cell-Specific Signal Transduction Pathways (New Paradigm for the Development of Potent anti-angiogenic Therapies) *Shigeru Kanda, Yasuyoshi Miyata and Hiroshi Kanetake*	**43**
Chapter III	Hormonal Effects on Endometrial Angiogenesis *Gareth C Weston, Jane E Girling, Caroline E Gargett and Peter AW Rogers*	**71**
Chapter IV	Software-Supported Quantification of Angiogenesis in an in vitro Culture System. Examples of Applications in Studies of Basic Research, Biocompatibility and Drug Discovery *Kirsten Peters, Harald Schmidt, Günter Kamp, Ronald E. Unge, Bettina Hoffmann, Frauke Stenzel, Günter Ziegler, Manfred Jung, Susanne Stumpf and C. James Kirkpatrick*	**103**
Chapter V	Restin, A Potent Angiogenesis Inhibitor Derived from Type XV Collagen *Ren Xu and Ren-Bao Gan*	**125**
Chapter VI	Endothelial Cell Adhesion Molecules, Inflammation and Atherosclerosis in Chronic Renal Failure *Aikaterini Papagianni and Dimitrios Memmos*	**139**
Chapter VII	The Effects of the Endothelins - An Angiogenic Family of Molecules - In Solid Cancers *Matthew J. Grimshaw*	**153**

Chapter VIII Vascular Endothelial Growth Factor and Breast Cancer **183**
Danila Coradini and Maria Grazia Daidone

Chapter IX Involvement of Erythropoietin in Angiogenesis of Normal and Malignant Tissues of Female Reproductive Organs **211**
Yoshiko Yasuda

Index **243**

PREFACE

The development of a neovasculature is vital for tumour growth and metastasis and has been a major target for novel drugs. Much research in the last decade has focused on the identification of endogenous angiogenesis inhibitors and to date more than half of those identified have been cryptic proteolytic fragments of extracellular matrix proteins. In Chapter I, the authors describe the proteolytic pathways generating these angiogenic regulators and summarise the research that has been conducted elucidating their potential mechanisms of action.

Angiogenesis plays pivotal roles in pathophysiological conditions, such as solid tumor growth, ischemic retinopathy, and collateral formation after the occlusion of arteries. Inhibition of angiogenesis is anticipated to control human advanced malignant tumors. In animal studies, various anti-angiogenic strategies significantly reduce the size of preexisting, transplanted tumors, or retard the growth of tumors, leading to the extension of survival of tumor-bearing animals. However, in humans, almost no anti-angiogenic agent has solely been reported to cause regression of advanced tumors and only a few clinical studies showed enhanced survival of patients. In Chapter II, the authors discuss the impact of attenuation of the anti-angiogenic actions by particular agents and the possible studies that could solve these problems.

Angiogenesis in the endometrium occurs in a cyclic manner under the influence of the steroid hormones estrogen and progesterone. Whether effects by these hormones on the endothelial cells are direct, indirect, or a combination of both, is unclear. In addition, little is known of the mechanisms by which estrogen and progesterone influence angiogenesis in the endometrium. In Chapter III, the authors describe their work examining possible direct and indirect effects of these hormones on endometrial angiogenesis.

Angiogenesis is regulated by complex interactions between endothelial cells and other cell types such as macrophages, fibroblasts, and smooth muscle cells. These intercellular interactions are mediated by cellular compounds such as cytokines, growth factors and extracellular matrix molecules. Although a large number of angiogenic and anti-angiogenic factors have been identified, knowledge concerning the regulation of the dynamic, highly complex and multi-step angiogenic process is incomplete. Due to this complexity studies on angiogenesis in vivo often do not allow insight into cell-specific aspects and a distinction between direct and indirect effects of possible modulators cannot be accurately made. In

Chapter IV, the authors describe examples of the application of this model system to examine the effects of biological factors, the effects of pharmacological compounds and the use of this model system in biocompatibility testing.

As reported in Chapter V, extracellular matrix (ECM) has been found to be involved in the regulation of angiogenesis, thus making ECM a candidate source of angiogenesis inhibitors. Recently several angiogenesis inhibitors have been identified from ECM components, including endostain, restin, tumstatin, canstatin, and vastatin. These data indicate that restin is able to inhibit angiogenesis both in vitro and in vivo, and that it also has a potential anti-tumor activity.

Atherosclerotic cardiovascular disease is greatly increased in patients with chronic renal failure (CRF) and contribute to the high mortality rate observed in these patients. The prevalence of atherosclerotic disease is especially marked in patients undergoing renal replacement therapy but the probable effect of hemodialysis (HD) treatment is not yet established. In Chapter VI, the authors report the research results of adhesion molecule ICAM-1, VCAM-1 and E-selectin levels and atherosclerotic vascular changes, as assessed by high resolution ultrasonography of the common carotid arteries, in patients with stage 5 CRF prior to the start of renal replacement therapy. Further research aimed at identifying novel markers of atherosclerosis would provide additional targets for preventive and therapeutic interventions in this high-risk population.

Endothelins are a family of small, structurally related, vasoactive peptides that have a variety of physiological roles in many tissues. The association between endothelins, poor prognosis and angiogenesis may mean that the endothelin axis is a valid therapeutic target for the treatment of several types of solid tumours. Chapter VII summarises the authors current knowledge of the role of endothelins in angiogenesis in solid tumours and discusses the potential further directions of such research as well as the possibility of anti-endothelin-based therapy of cancer.

Angiogenesis is a complex multi-step process leading to the formation of new blood vessels from the existing vascular network. It is normally well regulated in the adult, where angiogenesis occurs transiently only during development, wound healing and in the female reproductive cycle. Otherwise, abnormal angiogenesis can occur during the pathogenesis of certain chronic diseases such as diabetes, rheumatoid arthritis, psoriasis and tumor, including breast cancer. In Chapter VIII, the authors first discuss the biological role of hypoxia- or estrogen-dependent angiogenesis on breast cancer development and the relationship between some angiogenesis-related biomarkers with some other important pathobiologic characteristics of the tumor including histotype, hormone-responsiveness, cell proliferation and expression of pro- and anti-apoptotic factors.

There is increasing evidence that the glycoprotein erythropoietin plays a role other than in erythropoiesis. We have found that erythropoietin and its receptor are expressed in human malignancies and that the signaling promotes not only tumorigenesis but also angiogenesis. In Chapter IX, four items are described to analyze the role of erythropoietin in normal and malignant ovarian and uterine tissues with special reference to the vascular formation.

In: Trends in Angiogenesis Research
Editor: Roberta V. Zubar, pp. 1-41

ISBN 1-59454-452-2

Chapter I

PROTEOLYTIC FRAGMENTS OF EXTRACELLULAR MATRIX COMPONENTS AS ANGIOGENIC REGULATORS

A. R. Clamp* and G. C. Jayson
Cancer Research UK Department of Medical Oncology, Christie Hospital, Manchester, United Kingdom

ABSTRACT

The development of a neovasculature is vital for tumour growth and metastasis and has been a major target for novel drugs. Much research in the last decade has focused on the identification of endogenous angiogenesis inhibitors and to date more than half of those identified have been cryptic proteolytic fragments of extracellular matrix proteins. These include angiostatin, a fragment of plasminogen, products derived from fibronectin and thrombospondin and a series of fragments cleaved from the non-collagenous domains of basement membrane collagens. In this chapter, we will describe the proteolytic pathways generating these angiogenic regulators and summarise the research that has been conducted elucidating their potential mechanisms of action. Using endostatin, a C-terminal fragment of collagen XVIII, as a paradigm we will then discuss possible reasons for the relative lack of anti-tumour activity of these molecules in early clinical trials compared to results obtained in the laboratory.

Key words: Angiogenesis, Clinical trials, Collagen XV, Collagen XVIII, Endostatin, Extracellular matrix, Tumstatin

---

* Correspondence concerning this article should be addressed to Dr. AR Clamp, Cancer Research UK Department of Medical Oncology, Christie Hospital, Wilmslow Road, Manchester, M20 4BX, United Kingdom.

1. Introduction

Angiogenesis, the development of a neovasculature from pre-existing blood vessels is vital for tumour growth and metastasis. Without a blood supply, neoplastic deposits remain dependent on diffusion for nutrients, oxygenation and the removal of waste metabolites. Their growth is therefore restricted to a maximum of 1-2mm^3 and they remain clinically quiescent[1].

Interactions between the extracellular matrix (ECM) and endothelial cells play key roles in angiogenesis and it is of particular interest that cryptic proteolytic fragments of ECM proteins have been identified as endogenous angiogenesis inhibitors. Fragments of fibronectin[2], perlecan[3], thrombospondin[4] and most importantly the basement membrane collagens IV, VIII, XV and XVIII[5] inhibit endothelial cell proliferation and migration and many of these molecules have shown anti-tumour activity in *in vivo* model systems.

However, the mechanisms of action and cell surface receptors recognised by many of these molecules are poorly elucidated and in the case of endostatin, the cleaved first non-collagenous domain of collagen XVIII, despite extensive research many potential mechanisms and binding partners have been proposed.

In this review we will discuss the current research findings detailing angiogenesis inhibitors derived from ECM proteins and their mechanisms of action. We will then focus on the development of endostatin as a 'drug' and try to highlight possible reasons for the low levels of activity seen in the early phase clinical trials that have been reported to date.

2. Physiological Versus Tumour Angiogenesis

Physiological angiogenesis only occurs in areas of active wound healing and during menstruation. After initial vasodilatation and subsequent increased vascular permeability of an existing vessel, there is proteolysis of the underlying basement membrane and interstitial matrix, loss of endothelial cell adhesion and subsequent cell proliferation and migration. This process is assisted by the influx of endothelial cell precursors from the bone marrow (vasculogenesis). Finally, the endothelial cells re-adhere to form capillary tubes which mature by synthesis of a new basement membrane and recruitment of pericytes and smooth muscle cells. These tubes then anastomose to form part of the functional circulation[6,7].

This process is tightly controlled by a series of pro-angiogenic and anti-angiogenic factors that are normally balanced holding the angiogenic switch in an off position[8]. Tumour angiogenesis is however characterised by the uncoordinated secretion of a multiplicity of proangiogenic factors[9]. This results in the tumour vasculature being structurally and functionally abnormal. The vessels are tortuous and dilated with excessive branching and shunts and often lack functional perivascular cells. It has also been reported that up to 15% of cells lining vessels in xenografted tumours and spontaneous human colon carcinomas are tumour-derived. Whether this is due to apoptosis of host endothelial cells or the adoption of a vascular phenotype ('vasculogenic mimcry') by malignant cells is unclear[10-12].

2.1. Angiogenesis and the Extracellular Matrix

The ECM is composed of secreted proteins and polysaccharides that assemble into an organised meshwork. Whilst the main structural integrity of the ECM is provided by a family of more than 20 collagens and proteoglycans, connections between these molecules and the cell surface are also facilitated by tenascins and fibronectin amongst others[13]. Transmembrane signalling through integrins then enables the ECM to play crucial roles in controlling cell development, proliferation, migration and function[14]. Of key interest with respect to angiogenesis is the vascular basement membrane (VBM). This thin sheet of highly specialized ECM exists at the endothelial/ mesenchymal interface and consists primarily of interacting but independent scaffolds of laminins and type IV collagens[15,16]. These two networks are bridged by nidogens/entactins but also interact with the heparan sulfate proteoglycan perlecan[17] and other minor components of the VBM such as the fibulins and type XV and XVIII collagens[15]. Many different isoforms of these proteins exist- for instance there are at least 6 different type IV collagen α chains [5] and 12 different laminins[13]. These isoforms have overlapping but distinct properties which means that their patterns of expression can be used to control organ-specific endothelial cell behaviour.

Whilst in contact with mature VBM, endothelial cells are quiescent, indicating that signals arising from this highly crosslinked structure inhibit proliferation and facilitate cell-cell adhesion[15]. In the presence of pro-angiogenic growth factors- for instance vascular endothelial growth factor (VEGF) or fibroblast growth factor-2 (FGF-2), there is production of enzymes- in particular the matrix metalloproteases (MMPs) [18] and heparanase[19] by activated stromal and endothelial cells. As well as degrading the VBM, so removing a physical barrier to endothelial cell migration, these enzymes release sequestered ECM stores of VEGF and FGF-2 further stimulating the angiogenic process and expose cryptic epitopes on VBM proteins to endothelial cells. These epitopes, which may remain *in situ* as part of the degraded protein within the VBM or be released as proteolytic fragments, can have pro- or anti-angiogenic effects. For example, a monoclonal antibody directed against a pro-angiogenic epitope in proteolytically-denatured type IV collagen binds to the VBM in tumour blood vessels and effectively inhibits angiogenesis *in vivo* possibly by blocking an $\alpha_v\beta_3$ integrin- binding site not exposed in native type IV collagen[20]. More than 20 laminin sequences have also been identified as having angiogenic modulating properties when assayed as synthetic peptides[21]. Whether these all have physiological roles as cryptic epitopes is not yet clear and it should be noted that many of these sequences have been generated from laminin-1 rather than laminins-8 and -10 the major VBM laminins[22].

Whilst the identification of cryptic epitopes *in situ* within the ECM has proven difficult, many proteolytic fragments of both ECM and other proteins have been shown to have anti-angiogenic properties and these will be discussed below.

2.2. Proteolytic Fragments as Angiogenesis Inhibitors

The isolation of internal proteolytic fragments with the ability to inhibit angiogenesis derived from proteins without physiological effects on endothelial cells has been a fruitful field of research in the last twenty years. In 1985, Homanberg et al isolated 29 and 40kDa fibronectin fragments that inhibited endothelial cell proliferation[23] and subsequently a 16kDa N-terminal proteolytic fragment of prolactin was also shown to inhibit angiogenesis in the chick chorioallantoic membrane assay[24].

The first truly endogenous inhibitor of angiogenesis, angiostatin was isolated in 1994[25]. This 38kDa internal fragment of plasminogen was identified based on the hypothesis that in certain clinical cases and *in vivo* tumour model systems, the presence of a large primary tumour prevents the appearance of symptomatic metastases by secreting angiogenesis inhibitors into the circulation. Whereas the production of short-lived proangiogenic agents supports the development of a functional vasculature in the primary tumour, the production of a circulating anti-angiogenic molecule with a significantly longer half-life prevents the neovascularisation of neoplastic deposits at distant sites as these microscopic colonies cannot initiate the local production of sufficient angiogenic stimulators to overcome this inhibition.

Subsequent work has proven that the first 3 Kringle domains of plasminogen have the most significant anti-angiogenic activity, inhibiting both endothelial cell proliferation and migration[26,27]. Four possible cell surface receptors for angiostatin have been identified; ATP synthase- which has been shown to play an important role in maintaining intracellular pH in endothelial cells[28,29], $\alpha_v\beta_3$ integrin[30], c-met[31] and angiomotin[32]. Analysis of the crystal structure of angiostatin supports binding to the first two of these targets via interactions with the second and third kringle domains[26].

Since the isolation of angiostatin, proteolytic fragments of several other coagulation pathway proteins have also been demonstrated to have antiangiogenic activity[33] identifying a second common and previously unidentified functional theme within this protein family. These proteins are summarised in table 1.

Table 1. Proteolytic fragments of coagulation pathway and other plasma proteins with antiangiogenic activity.

Proteolytic fragment	Plasma protein	Anti-tumour activity in animal models	Clinical trials	References
Angiostatin	Plasminogen	Y	Y	[25,182,183]
Kringle domain 5	Plasminogen	N	N	[184-186]
Fragment 2 (Kringle domain 2)	Prothrombin	Y	N	[187,188]
Cleaved form	Antithrombin	Y	N	[189]
E fragment	Fibrinogen	Y	N	[190,191]
Kininostatin (domain 5)	High molecular weight kininogen	N	N	[192]
140kDa fragment (Second and third type I repeats)	Thrombospondin-1	Y	Y	[33,64]

2.3. VBM Collagen Fragments as Anti-Angiogenic Molecules

Research has also identified several protease-resistant fragments of VBM collagens as antiangiogenic agents. The properties of these are summarised in table 2 and discussed below.

Table 2. Anti-angiogenic fragments of VBM collagens.

Proteolytic fragment	Collagen chain (NC1 domain)	Putative cell surface receptor(s)	Possible mechanisms of action	References
Arresten	α1 collagen IV	$\alpha_1\beta_1$ integrin and HSPG	Interference with Ras-Shc-MAPK signalling	[35,36]
Canstatin	α2 collagen IV	?$\alpha_v\beta_3$ integrin	Downregulation of FLIP Inhibition of PI-3K/Akt signalling	[35,38,42]
Tumstatin	α3 collagen IV	$\alpha_v\beta_3$ integrin $\alpha_6\beta_1$ integrin	Inhibition of protein synthesis via inhibition of PI-3K/Akt signalling	[43,44,51]
α6 NC1	α6 collagen IV	$\alpha_v\beta_3$ integrin	?	[35]
Vastatin	α1 Collagen VIII	?	?	[193]
Restin	α1collagen XV	?	?	[92]

3. Collagen IV

Type IV collagen is a major component of the VBM. Six genetically distinct gene products encode 6 α-chains. These chains all possess an amino terminus 7S domain followed by a long collagenous domain (about 1400 amino acids) and a C-terminal first non-collagenous (NC1) domain of c.230 amino acids. These α-chains then assemble into triple helical protomers. Although many possible combinations exist, only 3 triple helices have been identified in vivo- α1.α1.α2(IV), α3.α4.α5(IV) and α5.α5.α6(IV)[34]. These protomers then assemble into networks via interactions involving the 7S- amino termini that form tetramers and the NC1 domains which promote lateral association and dimerisation of triple helices.

The importance of basement membranes for cell differentiation and morphogenesis in diverse and ancient organisms such as Hydra vulgaris and the biological activity of collagen IV fragments in these organisms (summarised in[5]) led to the investigation of these molecules as potential antiangiogenic agents. Initial in vitro screening of all six human collagen IV NC1 domains expressed as recombinant proteins in the mammalian HEK293 cell system identified anti-angiogenic properties for the NC1 domains of the α2, α3 and α6 chains.[35] These molecules supported human umbilical vein endothelial cell (HUVEC) adhesion and migration and also decreased FGF-2-induced angiogenesis in the chick chorioallantoic membrane (CAM) assay. Growth of CS-1 melanoma cells applied to CAMs was also retarded by c.60% by a single injection of these protein fragments associated with decreased vascularity of the subsequent tumour nodules. NC1 domains of the α1, α4 and α5 chains failed to affect HUVEC behaviour or angiogenesis in this study.

3.1. Arresten and Canstatin

Further studies investigating collagen IV NC1 domains have subsequently been conducted. Arresten, the NC1 domain of collagen IV α1 when expressed as a soluble His-tagged protein in E. coli specifically inhibits calf pulmonary artery endothelial (CPAE) cell proliferation in vitro and inhibits endothelial tube formation in the Matrigel assay system in a dose-dependent manner. Further in vivo experiments showed decreased vascularisation of a matrigel plug in C57/BL6 mice and decreased growth of established tumour xenografts in response to repeated arresten administration[36]. These findings are in contrast to those documented above with a α1 NC1 expressed in a mammalian system[35]. A Scatchard analysis performed using radio-iodinated arresten on CPAE cells identified 2 binding sites, a low affinity high capacity site suggested to be cell surface heparan sulfate proteoglycan (HSPG)[37] and a high affinity low capacity site. Preincubation of HUVECs with function-blocking anti-α_1 and anti-β_1 integrin antibodies decreased arresten binding by 60-70% indicating that $\alpha_1\beta_1$ integrin may be the high affinity cell surface receptor[36]. As this integrin is involved in activation of the Ras-Shc-MAPkinase pathway this may be a possible mechanism of action for arresten.

Canstatin, the NC1 domain of the α2 chain of collagen IV has also been demonstrated to specifically inhibit endothelial cell migration and proliferation as well as tube formation in the Matrigel assay[38]. It also inhibits the growth of established tumour xenografts associated with a decrease in CD31-positive tumour-associated vasculature. Initial investigations indicated that canstatin promotes endothelial cell apoptosis,[38] a function that appears to be controlled by the N-terminal 89 amino acids[39]. It has now been demonstrated that this is associated with a decrease in cytoplasmic levels of FLIP, an anti-apoptotic protein that is a structural homologue of procaspases 8 and 10. FLIP competes with these proteases for recruitment to the cell membrane but lacks a critical cysteine residue[40] in its active site and so does not induce the downstream events that lead to apoptosis but activates pathways associated with apoptosis resistance[41]. FLIP downregulation by canstatin is caused by both decreased gene expression and also decreased protein synthesis[42]. Whereas the interactions with cell surface integrins is not as clearly delineated for canstatin as for arresten, HUVEC binding to immobilised collagen IV α2 NC1 domain is markedly inhibited by coincubation with anti- $\alpha_v\beta_3$ integrin antibodies and to a lesser extent by anti-$\alpha_v\beta_5$, anti-β_1 and anti-α_1 antibodies[35] suggesting that cell-surface canstatin-integrin interactions may be important for its actions.

Of note both a 26kDa form of arresten[35] and a 24kDa form of canstatin[38] have been purified from human placenta indicating that they may have a physiological role as proteolytic fragments.

3.2. Tumstatin

The most investigated anti-angiogenic proteolytic fragment of collagen IV is the 232 amino acid NC1 domain of the α3 chain, designated tumstatin[43]. Physiological expression of the α3 chain is limited to the glomerular, cochlear, ocular, ovarian and testicular basement membranes as well as the alveolar capillary VBM[44]. Previous experimental data indicated that a synthetic peptide incorporating residues 185-203 of the α3 chain inhibited the proliferation of melanoma and carcinoma cells in vitro[45] and their production of matrix metalloproteinases[46].

Investigation of the whole NC1 fragment expressed in E. coli demonstrated that this inhibits CPAE proliferation and tubule formation in the Matrigel assay system but had no effect on melanoma cell proliferation[43]. Higher concentrations of tumstatin induced endothelial cell apoptosis in vitro as indicated by annexin V binding and increased caspase-3 activity. This property was also demonstrated in vivo within established tumour xenografts in nude mice. Subsequent solid phase binding assays of CPAEs and HUVECs to tumstatin coated plates indicate that tumstatin binding occurs via $\alpha_v\beta_3$ and $\alpha_6\beta_1$ integrins[47]. However, this did not appear to involve the RGD sequence present at the N-terminus of tumstatin as cell binding was not inhibited by co-incubation with cyclic RGD peptide and endothelial cells failed to adhere to plates coated in T1-peptide (derived from the N-terminal 20 amino acids of tumstatin). A recent study has however questioned some of these findings, Pedchenko et al[48] used recombinant proteins/ chimaeras derived from the NC1 domains of the α3 and α1 collagen IV chains, the latter of which does not contain an RGD sequence. These were expressed in mammalian cell systems to ensure correct protein folding. This study implicated both the proximal RGD site and non-RGD sites as being important for integrin-binding of tumstatin when it is in it's native conformation.

The anti-angiogenic properties of tumstatin have subsequently been shown to depend on the central portion of the molecule. A series of overlapping tumstatin-derived peptides were generated. Initially T-5 peptide (amino acids 54-132) was demonstrated to bind both $\alpha_v\beta_3$ integrin, predominantly via the β3 subunit, inhibit endothelial cell proliferation and suppress the growth of tumour xenografts. In nude mice, T-5 peptide appeared to be ten times as potent as endostatin[49]. Subsequent work with shorter peptides identified amino acids 74-88 as the critical sequence for anti-angiogenic activity[50]. The elimination of the N-terminal region of tumstatin without loss of anti-angiogenic activity is an important consideration for potential clinical development of this molecule as the epitope recognised by the pathogenic auto-antibodies in Goodpastures syndrome (GPS)- a condition characterised by rapidly progressive glomerulonephritis and pulmonary haemorrhage is located at the N-terminus of the NC1 domain of the α3 collagen IV chain[34].

Tumstatin and T-5 peptide have been demonstrated to inhibit protein synthesis specifically in endothelial cells. In an elegant study by Maeshima et al[51], tumstatin was shown to inhibit FAK phosphorylation induced by attachment to vitronectin in endothelial cells with downstream inhibition of the PI-3K/ Akt pathway. This results in decreased mTOR activity and subsequent decreased phosphorylation of eukaryotic initiation factor 4E-binding protein (eIF-4EBP) leading to its increased interaction with eIF-4E preventing protein translation in a CAP-dependent manner. This mechanism of action was noted to be absolutely dependent on the expression of cell-surface β_3 integrin.

Whilst the studies detail the anti-angiogenic properties and mechanism of action of tumstatin in vitro or when administered in murine model systems at pharmacological doses, they give little information about any physiological role for this protein fragment. The development of Col IVα3 knockout mice has allowed this to be addressed. These mice on a C57BL/6 background are viable and although they develop progressive renal failure associated with glomerular basement membrane (GBM) abnormalities, their median life expectancy is about 40 weeks[52]. When Lewis lung carcinoma cells are implanted subcutaneously into these mice, they grow at the same rate as in wild type C57BL/6 mice until 500mm^3 in size but then at an accelerated rate due to an increased angiogenic response[44]. The exogenous administration of tumstatin to obtain physiological serum concentrations prevented this accelerated tumour growth but had no effect on wound healing. Differential expression of integrins was proposed as a potential explanation for this observation as $\alpha_v\beta_3$ integrin expression was seen on 40% of proliferating capillaries in tumour explants but not on capillaries in healing skin wounds.

In vivo generation of tumstatin appears to be predominantly mediated by MMP-9[44]. Tumstatin is liberated from GBM in vitro more effectively by MMP-9 than MMP-2/-3/-13. MMP-9 knockout mice have 60% lower circulating tumstatin levels than wild-type and subcutaneous tumour implants grow faster on a MMP-9 -/- background.. The research on tumstatin identifies it as a promising and specific anti-angiogenic molecule in vitro and in murine models. It also defines cell surface receptors and downstream signalling pathways. Whilst a physiological role has been proposed in mice, no research has yet been published focusing on tumstatin in cancer patients or other human subjects. This is a clear gap that needs to be addressed before clinical trials with this molecule can be planned. One further caveat that needs to be considered is the association between GPS and tumstatin. The generation of animal models of GPS by immunisation with the α3 NC1 domain of collagen IV[53] suggests that repeated administration of tumstatin will carry at least a theoretical risk of inducing a GPS-like condition and so will need to be monitored for closely. The use of tumstatin peptides that do not contain the GPS epitope may however circumvent this problem.

4. Fragments of other ECM Proteins

Several other proteolytic fragments of ECM and VBM proteins have been shown to have antiangiogenic properties and the most interesting of these are discussed below.

4.1. Perlecan and endorepellin

Perlecan is a large modular HSPG that is expressed in all VBMs. It plays essential roles in vasculogenesis and angiogenesis[17]. Whereas perlecan knockout mice die in utero at embryonic day 10.5 from intra-pericardial haemorrhage and cardiac developmental abnormalities[54], mice with a directed knockout of the perlecan HS attachment sequence develop normally but have significantly delayed wound healing and FGF-2 induced tumour angiogenesis[55].

Using domain V of perlecan as a probe for physiological binding partners in a yeast two-hybrid system, Mongiat and colleagues[3] identified that as well as binding the endostatin-containing NC1 domain of collagen XVIII, the perlecan protein fragment which they designated endorepellin also had significant endogenous anti-angiogenic properties. It inhibited endothelial cell migration, collagen-induced capillary formation and angiogenesis in both the CAM and Matrigel plug assays. Subsequent work has shown that these anti-angiogenic properties reside in the LG3 domain of endorepellin and are secondary to endothelial cell specific disruption of actin stress fibres induced by endorepellin binding to cell surface $\alpha 2\beta 1$ integrin with subsequent increase in intracellular cAMP concentrations and upregulation of PKA and FAK activity[56]. As the endorepellin LG3 domain has relatively few predicted interactions with other VBM components it is likely to be accessible to extracellular proteases and therefore be susceptible to release by proteolytic cleavage in vivo.

4.2. Fibronectin, Heparin-Binding Fragments and Anastellin

Fibronectin is a large modular glycoprotein that is a critical ECM component. In 1985, two heparin-binding proteolytic fragments were noted to inhibit endothelial cell proliferation[23]. Subsequent work has identified a 76 amino acid fragment containing the first type III repeat as having significant ability to inhibit tumour growth and metastasis in murine xenograft models[2]. This fibronectin fragment, named anastellin induces polymerisation of fibronectin and fibrinogen in solution and derives its antineoplastic activity from an antiangiogenic effect. This effect has been shown to be dependent on the presence of serum fibronectin in a conditional mouse knockout where Cre expression is under the control of the albumin promoter so eliminating hepatic fibronectin expression[57]. It has been suggested that the formation of soluble polymers of adhesion proteins such as those induced by anastellin may be a common mechanism of action of anti-angiogenic protein fragments as many of these are known to bind such proteins in plasma.

4.3. Matrix Metalloproteinase-2 and PEX

MMP-2 is the most widely distributed MMP and has significant activity against collagen IV. Levels of MMP-2 expression correlate with tumour invasiveness and angiogenesis[58,59]. MMPs are secreted as proenzymes and activated extracellularly. In the case of MMP-2 this activation process involves interaction with $\alpha_v\beta_3$ integrin at the cell surface. It has recently been demonstrated that a 29kDa proteolytic fragment of MMP-2-PEX, that contains the C-terminal hemopexin-like domain inhibits angiogenesis by preventing MMP-2 binding to $\alpha_v\beta_3$ integrin so blocking its cell-surface collagenolytic activity[60]. Importantly, PEX is detectable in vivo and is likely to act as a negative regulator of retinal neovascularization during murine development.

PEX has subsequently been shown to retard the growth of human melanoma xenografts in nude mice by decreasing angiogenesis when transfected into peritumoral tissue using a lentiviral vector[61] and cause prolonged inhibition of glioma progression when administered in combination with metronomic chemotherapy[62].

Whilst laboratory results with PEX to date have been promising, it should be noted that the clinical development of small molecular MMP inhibitors has been uniformly disappointing despite promising preclinical data[58,59] indicating that the actions of the MMP system in human cancer may be more complex than first thought.

4.4. Thrombospondin-1 fragments

Thrombospondin-1 is a trimeric multi-domain matricellular protein with multiple physiological functions[33]. It can promote or inhibit angiogenesis depending on other microenvironmental inputs- for instance transforming growth factor-β1 levels or relative protease levels[33,63]. A naturally-occurring 140kDa N-terminal fragment of thrombospondin has been shown to inhibit angiogenesis[64], possibly by activating p38 MAPKinase and downregulating MMP-2 and -9 activities[63]. These anti-angiogenic properties reside in the second and third type I repeats[65] and are mimicked by a synthetic nonapeptide, ABT-510 that is under clinical evaluation. This agent has been well-tolerated in early clinical trials as both a single agent and in combination with chemotherapy[66,67]. Early signs of anti-tumour activity have also been seen particularly in soft tissue sarcoma[68] and the results of further phase II clinical trials are eagerly awaited.

5. Endostatin-Preclinical Studies

The most investigated anti-angiogenic proteolytic fragment is endostatin, a 20kDa polypeptide derived from the NC1 domain of collagen XVIII. Endostatin was initially isolated in 1997 from the conditioned media of EOMA cells, a non-metastatic murine haemangioendothelioma cell line. Initial experiments demonstrated that it inhibited FGF-2 stimulated proliferation of bovine capillary endothelial cells in a dose-dependent manner but had no effect on the growth of a panel of human tumour cell lines in vitro. Endostatin dramatically induced regression of established tumour xenografts and metastases in a murine model due to inhibition of angiogenesis[69] and repeated cycles of endostatin treatment lead to tumour dormancy even after withdrawal of endostatin in the same mouse models[70].

5.1. Collagen XVIII, Knobloch Syndrome and Development

Endostatin's parental molecule, collagen XVIII is a highly evolutionarily conserved member of the mutiplexin family of collagens which are characterised by multiple triple helical domains interrupted by non-helical regions that allow molecular flexibility within the basement membrane[71]. The presence of several Ser- Gly- Gly sequences within collagen XVIII indicate that it is a major HSPG[72].

Three human isoforms of collagen XVIII exist and whilst the expression of these are distributed widely within basement membranes, there are organ-specific patterns[5,73,74].

Clinically, the importance of the short isoform is illustrated by the demonstration of pathological truncation mutations in the human collagen XVIII gene on Chr 21q22.3 in the rare autosomal recessive Knobloch syndrome[74,75]. This is characterised by high myopia, vitreoretinal degeneration with retinal detachment, macular abnormalities and also occipital encephalocoele- indicating important roles in ocular development and possibly in neural tube closure. The physiological importance of collagen XVIII/endostatin in retinal development is reinforced by the ocular phenotype seen in collagen XVIII knockout mice. There is delayed regression of blood vessels from the vitreous humour in utero and abnormal outgrowth of retinal vasculature after birth[76]. As these mice age, their visual function deteriorates associated with the massive accumulation of excess basement membrane material under the retinal pigment epithelium[77].

The importance of collagen XVIII in neural development is exemplified by studies on model organisms. The C.elegans orthologue cle-1, accumulates at high levels in the developing nervous system and its deletion results in organisms which have defects in axonal migration[78]. Analysis of collagen XVIII gene expression during zebrafish[79] and Xenopus laevis[80] development indicates high expression in the developing nervous system and eyes as well as in the endothelium of intersomitic arteries.

However, despite its key roles in retinal function and neural development, no significant defects can be detected in epithelial or endothelial basement membrane functions elsewhere. Notably neither the collagen XVIII- knockout mice nor Knobloch syndrome sufferers have been noted to have cancer predisposition.

5.2. Endostatin: Cleavage and Structure

Analysis of the 38kDa C-terminal domain (NC1) of collagen XVIII indicates that it consists of an N-terminal association domain separated from the endostatin moiety by a protease- sensitive hinge region. The 5kDa association domain allows non-covalent trimerisation of NC1 and, in vivo, both endostatin monomers and trimeric NC1 domains have been identified separate from their parent collagen XVIII molecule[81].

Endostatin can be proteolytically cleaved from collagen XVIII by the action of multiple proteases in vitro. In EOMA cell culture, endostatin cleavage is catalysed by cathepsin L [82]. This processing is most effective at a moderately acidic pH as would be found in the pericellular milieu in tumours. Although, it has been suggested that elastase may also play a role in this process[83], the significance of this in vivo is not yet established and indeed, EOMA cells do not express elastase. Several other proteases including the cysteine proteinases, cathepsins B and K, matrix metallproteinases and the aspartic proteinase, cathepsin D have also been shown to generate endostatin-like fragments from recombinant human Collagen XVIII NC1 domain, although at varying efficiencies[81,84].

Several X-ray crystal models of endostatin have been reported[85-87]. Murine endostatin crystallised from ammonium phosphate at pH5.5[86] folds into a compact globular molecule with the most prominent features being a highly twisted 7- stranded mixed β-sheet, two intramolecular disulphide bridges and a putative heparin- binding region. This latter region consists of eleven surface exposed arginine residues, divided into two clusters that are conserved between murine and human endostatin.

Crystal models of endostatin produced at alkaline pH have also demonstrated ligation of a zinc ion in a tetrahedral configuration at the N-terminus[85,87]. This binding of zinc fails to impinge significantly on endostatin structure outside of the N-terminus and the demonstrated degree of structural heterogeneity with respect to the position of the zinc ion and its binding residues suggests that it acts more to stabilise general molecular structure rather than having a direct functional role. This is confirmed by in vitro data. Although initial site-directed mutagenesis experiments using E. coli-derived insoluble endostatin suggested that zinc-binding was important for its anti-angiogenic function[88], subsequent work using soluble endostatins has not confirmed this. The deletion of the N-terminal 5 amino acids of human endostatin eliminated zinc binding but failed to impinge on its ability to inhibit HUVEC migration or inhibit RC-9 renal cell carcinoma xenograft growth[89]. Alanine mutagenesis of the zinc-binding histidine residues also failed to reduce the ability of endostatin to inhibit FGF-2 induced angiogenesis in the CAM assay[90].

5.3. Collagen XV and Restin- High Sequence Homology with Endostatin

By using the endostatin sequence as a probe in databanks, it was noted to have 61% sequence identity with the first non-collagenous domain of collagen XV which was named restin[91]. Of note, collagen XV is the second member of the mutiplexin subfamily of collagens and also has predominant basement membrane expression. Subsequent structural analysis by X-Ray crystallography indicated a similar overall fold pattern to endostatin[92]. However, no zinc-binding site is present and restin also fails to bind heparin, probably due to the lack of conservation of two critical surface-exposed arginine residues.

Functional analysis has revealed that restin retains some anti-angiogenic activity despite its inability to bind zinc or heparin. Although restin was unable to inhibit the proliferation of CPAE cells in response to FGF-2, it inhibited migration of ECV304 cells in response to FGF-2 in a dose-dependent manner[91]. In the CAM assay, restin inhibited angiogenesis in response to VEGF whereas the longer NC1 domain was required to prevent FGF-2 stimulated neovascularization[92]. Interestingly, the hinge region of the NC1 domain in collagen XV is shorter than collagen XVIII rendering it much more protease resistant and restin could not be identified in murine tissues by immunoblotting.

The creation of a collagen XV knockout mouse has also identified a distinct phenotype compared to the collagen XVIII knockout. COL15A1 knockouts are viable but rather than demonstrating an ocular phenotype, have progressive myopathic changes in skeletal muscle that are exacerbated by exercise. Cardiac muscle is also affected and ultrastructural analysis of cardiac / skeletal muscle capillaries revealed degenerate endothelial cells with narrowed capillary lumens[93]. These findings suggest a structural role for type XV collagen in muscle microvessels. Notably the recent generation of a double collagen XV/ XVIII knockout mouse failed to detect any further phenotypic changes indicating that the two multiplexins do not compensate functionally for each other in vivo[94].

5.4. Endostatin: Putative Cell Surface Receptors and Mechanism of Action

Initial studies on the binding partners for endostatin focussed on extracellular matrix proteins. Sasaki et al[81] demonstrated binding to the microfibrillar proteins fibulin-1 and -2 and also showed binding of the NC1 domain of collagen XVIII to sulfatides and laminin-1 in solid phase binding assays. Subsequently, Karumanchi et al[95] probed the binding of alkaline-phosphatase-tagged endostatin to CPAE cells by Scatchard analysis. This identified 2 cell surface binding sites designated high (Kd = 18pM) and low (Kd = 200pM) affinity. By screening a HUVEC cDNA library in NIH 3T3 fibroblasts which do not bind endostatin, they identified a transcript that restored binding. This was identified as encoding the HSPG glypican-4. Expression of glypican-1, the most common endothelial HSPG also restored binding and subsequent experiments confirmed that endostatin was binding to the HS side-chains in these cells.

5.5. Endostatin and Heparan Sulfate

The identification of HS as a cell-surface binding site reinforced the crystallography data described above[85-87] and site-directed mutagenesis experiments conducted by Sasaki et al [90]. The mutation of surface exposed arginines that make up the putative primary and secondary heparin-binding sites was demonstrated to reduce heparin affinity in filter-trapping assays and also abrogate the ability of endostatin to inhibit FGF-2- induced angiogenesis in the chick CAM assay. However, previous studies had shown endostatin heparin-binding mutants could still inhibit VEGF-induced migration in HUVECs [89] and that low concentrations of endostatin still bind to human tissue sections after treatment with heparitinases[96]. Whilst the latter findings may well be explained by endostatin binding to other tissue components- in particular the fibulins, it is still not clear that HS binding is absolutely required for all the anti-angiogenic actions of endostatin- at least in in vitro systems.

Heparan sulfate is initially synthesised as a complex polymer of repeating N-acetyl glucosamine (GlcNAc) and glucuronic acid (GlcA) residues. This backbone is then partially enzymatically modified on passage through the Golgi apparatus by N-deacetylation/ sulfation of GlcNAc residues followed by epimerisation of GlcA to iduronic acid (IdoA) and subsequent O-sulfation at the 2-O- position of IdoA or GlcA and 6-O-position and 3-O-positions of GlcN residues[97,98]. The pattern of these modifications is dependent partly on the tissue of origin and determines the repertoire of protein ligands bound by HS. Much work has focussed on the pattern of GAG sulfation that supports endostatin binding. Initial studies utilised size-defined and chemically modified oligosaccharides derived from the uniformly sulfated GAG heparin, and in biophysical assays identified oligosaccharides of at least ten sugar residues in length as having optimal affinity for binding[90,99]. Desulfation experiments have also indicated that N- and 2-O-sulfation in particular are critical for the interaction of endostatin with heparin[90,95,99]. Subsequent experiments have used the physiologically relevant ligand HS. Work in our laboratory[100] using HS derived from endothelial cells largely confirmed the size requirements for endostatin although suggested that N- and 6-O- sulfation were most important for binding and that lack of 2-O-sulfation could be compensated for by increases in sulfation at other sites. Interestingly, it was noted that long HS fragments derived largely from unsulfated regions but with short sulfated sequences at either end could bind endostatin with equal affinity to short highly sulfated oligosaccharides. This suggests that the structural motif required for endostatin binding need not consist of a contiguous sulfated sequence provided that negatively charged domains are present that can interact with the primary and secondary heparin-binding sites simultaneously.

This result confirms the findings of Kreuger et al[101], who identified a region composed of two short sulfated domains separated by a single unsulfated disaccharide ('SAS' domain) as being the likely physiologically relevant ligand for endostatin.

Whilst these studies take us closer towards understanding the HS- binding sequence for endostatin, they do not explain how HS binding results in its anti-angiogenic properties. Many pro-angiogenic growth factors including FGF-2 and some VEGF isoforms need to bind cell-surface HS for their activity and initial hypotheses were that endostatin functioned by competing for these HS binding sites[90]. However, HS oligosaccharides that bind FGF-2 strongly fail to bind endostatin[101] and it seems more likely that endostatin forms a trimolecular complex with HS and another higher affinity receptor at the cell surface[95]. The identity of this second receptor however remains to be firmly established although many candidates have been proposed.

5.6. Endostatin and Integrins

The initial observation of an interaction between endostatin and integrins came from the demonstration that anti-integrin antibodies prevented HUVEC spreading and focal adhesion formation on endostatin-coated plates. This inhibition of an adhesive phenotype was particularly marked with antibodies against the α_5 and β_1 integrin chains[102] and these molecules were also noted to inhibit HUVEC migration towards immobilised endostatin.

Subsequently further work indicated that treatment of endothelial cells with soluble endostatin modulates the pattern of focal adhesion formation in a manner dependent on the cell line and cytokine milieu[103,104] further implicating integrin signalling in the actions of endostatin. This signalling pathway has since been elucidated (see Figure 1). In HDMECs, soluble endostatin induces clustering of $\alpha_5\beta_1$ integrins within lipid rafts in the cell membrane. This clustering results in the activation of Src kinases which, via negative regulation of RhoA activity, result in the downregulation of focal adhesions and actin stress fibres in a manner dependent on tyrosyl phosphatases[105,106]. Of note, the enzymatic removal of cell surface HS prevents the translocation of $\alpha_5\beta_1$ integrin-bound endostatin to lipid rafts suggesting that HSPGs may play a critical role in moving potential endostatin signalling complexes into membrane microdomains where they can engage with their downstream signalling partners[106].

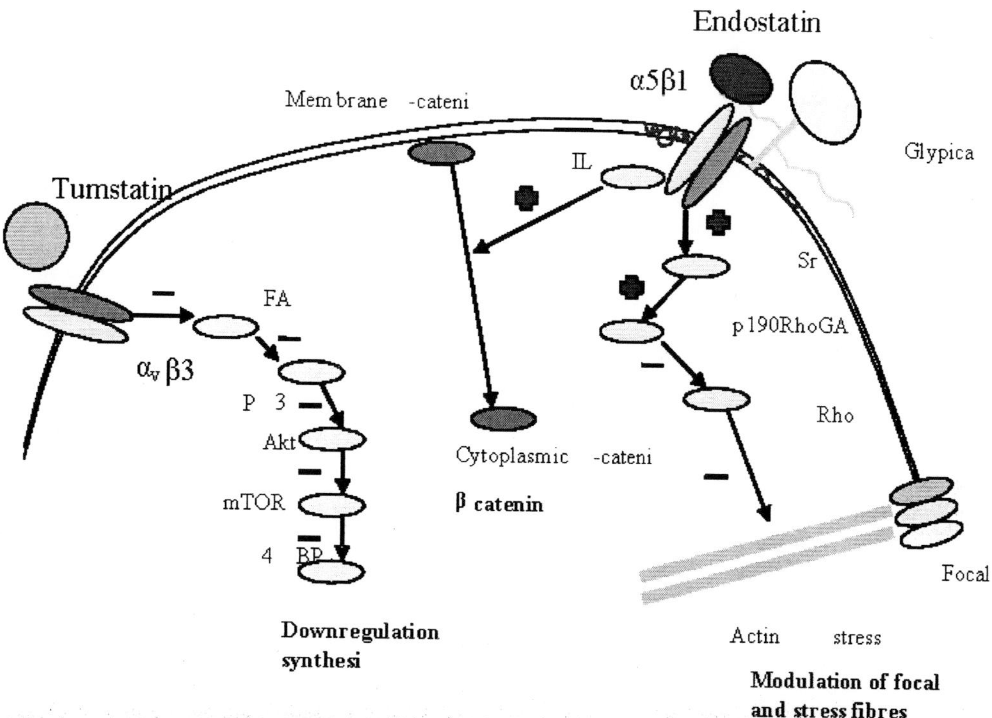

Figure 1. Putative integrin-dependent signalling pathways for the endogenous angiogenesis inhibitors endostatin and tumstatin. Tumstatin binds to $\alpha_v\beta_3$ integrin at the cell surface resulting in downregulation of CAP-dependent protein synthesis. Endostatin has been demonstrated to bind to $\alpha_5\beta_1$ integrin and glypican heparan sulfate at the cell surface causing translocation of these molecules to lipid rafts. Downstream signalling pathways result in modulation of actin stress fibre and focal adhesion formation. It has also been suggested that endostatin causes degradation of cytoplasmic β-catenin potentially via the actions of integrin-linked kinase (ILK). For abbreviations see main text.

Notably however, endostatin, lacks a consensus RGD integrin-binding sequence although it appears to bind to $\alpha_5\beta_1$ integrin in an RGD-motif dependent manner[107]. Recent work has utilised five peptides derived from regions of endostatin encompassing surface-exposed basic amino acids identified by crystallography data. A peptide containing amino acids 60-70 (and arginines 62, 63, 66) retained many of the biological functions of full-length endostatin in a manner that was dependent on its positive charge. Of note, both heparin and an anti-β1 integrin antibody prevented endothelial cell binding to this peptide when it was immobilised suggesting that this region contains both the heparin and integrin binding sites of endostatin[108]. However such results must be considered with caution as such a short peptide may not conform to the secondary/ tertiary structure that it adopts within its parental molecule.

Intriguingly results of experiments using endostatin as an antiangiogenic agent in vitronectin–null mice and conditional mice knockouts lacking circulating fibronectin may provide further support for the role of endostatin-integrin interactions. Endostatin was unable to inhibit FGF-2 –induced angiogenesis in a Matrigel plug assay in mice without plasma fibronectin and had decreased activity in the vitronectin knockout system[57]. Whilst endostatin fails to bind either of these proteins directly, it may form soluble complexes via interactions with circulating fibulins. These complexes could then mediate signals via interactions with integrins to induce endothelial cell apoptosis or prevent recruitment of circulating endothelial cell precursors.

5.7. Endostatin and other Cytoskeletal Ligands

The research exploring endostatin's interactions with integrins and HSPGs at the cell surface has implicated modulation of endothelial cell cytoskeletal architecture as a critical pathway for endostatin's antimigratory properties and several other cytoskeletal proteins have also been identified as potential endostatin ligands. Tropomyosin isoform 3, a protein that binds the α- helical groove of actin microfilaments stabilising the polymerised form has been shown to bind endostatin and the 2 proteins co-localise in endothelial cells [109] and Kaposi's sarcoma cells[110]. Of note, a peptide that blocks endostatin binding to tropomyosin prevents endostatin from inhibiting the development of pulmonary metastases in a murine melanoma model[109].

Further work utilising a simple proteomics assay[111] has suggested that endostatin induces phosphorylation of cofilin; a regulator of actin depolymerisation; and hsp27 which can modulate the cytoskeleton by capping actin microfilaments. These changes were also noted in endothelial cells treated with other angiogenesis inhibitors including thrombospondin-1. However, in this study incubation of endothelial cells with endostatin resulted in prolonged upregulation of both actin stress fibres and focal adhesions in contrast to those studies discussed earlier.

5.8. Endostatin and Modulation of Extracellular Protease Activity

For activated endothelial cells to invade surrounding tissues as a prelude to new blood vessel development, degradation of the extracellular matrix by proteases is vital. These enzymes are therefore another potential target for anti-angiogenic molecules. Endostatin has been shown to decrease HUVEC invasion by inhibiting both the activity of MMP-2 and the proteolytic processing of its precursor[112]. This inhibition is likely to be due to endostatin's ability to bind directly to the active site of MMP-2 as suggested by both immunoprecipitation experiments and direct surface plasmon resonance binding assays[113].

Endostatin has also been shown to downregulate uPA secretion from endothelial cells and causes redistribution of cell membrane-associated uPA from the invasive cell edge to a diffuse pattern that is associated with a marked decrease in focal adhesion formation[103].

5.9. Endostatin, Apoptosis and the Cell Cycle

Endostatin induces apoptosis in endothelial cells in vitro in several studies[114,115]. The degree of apoptosis induced appears to be higher when cells are undergoing active cell division which may partly explain the specificity for active tumour vasculature in vivo. It has been variously suggested that the pro-apoptotic effects of endostatin are due to downregulation of the anti-apoptotic protein Bcl-2[115] or due to an increase in phosphorylation of the Shb adaptor protein[114].

Endostatin also causes G1 cell cycle arrest in growth factor-stimulated endothelial cells[114,116]. This occurs secondary to a downregulation of cyclin D1 mRNA synthesis due to the interaction of a transcriptional inhibitor with a LEF-1 binding site in the promoter region of the cyclin D1 gene[116]. Interestingly other work has indicated that c-myc gene expression is also inhibited by endostatin probably via a LEF1 binding site[117].

5.10. Endostatin, Wnt Signalling and Beta-Catenin

The identification of gene downregulation secondary to effects on LEF transcriptional elements suggests that β-catenin may be involved in endostatin signalling. Other research has reinforced this possibility. Hanai et al[118] assessed the effect of endostatin overexpression in the Xenopus model of embryogenesis as a means of assessing possible signal transduction pathways. They demonstrated that endostatin mRNA injection into the ventral blastomere induced formation of an ectopic cement gland, a phenotype also seen with inhibition of the Wnt signalling pathway. B-catenin is an essential downstream mediator of this pathway and indeed endostatin overexpression prevents axis duplication in Xenopus embryos induced by β-catenin overexpression. Further experiments confirmed that endostatin induces β-catenin downregulation not only in Xenopus embryos but also in HUVEC lines in vitro. This occurs via a novel pathway as it is independent of the standard GSK-3-dependent β-catenin degradation pathway. Whilst these results need to be interpreted cautiously due to the large doses of endostatin used the role of β-catenin as an effector protein for endostatin is supported by work exploring another of β-catenin's functions. In quiescent endothelial cells, β-catenin forms part of a multiprotein complex at cell-cell adherens junctions. It is released from these when it is tyrosine phosphorylated in response to growth factor stimulation resulting in increased cell motility. Exogenous endostatin can transiently increase or decrease β-catenin's phosphorylation status and hence intracellular distribution dependent on whether endothelial cells are stimulated by FGF-2 or quiescent[104]. Of note, integrin-linked kinase coupled to β1-integrin can also increase cytoplasmic concentrations of stabilised β-catenin[119] so indicating a potential convergence of putative endostatin signalling pathways.

5.11. Endostatin and Interference with VEGF Signalling

Many studies have demonstrated the ability of endostatin to inhibit VEGF-induced endothelial cell proliferation, survival and in particular migration. The pattern of these effects in vitro appears to be to some extent dependent on endostatin concentration, cell line used and experimental conditions. It has been suggested that endostatin may inhibit VEGF by binding to its main signalling receptor KDR[120]. Whilst endostatin inhibited VEGF-induced KDR and Erk phosphorylation in HUVEC cells and bound directly to KDR in solid phase assays in this study, it should be noted that endostatin was still able to inhibit signalling from a chimaeric receptor containing the intracellular domain of KDR fused to the extracellular portion of EGFR [95] indicating that direct binding of endostatin to KDR is not the sole mode of action for its anti-angiogenic effects.

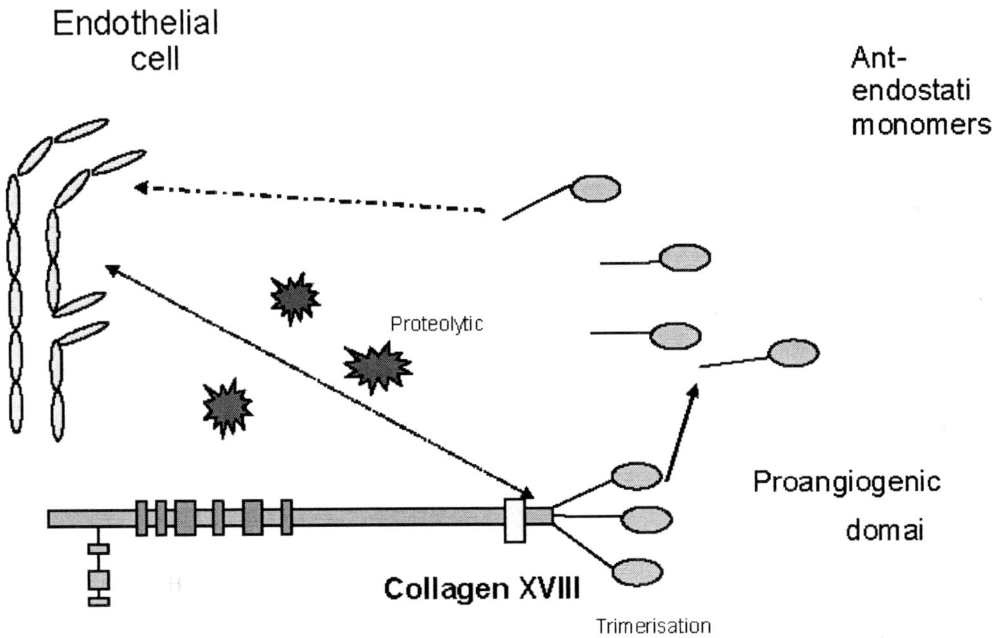

Figure 2. The putative endostatin negative autoregulatory loop. The NC1 domain of collagen XVIII is motogenic for endothelial cells. Proteolytic processing result in the formation of monomeric endostatin which is anti-migratory and anti-proliferative for endothelial cells. Such a process could promote angiogenesis in areaas of wounding but limit the time and location of pro-angiogenic signalling.

Interestingly, adenoviral transfection of endostatin into endothelial cells and 2 tumour cell lines resulted in reduction in VEGF production by these cell lines although the mechanism for this was not elucidated[121].

Other research has focused on one of the main downstream effectors of VEGF signalling. Endothelial Nitrous oxide synthase (eNOS) is activated on cell stimulation with VEGF by phosphorylation at serine 1177 resulting in cell proliferation and migration[122]. In vitro, low concentrations (10-100ng/ml) of endostatin have been shown to inhibit VEGF-induced NO release due to specific serine 1177 dephosphorylation of eNOS possibly via activation of protein phosphatase 2A[123]. Interestingly, further research has shown that endothelial endostatin synthesis and release may be stimulated by high NO concentrations suggesting a potential negative feedback loop[124]. Although this mechanism may have physiological relevance for the actions of endostatin, it is unclear how important this system would be in the intratumoral setting where high levels of inducible NO synthase may be expressed[125].

It has also been shown that the administration of endostatin can reduce the number of circulating endothelial progenitors in mice[126] and that this is via the inhibition of VEGF-induced mobilisation of this cell type from the bone marrow[127]. This indicates another novel anti-angiogenic, specifically anti-VEGF property of endostatin.

5.12. Other Signalling Pathways and Endostatin

Several other studies have provided insight into potential signalling pathways for endostatin. Endostatin induces a three-fold increase in intracellular calcium ion concentration in BAECs primarily via inositol-3-phosphate- mediated release of calcium from intracellular stores[128] although there is a minor contribution from extracellular calcium influx[117].

Interestingly, Eriksson et al[129] failed to demonstrate any changes in the activation status of multiple intracellular signal transduction pathways in HDMECs coincubated with endostatin despite its ability to inhibit their migration in response to VEGF/ FGF-2 indicating that a novel pathway may be involved.

Work has also implicated endothelial cell surface E-selectin as vital for the in vivo anti-angiogenic properties of endostatin[130]. E-selectin is an endothelial-specific membrane glycoprotein which when upregulated functions to recruit leukocytes to areas of active inflammation. Endostatin is inactive in the corneal pocket angiogenesis assay in E-selectin knockout mice and the sensitivity of HDMECs to endostatin can be increased markedly by transfection with the E-selectin gene. However, endostatin itself does not bind E-selectin in solid phase assays or on the surface of activated endothelial cells so the precise role of E-selectin in endostatin's anti-angiogenic activity remains unclear.

One further novel proposal for the mechanism underpinning endostatin's anti-angiogenic actions relates to the ability of partially denatured endostatin to form amyloid fibrils[131]. These fibrils may be directly toxic to endothelial cells and also activate tissue plasminogen activator leading to degradation of basement membrane proteins which could remove endothelial cell survival signals[132].

5.13. Gene Expression Profiling and Endostatin

The discussion above indicates the bewildering arrays of possibilities by which endostatin mediates its anti-angiogenic effects. Recently several studies have focussed on a more global assessment of the effects of endostatin on endothelial cell biology by using gene expression profiling. One initial study[117] assessed a panel of 31 candidate genes by quantitative rtPCR. Although a subset of these genes were downregulated on endostatin exposure in endothelial cells but not in fibroblasts or a gastric carcinoma cell line, the pattern of downregulation varied somewhat between the endothelial cell lines investigated and did not reflect the absolute level of active protein present indicating some of the problems of gene expression assessments.

Subsequent studies have used more sophisticated microarray technology. Cline et al[133] using a chip consisting of over 9000 expressed sequences identified 120 whose expression varied more than 3-fold when HMVECs were incubated with 3nM endostatin for 4 hours. Notably a specific genomic profile could be identified for endostatin compared to 4 other anti-angiogenic agents tested and this predicted synergistic activity in in vitro and in vivo models.

Most recently, Abdollahi et al[134] analysed the genomic and phosphoproteomic profiles induced by the stimulation of HDMECs with 200ng/ml endostatin for 2 hours. Notably, they demonstrated at least 2-fold changes in expression of almost 12% of the genome. They subsequently confirmed endostatin dose and time-dependent downregulation of 15 candidate genes by quantitative rtPCR. Phosphoproteomic analysis of the same cell pool by antibody array analysis identified 19 proteins that were differentially phosphorylated. Whilst several of these targets of endostatin had been previously identified- for instance cell cycle regulators such as cyclins D, B and A- 8 signalling cascades were noted to be modulated by endostatin stimulation (see table 4). This co-ordinated regulation of a diverse angiogenic network (the upregulation of anti-angiogenic effectors and concurrent downregulation of pro-angiogenic agents) by a single anti-angiogenic effector is remarkable.

However, certain caveats need to be borne in mind when interpreting the large amount of data generated. This study involves the stimulation in vitro of a single endothelial cell line with a single dose of endostatin with the effects determined at a single timepoint. Most of the data are only analysed at the transcriptional level and it should be noted that other studies have failed to detect any effects on, for instance, intracellular protein levels of HIF-1α[135] or JNK phosphorylation[104,117]. As endostatin may also partly function via direct binding to KDR[120] it is feasible that part of the change in expression profile seen is due to removal of a pro-angiogenic signal rather that a specific anti-angiogenic one. Clearly further work needs to be done utilising other endothelial cell lines and also assessing whether tumour endothelial cells differ in response to endostatin in comparison to those in normal tissues. It is also of concern that the study by Cline et al[133] failed to identify any of the angiogenic genes detailed by Abdollahi. Nevertheless this study may alter our thinking as to how angiogenesis is controlled[136] and certainly generates many hypotheses with respect to endostatin's effects.

5.14. Further Complicating the Endostatin Story

Whereas most initial research focused on endostatin as a monomer functioning as an endothelial-cell specific anti-angiogenic agent, this concept has been challenged recently as studies have demonstrated direct effects on cancer cell lines and identified oligomeric endostatin as a promigratory stimulus for endothelial cells.

Monomeric endostatin has been shown to directly inhibit the growth of and promote apoptosis in two colon cancer cell lines in vitro[137]. It also inhibits the invasive characteristics of a human tongue carcinoma cell line by inhibiting the activity of MMP-9 and -2[138] although higher doses were required than in studies using endothelial cell lines[139].

A role for endostatin in normal renal development has also been proposed. Endostatin binds to renal tubular epithelial cells in a glypican-dependent manner[95] and has been shown to inhibit the branching morphogenesis of both renal tubular cell lines and ureteric buds in an ex vivo model[140]. Notably ureteric bud branching could be increased in this model by co-incubation with a polyclonal anti-endostatin antibody indicating a role for endogenously produced endostatin.

Endostatin, as part of the NC1 domain of collagen XVIII can trimerise physiologically[81] and high molecular weight bands have been detected by Western blotting in the sera of renal cell carcinoma patients suggesting the existence of circulating oligomers[141]. Recent research has shown that trimeric collagen XVIII NC1 and an artificially synthesised endostatin dimer are promigratory for endothelial cells causing disaggregation of pre-formed tubules on a Matrigel substratum[142]. This effect is dependent on prolonged activity of MAPKinase and occurs via interaction of oligomeric endostatin with laminin within the substratum[143] and heparan sulfate at the cell surface (Clamp et al unpublished observations). These motogenic properties of oligomeric endostatin are not specific to endothelial cells but are also apparent on stimulation of cancer cell lines and the NC-1 domain of the C. elegans collagen XVIII orthologue, cle-1 is important in neuronal migration[78]. Of note the effects of oligomeric endostatin can be inhibited by cellular pre-incubation with monomeric endostatin suggesting a negative autoregulatory loop with potential far-reaching functions in directing cell migration over basement membranes.

5.15. Endostatin: Summary of Pre-Clinical Studies

The extensive research discussed above has highlighted many potential mechanisms of action for endostatin (see table 3). Whilst some may only have significance in vitro, it is likely that no one pathway solely defines the anti-angiogenic properties of endostatin. This is borne out by the gene expression profile studies that have been conducted[133,134] (table 4). The profound cytoskeletal alterations often seen in endothelial cells on endostatin stimulation and studies on renal development indicate that cell surface integrins, in particular $\alpha_5\beta_1$, and HSPGs are important candidates for endostatin binding. The role for integrins is further reinforced by the identification of these as receptors for other proteolytic anti-angiogenic fragments.

Future studies need to identify the relative importance of the signalling pathways identified for endostatin's biological activity and whether the activity of these vary between tumour- and normal endothelial cells in vivo.

Table 3. The potential anti-angiogenic mechanisms of action of endostatin.

Cytoskeletal reorganisation Downregulation of actin stress filaments and FAs	$\alpha_5\beta_1$ integrin and glypican-1 dependent translocation to lipid rafts with downstream Src-dependent deactivation of RhoA
Persistence of FAs	Cofilin/ hsp27 phosphorylation Tropomyosin-binding
Reorganisation of actin stress filaments and FAs dependent on FGF-2 stimulation	FAK, paxilin and β-catenin
Blockade of VEGF signalling	Direct competition for KDR Akt-independent dephosphorylation of eNOS Downregulation of VEGF synthesis by endothelial cells Inhibition of VEGF-induced of circulating endothelial progenitors
Induction of apoptosis	Bcl-2 downregulation Induction of Shb-dependent tyrosine kinase activity
Downregulation of TCF/LEF- dependent gene transcription	Degradation of β-catenin by GSK-3-independent pathway
Increase in intracellular calcium ion concentration	Primarily via release of calcium from IP_3- sensitive intracellular stores
Formation of amyloid fibrils	Induction of apoptosis and activation of tPA

Table 4. Signalling cascades down-regulated by endostatin identified by gene expression profiling (Abdollahi et al 2004).

Id- signalling Downregulation of Id-1 and Id-3- decreased endothelial cell proliferation
Hypoxia- inducible factor 1α signalling Downregulation of HIF-1α and upregulation of its antagonist, HIF1AN- required for hypoxia and metabolic adaptation
Ephrin and TNF-α signalling
Nuclear factor –κB signalling Downregulation of NF-κB mRNA expression and phosphorylation
STAT signalling
AP-1 signalling Downregulation of both Jun and Fos families and dephosphorylation of JNK
Ets-1 signalling
Coagulation cascade Downregulation of thrombin receptors, tissue factor, Factors VII, X, XI, XII

6. The Clinical Development of Endostatin

The marked anti-angiogenic effects of endostatin in animal models in vivo and the observation of tumour dormancy after prolonged endostatin administration (summarised in [119]) resulted in great enthusiasm for the development of endostatin as a therapeutic agent in both the scientific community and the media[144]. The disappointing results of Phase I/II studies conducted in the last 3-4 years have however dampened the optimism surrounding endostatin significantly. In this section we will discuss the results of studies focusing on endostatin in human cancer patients and present some of the possible reasons for the lack of therapeutic efficacy seen with endostatin in clinical trials.

6.1. Circulating Endostatin and Cancer

Endostatin is detectable in the plasma/ serum of the normal population at levels of 15-30ng/ml (see table 5 for references) secondary to low levels of collagen XVIII degradation within basement membranes. Patients with Down's syndrome who have chromosome 21 trisomy, and therefore three copies of the Collagen XVIII gene, have been reported to have endostatin levels 50-100% higher than control patients[145]. This is of particular interest as Down's syndrome patients have a much lower risk of death from malignant neoplasia than the rest of the population. In an analysis of data from US death certificates from 1983-1997, the standardised mortality odds ratio for all malignancies apart from acute leukaemia was 0.07[146] suggesting that the anti-angiogenic effects of circulating endostatin may protect against the development of clinically manifest cancers.

However, if circulating levels of endostatin are analysed in cancer patients, levels are generally significantly higher than in age-matched controls across a broad range of solid and haematological malignancies (see table 5). Of note, in many tumour types, a raised endostatin level at presentation is an independent poor prognostic factor. This has been demonstrated for relapse-free survival in soft tissue sarcomas[147], transitional cell carcinoma of the bladder[148] and node negative breast carcinoma[149] and for overall survival in Non-Hodgkin's lymphoma[150], renal cell carcinoma (RCC)[151], acute myeloid leukaemia (AML)[152] and non-small cell lung carcinoma (NSCLC)[153]. Whilst many of these studies were retrospective in design and variable cut-offs were used to assign patients to high and low endostatin subgroups, a recurrent theme has clearly emerged.

It is unclear as to whether these elevated endostatin concentrations are due to direct intratumoral production or a coordinated 'host' response to pro-angiogenic stimuli produced by the tumour. Elevated endostatin gene expression has been noted in ovarian carcinoma[154] and positive intratumoral immunohistochemical staining for collagen XVIII has been shown to correlate with both serum endostatin levels and poor prognosis in NSCLC[155]. Whilst these results suggest that the cancer is the source of serum endostatin and are consistent with the hypothesis that removal of the primary tumour reduces the anti-angiogenic drive allowing more rapid growth of metastases, analysis of serum endostatin levels pre- and post surgical resection is not fully supportive of this. For instance, whilst serum endostatin levels fall after resection of hepatocellular carcinoma[156], no significant differences were noted in a series of 59 breast cancer patients[157]. Interestingly, in a prospective study of 66 RCC patients undergoing nephrectomy[151], serum endostatin actually rose after surgery and a rise of greater than 2-fold was associated with a significantly lower overall survival.

Table 5. Serum endostatin concentrations and prognosis in human cancer.

Tumour type	Prospective/ retrospective	No. Pts/ Control	Endo levels Pt/control (ng/ml)	Statistically significant difference	Adverse Prognostic indicator	Reference
HCC	P	108/20	35.0 (6.5-75.6) 31.6 (2.9-41.6)	No	No	[159]
Breast	P	59/59	40.0 (12.4-110.6) 15.3 (3.9-68)	Yes (p<.005)	No	[157]
Ovarian	R	61/29	18.5 (6.3-50.3) 18.4 (8.4-27.0)	No	Yes if >2S.D. above mean	[194]
NHL	R	143/24	29.6 (4.5-116) 16.4	Yes	Yes (RR of death=1.8)	[150]
Various (hepatic metastases)	?	25/12/15	18.8 /23.9/17.1	No	NA	[195]
TCC bladder	?	53/32	46.8 30.6	Yes (p<.001)	Yes (risk of metastases)	[148]
Myeloma	R	84/13	58 40	Yes (p=.015)	No	[196]
HCC	P	33/-	17.2 (4.8-113.5)	NA	No? assoc with better prognosis	[156]
RCC	P	66/32	29.1 22.2	Yes (p=.05)	Yes (raised post-nephrectomy levels assoc with poor Px)	[151]
AML/MDS	P	71/43/12	29.9 (4-78) 34.4 (10.4-92.4) 30.4 (14.0-63.6)	No	Yes	[152]
NSCLC (resectable)	P	99/17	42.4/ 16.3	Yes (p=.0003)	Yes	[153]
Colorectal (hepatic mets)	R	30/?		Yes (p<.0001)	Elevated level on F/U assoc with relapse	[197]
Endometrial	R	72/30	I-320 III/IV-1250 Cont-13	Yes	NA	[198]
STS	R	25/34	43.0/25.8	Yes (p=.0002)	Yes (recurrence)	[147]
Breast Ca	?	183/221		Yes (p<.01)	Yes in node negative disease	[149]
RCC (clear cell)	R	15/18	24.6(15.1-54) 14.1 (1.0-19.3)	Yes (p<.0001)	NA	[141]
Vulvar Ca	R	41/35	52.3(25.5-128.2) 49.8 (25.7-115.2)	No	No	[199]
HCC	R	42/10	18.2 (2.0-35.3) 15.2 (2.2-54.3)	No	NA	[200]

Abbreviations; P- prospective, R- retrospective, HCC- hepatocellular carcinoma, RCC- renal cell carcinoma, STS- soft tissue sarcoma, NSCLC- non-small cell lung cancer, AML- acute myeloid leukaemia, MDS- myelodysplastic syndrome, TCC- transitional cell carcinoma, NHL- Non-Hodgkin's lymphoma NA- not assessed.

In the only study to analyse endostatin levels after cytotoxic chemotherapy, Glenjen et al[158] found no difference in levels before and after intensive induction/ consolidation treatment for AML indicating that the leukaemic blasts were not the source of circulating endostatin.

Several of these studies have assessed circulating concentrations of pro-angiogenic cytokines as well as endostatin. Many of these demonstrated weak-to-moderate positive correlations with FGF-2[158] and VEGF[141,150,151,156,157,159] in particular. This may indicate that endostatin levels are secreted endogenously in a co-ordinated manner to counteract pro-angiogenic stimuli secreted by the tumour. As raised endostatin concentrations are associated with poor prognosis, it may be that in clinically manifest tumours, once the angiogenic switch has been tripped raising the levels of endogenous anti-angiogenic agents is not effective in resetting this. A further alternative explanation is that in effect these cancers are already at the top of the dose-response curve for endostatin and so have overcome its inhibitory effects. This possibility would have significant implications for the use of endostatin as a single agent in the therapeutic setting.

6.2. Endostatin Polymorphisms and Cancer

Over 20 polymorphisms have been identified in the COL18A1 gene in the general population[74]. One of these encodes a missense mutation in the endostatin domain. This alteration of a surface-exposed aspartic acid to an asparagine (D104N) has been associated with a 2.4-fold increased risk of prostatic adenocarcinoma in a case-control study undertaken in Brazil[160]. The mechanism behind this is unclear but molecular modelling suggests an altered conformation of lysine 106 in the mutant molecule suggesting potential changes in receptor binding. However, subsequent studies in multiple myeloma[161] and leukaemia[162] have not identified increased risk in these haematological malignancies associated with D104N. No published studies have reported on risk of other solid malignancies.

6.3. Phase I Trials

Three phase I trials have been published using recombinant human endostatin derived from a Pichia pastoris expression system in a total of 61 patients with advanced metastatic cancer[163-165]. These have administered endostatin at doses of 15 to 600 mg/m^2/day as short daily intravenous infusions. No significant endostatin-related toxicity was noted apart from mild skin rashes. Endostatin displayed linear pharmacokinetics that was consistent across all three studies and the area under the serum concentration-time curve reached levels associated with activity in animal models at doses of 300mg/m^2/day. No formal disease responses were seen in these studies although some evidence of anti-tumour activity was noted with one patient with metastatic pancreatic neuroendocrine tumour experiencing a minor response[163] and patients with metastatic melanoma and synovial sarcoma having mixed responses[164]. These suggestions of anti-neoplastic activity did not appear to be dose-related with the minor response occurring at the 30mg/m^2/day dose level. A subsequent phase II study of endostatin administered subcutaneously in metastatic neuroendocrine tumours used a dose of 60mg/m^2/day in two divided doses with dose escalation if trough levels were low. Forty-one patients were recruited but only 2 minor responses were noted[166].

One problem for the phase I development of all anti-angiogenic agents, and exemplified by endostatin is the difficulty in establishing the biologically effective dose (BED). Whereas myelosuppression and other toxicities can be utilised as surrogate markers for this with cytotoxic agents, endostatin is essentially non-toxic at clinically feasible doses. All three phase I studies utilised radiological and biopsy-based indicators of tumour angiogenesis to try and assess BED. No significant changes were noted with in vivo imaging with dynamic CT (marker of microvessel density), dynamic MRI (marker of tumour blood flow) or [^{18}F]-FDG-PET (measure of tumour glucose metabolism) in one study[165]. Paired pre- and 8-week post-treatment tumour biopsies from patients on this study also failed to demonstrate any changes in microvessel density, endothelial cell apoptosis, proliferation or vessel maturity although only 8 pairs of samples were available for analysis. Interestingly, a skin wound angiogenesis assay also noted no difference in wound healing during endostatin treatment[167].

Herbst et al[164], however, in their study of 26 patients demonstrated some subtle effects on tumour blood flow and biopsy biomarkers of tumour angiogenesis. Utilising [^{15}O]-H_2O PET as an in vivo marker of blood flow, they noted that this decreased by an average of 20% with endostatin treatment by day 28 at the 180mg/m^2/day dose level, subtle changes in intra-tumoral glucose metabolism were also noted at higher endostatin doses[168]. It should be noted however, that changes in these parameters only reached statistical significance if patients treated at the 30mg/m^2/day dose level were included. These patients did not have baseline PET imaging and so changes during cycle 2 instead of cycle 1 were used in the analysis for this cohort. Analysis of tumour microvessel density, endothelial cell apoptosis and nuclear localisation of HIF-1α as a marker of tumour hypoxia in biopsy specimens also suggested that endostatin was having a biological effect on human cancers in vivo[169]. Intriguingly, the use of a novel statistical analysis- the quadratic polynomial model indicated that these biological effects may have a U-shaped relationship with dose, being most apparent around 250mg/m^2/day. Whilst these exploratory analyses give us a potential insight into a BED for endostatin, it is possible that the analysis employed was highly dependent on the range of doses used and may be distorted by the presence of outlying values. It should also be noted that the seven patients (28%) with early progressive disease on study were excluded from these analyses as paired biopsies were not taken in these patients. Most importantly however, these signs of biological activity were not translated into clinical activity and the lack of information on the natural history of the parameters assessed in untreated malignancy means that it is impossible to rule out a contribution of tumour biology to the changes documented.

6.4. Considerations for Further Clinical Development

Overall, although the studies discussed above have confirmed the safety of endostatin as a pharmacological agent in humans the lack of activity seen is disappointing. Although some of the problems behind this have been already discussed, several other points need to be borne in mind when considering the future clinical development of endostatin and other endogenous angiogenesis inhibitors.

1) Trial design and patient selection- By necessity, most phase I studies are conducted in patients with bulky metastatic disease that has progressed despite multiple lines of chemotherapy. Such patients are not ideal for the assessment of anti-angiogenic agents as not only do the tumours already have an established vasculature but the cancer cells are likely to have adapted to become tolerant of hypoxia and other apoptosis-inducing signals. It may be more appropriate once toxicity data are available to assess these agents in patients with minimal residual disease.

The assessment of tumour response as a trial endpoint in phase II studies may also be inappropriate for endogenous angiogenesis inhibitors as such molecules may only result in disease stabilisation. A randomised discontinuation model[170] may be more sensitive to a biological effect. In this model all patients entering the study commence the novel therapy. After a set period those patients with disease stabilisation are randomised to continue or discontinue treatment. Time to disease progression in these two subgroups can then be assessed.

2) Pharmacokinetic considerations- Endostatin was administered as short daily intravenous infusions in the published phase I studies. However, initial animal data were generated using the subcutaneous administration of a poorly soluble form of endostatin that is likely to have acted as a depot[69,70] and subsequent work has shown that continuous infusion of endostatin is markedly more effective than bolus administration in animal models[171]. Many other methods of prolonged delivery of endostatin have been investigated in animal models including alginate beads and gene therapy.

3) Poorly-defined mechanism of action- At the time of the design of the endostatin trials very little was known about endostatin's mechanism of action. This paucity of knowledge clearly inhibited the scope of biomarker/ translational research that was incorporated. The complexity of signalling pathways subsequently identified as being affected by endostatin treatment of endothelial cells in vitro means that no single biomarker can be proposed with certainty for investigation in future trials although assessment of $\alpha_5\beta_1$ integrin expression and downstream signalling should be considered. The emerging evidence for a role of cell surface heparan sulfate binding in endostatin's function means that the use of heparin, particularly as a line-lock during clinical trials may inhibit its activity. Such treatment was specifically contra-indicated in only one study[164].

4) Potential immunogenicity- The administration of exogenous protein, albeit of human origin is associated with an immunogenic risk. Although no significant allergic reactions were seen with endostatin, many patients rapidly developed anti-endostatin IgG titres[164,165]. Whether these antibodies have function- neutralising properties is not clear but their rapid induction is clearly a concern for future studies.

5) Intravascular proteolysis/ modification- The rapid clearance of circulating proteins by plasma and extracellular matrix proteases is a potential concern with all endogenous anti-angiogenics. Analysis of serum- isolated endostatin in one phase I study[165] did not demonstrate extensive proteolytic degradation. However small shifts in mass spectrometry profiles were noted that could have been consistent with limited terminal proteolytic cleavage. Of note, no in vitro activity could be demonstrated for re-isolated endostatin in any of the three studies.

6) Overloaded system- As discussed above, serum levels of endostatin are raised in many untreated cancer patients and the degree of elevation is associated with prognosis (see table 5). It is as yet unclear whether further increasing serum endostatin levels will have significant anti- angiogenic effects as maximal endostatin inhibition may already be present in these patients.

7) Vasculogenic mimicry- Many established tumours have blood vessels lined in part or completely by tumour cells. In some cases these cells express surface markers normally confined to endothelial cells[10]. A recent study has indicated that tubular network formation by such cell lines is unaffected by endostatin treatment and other angiogenesis inhibitors[172] indicating that the vascular network in some tumours will be unaffected by even if optimal inhibition of endothelial cell function is achieved in vivo.

6.5. How can we Improve the Efficacy of Endostatin?

Even if we address the above caveats, other means may need to be adopted to improve the clinical utility of endostatin. One method could be to use endostatin in combination with conventional anti-cancer therapy. Endostatin has been shown to be additive to radiotherapy in some animal models[173,174] and to be synergistic with cytotoxic chemotherapy in others[175.176]. Importantly no exacerbation of treatment-related toxicity was seen in these studies.

More intriguingly several studies have demonstrated synergism between endostatin and other anti-angiogenic agents. In a murine ovarian cancer xenograft model using adeno-associated viral gene therapy injected into muscle as a long-term source of direct angiogenesis inhibitors, endostatin and angiostatin proved synergistic in preventing tumour growth and improving survival[177]. Rational combinations determined by analysis of the microarray data discussed above have also been tested successfully in animal models. Cline et al[133] noted markedly different gene expression profiles when endothelial cells were treated with TNP-470, a synthetic fumagillin analogue or endostatin and subsequently showed synergistic activity against Lewis lung carcinoma xenografts. The results of Abdollahi et al[134] indicated that endostatin downregulated many of the key mediators of VEGF signalling. Subsequent work has shown that endostatin and SU5416 a small molecule ty.rosine kinase inhibitor of KDR, are synergistic in inhibiting endothelial cell prolferation and the growth and vascularisation of tumour xenografts[178].

Another approach to improving the efficacy of endostatin has been to alter its molecular structure. A point mutation resulting in an alanine to proline substitution at position 125 (P125A) created an endostatin mutant with increased binding affinity for HUVEC cell membrane, increased localisation to tumour tissue in vivo and increased biological activity compared to the parental molecule[179]. The molecular mechanism for this increased activity is unclear but involves increased avidity for a cell surface receptor. Indeed the addition of an N-terminal RGD sequence providing a second integrin-binding site increased the biological activity of P125A endostatin still further[180]. Clearly these mutants and the mechanisms behind their increased activity need to be explored further.

Endostatin-derived peptides have also been investigated. Whereas considerably higher concentrations of the basic amino-acid rich short peptides generated by Wickström [108] were required for equivalent in vitro anti-angiogenic activity, the synthesis of larger peptides by Cattaneo et al [181] demonstrated superior activity for a peptide encoding amino-acids 6-49. This peptide was more effective at inhibiting endothelial cell proliferation and also at preventing FGF-2-stimulated vessel ingrowth into a Matrigel plug in vivo. However, heparin was administered concurrently which may have inhibited the actions of the heparin-binding parental endostatin. The synthesis of such peptides is significantly easier than full-length endostatin so this strategy requires further investigation.

7. Conclusions

The identification of a series of proteolytic fragments of extracellular matrix components as endogenous angiogenesis inhibitors has increased our understanding of physiological control of blood vessel development. The isolation of fragments from highly evolutionarily conserved proteins such as fibronectin and collagens IV and XV/XVIII and the demonstration of a role for the NC-1 domain of the collagen XV/XVIII homologue in neuronal migration in C. elegans indicates the fundamental importance of at least some of these molecules. It is intriguing that whilst integrin-dependent signalling pathways have emerged as critical downstream mediators of the anti-angiogenic properties of many of these fragments, endostatin, the most investigated moelcule has many proposed cell- surface binding partners and has been shown to have a profound wide-ranging effect on the angiogenic gene expression profile of endothelial cells.

The discovery of these molecules has also opened up a significant new avenue in the development of anti-neoplastic agents. Whilst the clinical development of endostatin as an anti-angiogenic drug has been disappointing, it has enabled us to learn a number of lessons which could improve the strategy used to take other fragments, for instance tumstatin through to the clinic. It is important that careful biological assays are conducted in a variety of systems and that a defined mechanism of action has been elucidated prior to clinical trials commencing so that appropriate candidate biomarkers can be selected for testing alongside conventional toxicity screening. The potential for unique toxicities, for instance a GPS-like syndrome with tumstatin, also needs to be identified in the pre-clinical setting. An increased knowledge of the pathophysiology of cancer with respect to circulating anti-angiogenic fragment profiles and the effects of manipulating these on cancer growth is also crucial to the further development of these molecules.

Overall our understanding of angiogenesis has changed markedly with the identification of these endogenous cryptic angiogenesis inhibitors. However, much further basic and translational research needs to be done before they can be fully evaluated as pharmacological agents.

References

[1] Folkman J: Tumor angiogenesis: therapeutic implications. *N Engl J Med 285*:1182-6., 1971

[2] Yi M, Ruoslahti E: A fibronectin fragment inhibits tumor growth, angiogenesis, and metastasis. *Proc Natl Acad Sci U S A 98*:620-4, 2001

[3] Mongiat M, Sweeney SM, San Antonio JD, et al: Endorepellin, a novel inhibitor of angiogenesis derived from the C terminus of perlecan. *J Biol Chem 278*:4238-49, 2003

[4] Sargiannidou I, Zhou J, Tuszynski GP: The role of thrombospondin-1 in tumor progression. *Exp Biol Med (Maywood) 226*:726-33, 2001

[5] Ortega N, Werb Z: New functional roles for non-collagenous domains of basement membrane collagens. *J Cell Sci 115*:4201-14., 2002

[6] Carmeliet P: Angiogenesis in health and disease. *Nat Med 9*:653-60, 2003

[7] Conway EM, Collen D, Carmeliet P: Molecular mechanisms of blood vessel growth. *Cardiovasc Res 49*:507-21., 2001

[8] Carmeliet P, Jain RK: Angiogenesis in cancer and other diseases. *Nature 407*:249-57., 2000

[9] Relf M, LeJeune S, Scott PA, et al: Expression of the angiogenic factors vascular endothelial cell growth factor, acidic and basic fibroblast growth factor, tumor growth factor beta-1, platelet-derived endothelial cell growth factor, placenta growth factor, and pleiotrophin in human primary breast cancer and its relation to angiogenesis. *Cancer Res 57*:963-9., 1997

[10] Hendrix MJ, Seftor EA, Meltzer PS, et al: Expression and functional significance of VE-cadherin in aggressive human melanoma cells: role in vasculogenic mimicry. *Proc Natl Acad Sci U S A 98*:8018-23., 2001

[11] Chang YS, di Tomaso E, McDonald DM, et al: Mosaic blood vessels in tumors: frequency of cancer cells in contact with flowing blood. *Proc Natl Acad Sci U S A 97*:14608-13., 2000

[12] Bergers G, Benjamin LE: Tumorigenesis and the angiogenic switch. *Nat Rev Cancer 3*:401-10, 2003

[13] Bosman FT, Stamenkovic I: Functional structure and composition of the extracellular matrix. *J Pathol 200*:423-8, 2003

[14] Hynes RO: Integrins: bidirectional, allosteric signaling machines. *Cell 110*:673-87, 2002

[15] Kalluri R: Basement membranes: structure, assembly and role in tumour angiogenesis. *Nat Rev Cancer 3*:422-33, 2003

[16] Erickson AC, Couchman JR: Still more complexity in mammalian basement membranes. *J Histochem Cytochem 48*:1291-306., 2000

[17] Jiang X, Couchman JR: Perlecan and tumor angiogenesis. *J Histochem Cytochem 51*:1393-410, 2003

[18] Egeblad M, Werb Z: New functions for the matrix metalloproteinases in cancer progression. *Nat Rev Cancer 2*:161-74, 2002

[19] Vlodavsky I, Friedmann Y: Molecular properties and involvement of heparanase in cancer metastasis and angiogenesis. *J Clin Invest 108*:341-7., 2001

[20] Xu J, Rodriguez D, Petitclerc E, et al: Proteolytic exposure of a cryptic site within collagen type IV is required for angiogenesis and tumor growth in vivo. *J Cell Biol 154*:1069-79, 2001

[21] Engbring JA, Kleinman HK: The basement membrane matrix in malignancy. *J Pathol 200*:465-70, 2003

[22] Patarroyo M, Tryggvason K, Virtanen I: Laminin isoforms in tumor invasion, angiogenesis and metastasis. *Semin Cancer Biol 12*:197-207, 2002

[23] Homandberg GA, Williams JE, Grant D, et al: Heparin-binding fragments of fibronectin are potent inhibitors of endothelial cell growth. *Am J Pathol 120*:327-32., 1985

[24] Clapp C, Martial JA, Guzman RC, et al: The 16-kilodalton N-terminal fragment of human prolactin is a potent inhibitor of angiogenesis. *Endocrinology 133*:1292-9., 1993

[25] O'Reilly MS, Holmgren L, Shing Y, et al: Angiostatin: a novel angiogenesis inhibitor that mediates the suppression of metastases by a Lewis lung carcinoma. *Cell 79*:315-28, 1994

[26] Geiger JH, Cnudde SE: What the structure of angiostatin may tell us about its mechanism of action. *J Thromb Haemost 2*:23-34, 2004

[27] Wahl ML, Moser TL, Pizzo SV: Angiostatin and anti-angiogenic therapy in human disease. *Recent Prog Horm Res 59*:73-104, 2004

[28] Moser TL, Stack MS, Asplin I, et al: Angiostatin binds ATP synthase on the surface of human endothelial cells. *Proc Natl Acad Sci U S A 96*:2811-6, 1999

[29] Moser TL, Stack MS, Wahl ML, et al: The mechanism of action of angiostatin: can you teach an old dog new tricks? *Thromb Haemost 87*:394-401, 2002

[30] Tarui T, Miles LA, Takada Y: Specific interaction of angiostatin with integrin alpha(v)beta(3) in endothelial cells. *J Biol Chem 276*:39562-8, 2001

[31] Wajih N, Sane DC: Angiostatin selectively inhibits signaling by hepatocyte growth factor in endothelial and smooth muscle cells. *Blood 101*:1857-63, 2003

[32] Troyanovsky B, Levchenko T, Mansson G, et al: Angiomotin: an angiostatin binding protein that regulates endothelial cell migration and tube formation. *J Cell Biol 152*:1247-54, 2001

[33] Daly ME, Makris A, Reed M, et al: Hemostatic regulators of tumor angiogenesis: a source of antiangiogenic agents for cancer treatment? *J Natl Cancer Inst 95*:1660-73, 2003

[34] Hudson BG, Tryggvason K, Sundaramoorthy M, et al: Alport's syndrome, Goodpasture's syndrome, and type IV collagen. *N Engl J Med 348*:2543-56, 2003

[35] Petitclerc E, Boutaud A, Prestayko A, et al: New functions for non-collagenous domains of human collagen type IV. Novel integrin ligands inhibiting angiogenesis and tumor growth in vivo. *J Biol Chem 275*:8051-61, 2000

[36] Colorado PC, Torre A, Kamphaus G, et al: Anti-angiogenic cues from vascular basement membrane collagen. *Cancer Res 60*:2520-6, 2000

[37] Keller KM, Keller JM, Kuhn K: The C-terminus of type I collagen is a major binding site for heparin. *Biochim Biophys Acta 882*:1-5, 1986

[38] Kamphaus GD, Colorado PC, Panka DJ, et al: Canstatin, a novel matrix-derived inhibitor of angiogenesis and tumor growth. *J Biol Chem 275*:1209-15, 2000

[39] He GA, Luo JX, Zhang TY, et al: Canstatin-N fragment inhibits in vitro endothelial cell proliferation and suppresses in vivo tumor growth. *Biochem Biophys Res Commun 312*:801-5, 2003

[40] Irmler M, Thome M, Hahne M, et al: Inhibition of death receptor signals by cellular FLIP. *Nature 388*:190-5, 1997

[41] Kataoka T, Budd RC, Holler N, et al: The caspase-8 inhibitor FLIP promotes activation of NF-kappaB and Erk signaling pathways. *Curr Biol 10*:640-8, 2000

[42] Panka DJ, Mier JW: Canstatin inhibits Akt activation and induces Fas-dependent apoptosis in endothelial cells. *J Biol Chem 278*:37632-6, 2003

[43] Maeshima Y, Colorado PC, Torre A, et al: Distinct antitumor properties of a type IV collagen domain derived from basement membrane. *J Biol Chem 275*:21340-8, 2000

[44] Hamano Y, Zeisberg M, Sugimoto H, et al: Physiological levels of tumstatin, a fragment of collagen IV alpha3 chain, are generated by MMP-9 proteolysis and suppress angiogenesis via alphaV beta3 integrin. *Cancer Cell 3*:589-601, 2003

[45] Han J, Ohno N, Pasco S, et al: A cell binding domain from the alpha3 chain of type IV collagen inhibits proliferation of melanoma cells. *J Biol Chem 272*:20395-401, 1997

[46] Pasco S, Han J, Gillery P, et al: A specific sequence of the noncollagenous domain of the alpha3(IV) chain of type IV collagen inhibits expression and activation of matrix metalloproteinases by tumor cells. *Cancer Res 60*:467-73, 2000

[47] Maeshima Y, Colorado PC, Kalluri R: Two RGD-independent alpha vbeta 3 integrin binding sites on tumstatin regulate distinct anti-tumor properties. *J Biol Chem 275*:23745-50, 2000

[48] Pedchenko V, Zent R, Hudson BG: Alpha(v)beta3 and alpha(v)beta5 integrins bind both the proximal RGD site and non-RGD motifs within noncollagenous (NC1) domain of the alpha3 chain of type IV collagen: implication for the mechanism of endothelial cell adhesion. *J Biol Chem 279*:2772-80, 2004

[49] Maeshima Y, Manfredi M, Reimer C, et al: Identification of the anti-angiogenic site within vascular basement membrane-derived tumstatin. *J Biol Chem 276*:15240-8, 2001

[50] Maeshima Y, Yerramalla UL, Dhanabal M, et al: Extracellular matrix-derived peptide binds to alpha(v)beta(3) integrin and inhibits angiogenesis. *J Biol Chem 276*:31959-68, 2001

[51] Maeshima Y, Sudhakar A, Lively JC, et al: Tumstatin, an endothelial cell-specific inhibitor of protein synthesis. *Science 295*:140-3, 2002

[52] Miner JH, Sanes JR: Molecular and functional defects in kidneys of mice lacking collagen alpha 3(IV): implications for Alport syndrome. *J Cell Biol 135*:1403-13, 1996

[53] Borza DB, Hudson BG: Of mice and men: murine models of anti-GBM antibody nephritis. *Kidney Int 61*:1905-6, 2002

[54] Costell M, Carmona R, Gustafsson E, et al: Hyperplastic conotruncal endocardial cushions and transposition of great arteries in perlecan-null mice. *Circ Res 91*:158-64, 2002

[55] Zhou Z, Wang J, Cao R, et al: Impaired angiogenesis, delayed wound healing and retarded tumor growth in perlecan heparan sulfate-deficient mice. *Cancer Res 64*:4699-702, 2004

[56] Bix G, Fu J, Gonzalez EM, et al: Endorepellin causes endothelial cell disassembly of actin cytoskeleton and focal adhesions through alpha2beta1 integrin. *J Cell Biol 166*:97-109, 2004

[57] Yi M, Sakai T, Fassler R, et al: Antiangiogenic proteins require plasma fibronectin or vitronectin for in vivo activity. *Proc Natl Acad Sci U S A 100*:11435-8, 2003

[58] Chau I, Rigg A, Cunningham D: Matrix metalloproteinase inhibitors--an emphasis on gastrointestinal malignancies. *Crit Rev Oncol Hematol 45*:151-76, 2003

[59] Overall CM, Lopez-Otin C: Strategies for MMP inhibition in cancer: innovations for the post-trial era. *Nat Rev Cancer 2:*657-72, 2002

[60] Brooks PC, Silletti S, von Schalscha TL, et al: Disruption of angiogenesis by PEX, a noncatalytic metalloproteinase fragment with integrin binding activity. *Cell 92*:391-400, 1998

[61] Pfeifer A, Kessler T, Silletti S, et al: Suppression of angiogenesis by lentiviral delivery of PEX, a noncatalytic fragment of matrix metalloproteinase 2. *Proc Natl Acad Sci U S A 97*:12227-32, 2000

[62] Pluderi M, Lucini V, Caronzolo D, et al: Long-term inhibition of glioma growth by systemic administration of human PEX. *J Neurosurg Sci 47*:69-78, 2003

[63] Donnini S, Morbidelli L, Taraboletti G, et al: ERK1-2 and p38 MAPK regulate MMP/TIMP balance and function in response to thrombospondin-1 fragments in the microvascular endothelium. *Life Sci 74*:2975-85, 2004

[64] Good DJ, Polverini PJ, Rastinejad F, et al: A tumor suppressor-dependent inhibitor of angiogenesis is immunologically and functionally indistinguishable from a fragment of thrombospondin. *Proc Natl Acad Sci U S A 87*:6624-8, 1990

[65] Iruela-Arispe ML, Lombardo M, Krutzsch HC, et al: Inhibition of angiogenesis by thrombospondin-1 is mediated by 2 independent regions within the type 1 repeats. *Circulation 100*:1423-31, 1999

[66] De Vos FY, Hoekstra R, Gietema JA, et al: A phase I dose escalating of the angiogenesis inhibitor thrombospondin-mimetic (ABT-510) in patients with advanced cancer. *Proc Am Soc Clin Oncol 21*:324a, 2002

[67] De Vos FY, Hoekstra R, Eskens FA, et al: Dose-finding and pharmacokinetic study of ABT-510 with gemcitabine and cisplatin in patients with advanced cancer. *Proc Am Soc Clin Oncol 22*:3077a, 2004

[68] Gordon MS, Mendelson D, Guirguis MS, et al: ABT-510, an anti-angiogenic thrombospondin-1 (TSP-1) mimetic peptide, exhibits favorable safety profile and early signals of activity in a randomized phase IB trial. *Proc Am Soc Clin Oncol 22*:780a, 2003

[69] O'Reilly MS, Boehm T, Shing Y, et al: Endostatin: an endogenous inhibitor of angiogenesis and tumor growth. *Cell 88*:277-85., 1997

[70] Boehm T, Folkman J, Browder T, et al: Antiangiogenic therapy of experimental cancer does not induce acquired drug resistance. *Nature 390*:404-7., 1997

[71] Oh SP, Kamagata Y, Muragaki Y, et al: Isolation and sequencing of cDNAs for proteins with multiple domains of Gly-Xaa-Yaa repeats identify a distinct family of collagenous proteins. *Proc Natl Acad Sci U S A 91*:4229-33., 1994

[72] Halfter W, Dong S, Schurer B, et al: Collagen XVIII is a basement membrane heparan sulfate proteoglycan. *J Biol Chem 273*:25404-12., 1998

[73] Saarela J, Rehn M, Oikarinen A, et al: The short and long forms of type XVIII collagen show clear tissue specificities in their expression and location in basement membrane zones in humans. *Am J Pathol 153*:611-26., 1998

[74] Suzuki OT, Sertie AL, Der Kaloustian VM, et al: Molecular Analysis of Collagen XVIII Reveals Novel Mutations, Presence of a Third Isoform, and Possible Genetic Heterogeneity in Knobloch Syndrome. *Am J Hum Genet 71*:1320-9., 2002

[75] Sertie AL, Sossi V, Camargo AA, et al: Collagen XVIII, containing an endogenous inhibitor of angiogenesis and tumor growth, plays a critical role in the maintenance of retinal structure and in neural tube closure (Knobloch syndrome). *Hum Mol Genet 9*:2051-8., 2000

[76] Fukai N, Eklund L, Marneros AG, et al: Lack of collagen XVIII/endostatin results in eye abnormalities. *Embo J 21*:1535-44., 2002

[77] Marneros AG, Keene DR, Hansen U, et al: Collagen XVIII/endostatin is essential for vision and retinal pigment epithelial function. *Embo J 23*:89-99, 2004

[78] Ackley BD, Crew JR, Elamaa H, et al: The NC1/endostatin domain of Caenorhabditis elegans type XVIII collagen affects cell migration and axon guidance. *J Cell Biol 152*:1219-32., 2001

[79] Haftek Z, Morvan-Dubois G, Thisse B, et al: Sequence and embryonic expression of collagen XVIII NC1 domain (endostatin) in the zebrafish. *Gene Expr Patterns 3*:351-4, 2003

[80] Elamaa H, Peterson J, Pihlajaniemi T, et al: Cloning of three variants of type XVIII collagen and their expression patterns during Xenopus laevis development. *Mech Dev 114*:109., 2002

[81] Sasaki T, Fukai N, Mann K, et al: Structure, function and tissue forms of the C-terminal globular domain of collagen XVIII containing the angiogenesis inhibitor endostatin. *Embo J 17*:4249-56., 1998

[82] Felbor U, Dreier L, Bryant RA, et al: Secreted cathepsin L generates endostatin from collagen XVIII. *Embo J 19*:1187-94., 2000

[83] Wen W, Moses MA, Wiederschain D, et al: The generation of endostatin is mediated by elastase. *Cancer Res 59*:6052-6., 1999

[84] Ferreras M, Felbor U, Lenhard T, et al: Generation and degradation of human endostatin proteins by various proteinases. *FEBS Lett 486*:247-51, 2000

[85] Ding YH, Javaherian K, Lo KM, et al: Zinc-dependent dimers observed in crystals of human endostatin. *Proc Natl Acad Sci U S A 95*:10443-8., 1998

[86] Hohenester E, Sasaki T, Olsen BR, et al: Crystal structure of the angiogenesis inhibitor endostatin at 1.5 A resolution. *Embo J 17*:1656-64., 1998

[87] Hohenester E, Sasaki T, Mann K, et al: Variable zinc coordination in endostatin. *J Mol Biol 297*:1-6., 2000

[88] Boehm T, O'Reilly M S, Keough K, et al: Zinc-binding of endostatin is essential for its antiangiogenic activity. *Biochem Biophys Res Commun 252*:190-4, 1998

[89] Yamaguchi N, Anand-Apte B, Lee M, et al: Endostatin inhibits VEGF-induced endothelial cell migration and tumor growth independently of zinc binding. *Embo J 18*:4414-23., 1999

[90] Sasaki T, Larsson H, Kreuger J, et al: Structural basis and potential role of heparin/heparan sulfate binding to the angiogenesis inhibitor endostatin, *Embo J 18*: 6240-8., 1999

[91] Ramchandran R, Dhanabal M, Volk R, et al: Antiangiogenic activity of restin, NC10 domain of human collagen XV: comparison to endostatin. *Biochem Biophys Res Commun 255*:735-9, 1999

[92] Sasaki T, Larsson H, Tisi D, et al: Endostatins derived from collagens XV and XVIII differ in structural and binding properties, tissue distribution and anti-angiogenic activity. *J Mol Biol 301*:1179-90., 2000

[93] Eklund L, Piuhola J, Komulainen J, et al: Lack of type XV collagen causes a skeletal myopathy and cardiovascular defects in mice. *Proc Natl Acad Sci U S A 98*:1194-9, 2001

[94] Ylikarppa R, Eklund L, Sormunen R, et al: Double knockout mice reveal a lack of major functional compensation between collagens XV and XVIII. *Matrix Biol 22*:443-8, 2003

[95] Karumanchi SA, Jha V, Ramchandran R, et al: Cell surface glypicans are low-affinity endostatin receptors. *Mol Cell 7*:811-22., 2001

[96] Chang Z, Choon A, Friedl A: Endostatin binds to blood vessels in situ independent of heparan sulfate and does not compete for fibroblast growth factor-2 binding. *Am J Pathol 155*:71-6., 1999

[97] Sugahara K, Kitagawa H: Heparin and heparan sulfate biosynthesis. *IUBMB Life 54*:163-75, 2002

[98] Gallagher JT, Lyon M: *Heparan sulfate: Molecular structure and interactions with growth factors and morphogens*, in RV I (ed): Proteoglycans structure, biology and molecular interactions, Marcel Dekker Inc, 2000

[99] Ricard-Blum S, Feraud O, Lortat-Jacob H, et al: Characterization of endostatin binding to heparin and heparan sulfate by surface plasmon resonance and molecular modeling: role of divalent cations. *J Biol Chem 279*:2927-36, 2004

[100] Blackhall FH, Merry CL, Lyon M, et al: Binding of endostatin to endothelial heparan sulphate shows a differential requirement for specific sulphates. *Biochem J 375*:131-9 2003

[101] Kreuger J, Matsumoto T, Vanwildemeersch M, et al: Role of heparan sulfate domain organization in endostatin inhibition of endothelial cell function. *Embo J 21*:6303-11, 2002

[102] Rehn M, Veikkola T, Kukk-Valdre E, et al: Interaction of endostatin with integrins implicated in angiogenesis. *Proc Natl Acad Sci U S A 98*:1024-9., 2001

[103] Wickstrom SA, Veikkola T, Rehn M, et al: Endostatin-induced modulation of plasminogen activation with concomitant loss of focal adhesions and actin stress fibers in cultured human endothelial cells. *Cancer Res 61*:6511-6., 2001

[104] Dixelius J, Cross M, Matsumoto T, et al: Endostatin regulates endothelial cell adhesion and cytoskeletal organization. *Cancer Res 62*:1944-7., 2002

[105] Wickstrom SA, Alitalo K, Keski-Oja J: Endostatin Associates with Integrin alpha(5)beta(1) and Caveolin-1, and Activates Src via a Tyrosyl Phosphatase-dependent Pathway in Human Endothelial Cells. *Cancer Res 62*:5580-5589., 2002

[106] Wickstrom SA, Alitalo K, Keski-Oja J: Endostatin associates with lipid rafts and induces reorganization of the actin cytoskeleton via downregulation of RhoA activity. *J Biol Chem 278:*37895-901, 2003

[107] Sudhakar A, Sugimoto H, Yang C, et al: Human tumstatin and human endostatin exhibit distinct antiangiogenic activities mediated by alpha v beta 3 and alpha 5 beta 1 integrins. *Proc Natl Acad Sci U S A 100*:4766-71, 2003

[108] Wickstrom SA, Alitalo K, Keski-Oja J: An endostatin-derived peptide interacts with integrins and regulates actin cytoskeleton and migration of endothelial cells. *J Biol Chem 279:*20178-85 2004

[109] MacDonald NJ, Shivers WY, Narum DL, et al: Endostatin binds tropomyosin. A potential modulator of the antitumor activity of endostatin. *J Biol Chem 276*:25190-6., 2001

[110] Mallery SR, Morse MA, Wilson RF, et al: AIDS-related Kaposi's sarcoma cells rapidly internalize endostatin, which co-localizes to tropomysin microfilaments and inhibits cytokine-mediated migration and invasion. *J Cell Biochem 89*:133-43, 2003

[111] Keezer SM, Ivie SE, Krutzsch HC, et al: Angiogenesis inhibitors target the endothelial cell cytoskeleton through altered regulation of heat shock protein 27 and cofilin. *Cancer Res 63*:6405-12, 2003

[112] Kim YM, Jang JW, Lee OH, et al: Endostatin inhibits endothelial and tumor cellular invasion by blocking the activation and catalytic activity of matrix metalloproteinase. *Cancer Res* 60:5410-3., 2000

[113] Lee SJ, Jang JW, Kim YM, et al: Endostatin binds to the catalytic domain of matrix metalloproteinase-2. *FEBS Lett 519*:147-152., 2002

[114] Dixelius J, Larsson H, Sasaki T, et al: Endostatin-induced tyrosine kinase signaling through the Shb adaptor protein regulates endothelial cell apoptosis. *Blood 95*:3403-11., 2000

[115] Dhanabal M, Ramchandran R, Waterman MJ, et al: Endostatin induces endothelial cell apoptosis. *J Biol Chem 274*:11721-6., 1999

[116] Hanai J, Dhanabal M, Karumanchi SA, et al: Endostatin causes G1 arrest of endothelial cells through inhibition of cyclin D1. *J Biol Chem 277*:16464-9., 2002

[117] Shichiri M, Hirata Y: Antiangiogenesis signals by endostatin. *Faseb J 15*:1044-53., 2001

[118] Hanai J, Gloy J, Karumanchi SA, et al: Endostatin is a potential inhibitor of Wnt signaling. *J Cell Biol 158*:529-39., 2002

[119] Dixelius J, Cross MJ, Matsumoto T, et al: Endostatin action and intracellular signaling: beta-catenin as a potential target? *Cancer Lett 196*:1-12, 2003

[120] Kim YM, Hwang S, Pyun BJ, et al: Endostatin blocks VEGF-mediated signaling via direct interaction with KDR/Flk-1. *J Biol Chem 23*:23, 2002

[121] Hajitou A, Grignet C, Devy L, et al: The antitumoral effect of endostatin and angiostatin is associated with a down-regulation of vascular endothelial growth factor expression in tumor cells. *Faseb J 16*:1802-4, 2002

[122] Dimmeler S, Dernbach E, Zeiher AM: Phosphorylation of the endothelial nitric oxide synthase at ser-1177 is required for VEGF-induced endothelial cell migration. *FEBS Lett 477*:258-62., 2000

[123] Urbich C, Reissner A, Chavakis E, et al: Dephosphorylation of endothelial nitric oxide synthase contributes to the anti-angiogenic effects of endostatin. *Faseb J 16*:706-8., 2002

[124] Deininger MH, Wybranietz WA, Graepler FT, et al: Endothelial endostatin release is induced by general cell stress and modulated by the nitric oxide/cGMP pathway. *Faseb J 17*:1267-76, 2003

[125] Thomsen LL, Miles DW: Role of nitric oxide in tumour progression: lessons from human tumours. *Cancer Metastasis Rev 17*:107-18, 1998

[126] Capillo M, Mancuso P, Gobbi A, et al: Continuous Infusion of Endostatin Inhibits Differentiation, Mobilization, and Clonogenic Potential of Endothelial Cell Progenitors. *Clin Cancer Res 9*:377-382., 2003

[127] Schuch G, Heymach JV, Nomi M, et al: Endostatin inhibits the vascular endothelial growth factor-induced mobilization of endothelial progenitor cells. *Cancer Res 63*:8345-50, 2003

[128] Jiang L, Jha V, Dhanabal M, et al: Intracellular Ca(2+) signaling in endothelial cells by the angiogenesis inhibitors endostatin and angiostatin. *Am J Physiol Cell Physiol 280*:C1140-50., 2001

[129] Eriksson K, Magnusson P, Dixelius J, et al: Angiostatin and endostatin inhibit endothelial cell migration in response to FGF and VEGF without interfering with specific intracellular signal transduction pathways. *FEBS Lett 536*:19-24, 2003

[130] Yu Y, Moulton KS, Khan MK, et al: E-selectin is required for the antiangiogenic activity of endostatin. *Proc Natl Acad Sci U S A 101*:8005-10, 2004

[131] Kranenburg O, Kroon-Batenburg LM, Reijerkerk A, et al: Recombinant endostatin forms amyloid fibrils that bind and are cytotoxic to murine neuroblastoma cells in vitro. *FEBS Lett 539*:149-55, 2003

[132] Gebbink MF, Voest EE, Reijerkerk A: Do antiangiogenic protein fragments have amyloid properties? *Blood 104*:1601-5, 2004

[133] Cline EI, Bicciato S, DiBello C, et al: Prediction of in vivo synergistic activity of antiangiogenic compounds by gene expression profiling. *Cancer Res 62*:7143-8., 2002

[134] Abdollahi A, Hahnfeldt P, Maercker C, et al: Endostatin's antiangiogenic signaling network. *Mol Cell 13*:649-63, 2004

[135] Macpherson GR, Ng SS, Forbes SL, et al: Anti-angiogenic activity of human endostatin is HIF-1-independent in vitro and sensitive to timing of treatment in a human saphenous vein assay. *Mol Cancer Ther 2*:845-854, 2003

[136] Benezra R, Rafii S: Endostatin's endpoints-Deciphering the endostatin antiangiogenic pathway. *Cancer Cell 5*:205-6, 2004

[137] Dkhissi F, Lu H, Soria C, et al: Endostatin exhibits a direct antitumor effect in addition to its antiangiogenic activity in colon cancer cells. *Hum Gene Ther 14*:997-1008, 2003

[138] Nyberg P, Heikkila P, Sorsa T, et al: Endostatin inhibits human tongue carcinoma cell invasion and intravasation and blocks the activation of matrix metalloprotease-2, -9 and -13. *J Biol Chem 278:*22404-11, 2003

[139] Kim S, Bell K, Mousa SA, et al: Regulation of angiogenesis in vivo by ligation of integrin alpha5beta1 with the central cell-binding domain of fibronectin. *Am J Pathol 156*:1345-62., 2000

[140] Karihaloo A, Karumanchi SA, Barasch J, et al: Endostatin regulates branching morphogenesis of renal epithelial cells and ureteric bud. *Proc Natl Acad Sci U S A 98*:12509-14., 2001

[141] Feldman AL, Tamarkin L, Paciotti GF, et al: Serum endostatin levels are elevated and correlate with serum vascular endothelial growth factor levels in patients with stage IV clear cell renal cancer. *Clin Cancer Res 6*:4628-34, 2000

[142] Kuo CJ, LaMontagne KR, Jr., Garcia-Cardena G, et al: Oligomerization-dependent regulation of motility and morphogenesis by the collagen XVIII NC1/endostatin domain. *J Cell Biol 152*:1233-46., 2001

[143] Javaherian K, Park SY, Pickl WF, et al: Laminin modulates morphogenic properties of the collagen XVIII endostatin domain. *J Biol Chem 277*:45211-8, 2002

[144] Korata G: Hope in the lab: A special report; a cautious awe greets drugs that eradicate tumors in mice, New York Times. New York, 1998

[145] Zorick TS, Mustacchi Z, Bando SY, et al: High serum endostatin levels in Down syndrome: implications for improved treatment and prevention of solid tumours. *Eur J Hum Genet 9*:811-4., 2001

[146] Yang Q, Rasmussen SA, Friedman JM: Mortality associated with Down's syndrome in the USA from 1983 to 1997: a population-based study. *Lancet 359*:1019-25, 2002

[147] Feldman AL, Pak H, Yang JC, et al: Serum endostatin levels are elevated in patients with soft tissue sarcoma. *Cancer 91*:1525-9, 2001

[148] Guan KP, Ye HY, Yan Z, et al: Serum levels of endostatin and matrix metalloproteinase-9 associated with high stage and grade primary transitional cell carcinoma of the bladder. *Urology 61*:719-23, 2003

[149] Kuroi K, Tanaka C, Toi M: Circulating levels of endostatin in cancer patients. *Oncol Rep 8*:405-9, 2001

[150] Bono P, Teerenhovi L, Joensuu H: Elevated serum endostatin is associated with poor outcome in patients with non-Hodgkin lymphoma. *Cancer 97*:2767-75, 2003

[151] Feldman AL, Alexander HR, Jr., Yang JC, et al: Prospective analysis of circulating endostatin levels in patients with renal cell carcinoma. *Cancer 95*:1637-43., 2002

[152] Lai R, Estey E, Shen Y, et al: Clinical significance of plasma endostatin in acute myeloid leukemia/myelodysplastic syndrome. *Cancer 94*:14-7, 2002

[153] Suzuki M, Iizasa T, Ko E, et al: Serum endostatin correlates with progression and prognosis of non-small cell lung cancer. *Lung Cancer 35*:29-34, 2002

[154] Hata K, Fujiwaki R, Nakayama K, et al: Expression of the Endostatin gene in epithelial ovarian cancer. *Clin Cancer Res 7:*2405-9, 2001

[155] Iizasa T, Chang H, Suzuki M, et al: Overexpression of collagen XVIII is associated with poor outcome and elevated levels of circulating serum endostatin in non-small cell lung cancer. *Clin Cancer Res 10*:5361-6, 2004

[156] Dhar DK, Ono T, Yamanoi A, et al: Serum endostatin predicts tumor vascularity in hepatocellular carcinoma. *Cancer 95*:2188-95, 2002

[157] Zhao J, Yan F, Ju H, et al: Correlation between serum vascular endothelial growth factor and endostatin levels in patients with breast cancer. *Cancer Lett 204*:87-95, 2004

[158] Glenjen N, Mosevoll KA, Bruserud O: Serum levels of angiogenin, basic fibroblast growth factor and endostatin in patients receiving intensive chemotherapy for acute myelogenous leukemia. *Int J Cancer 101*:86-94., 2002

[159] Poon RT, Ho JW, Tong CS, et al: Prognostic significance of serum vascular endothelial growth factor and endostatin in patients with hepatocellular carcinoma. *Br J Surg 91*:1354-60, 2004

[160] Iughetti P, Suzuki O, Godoi PH, et al: A polymorphism in endostatin, an angiogenesis inhibitor, predisposes for the development of prostatic adenocarcinoma. *Cancer Res 61*:7375-8, 2001

[161] Ortega MM, Nascimento H, Teori MT, et al: A polymorphism in the angiogenesis inhibitor, endostatin, in multiple myeloma. *Leuk Res 27*:93-4., 2003

[162] Liu TC, Peng CT, Lin SF, et al: Assocation of endostatin D104N with leukemia. *Kaohsiung J Med Sci 19*:1-5, 2003

[163] Eder JP, Jr., Supko JG, Clark JW, et al: Phase I clinical trial of recombinant human endostatin administered as a short intravenous infusion repeated daily. *J Clin Oncol 20*:3772-84., 2002

[164] Herbst RS, Hess KR, Tran HT, et al: Phase I Study of Recombinant Human Endostatin in Patients With Advanced Solid Tumors. *J Clin Oncol 20*:3792-3803., 2002

[165] Thomas JP, Arzoomanian RZ, Alberti D, et al: Phase I pharmacokinetic and pharmacodynamic study of recombinant human endostatin in patients with advanced solid tumors. *J Clin Oncol 21*:223-31., 2003

[166] Kulke M, Bergsland E, Ryan DP, et al: A phase II open-label, safety, pharmacokinetic and efficacy study of recombinant human endostatin in patients with advanced neuroendocrine tumors. *Proc Am Soc Clin Oncol 22*:958a, 2003

[167] Mundhenke C, Thomas JP, Wilding G, et al: Tissue examination to monitor antiangiogenic therapy: a phase I clinical trial with endostatin. *Clin Cancer Res 7*:3366-74., 2001

[168] Herbst RS, Mullani NA, Davis DW, et al: Development of Biologic Markers of Response and Assessment of Antiangiogenic Activity in a Clinical Trial of Human Recombinant Endostatin. *J Clin Oncol 20*:3804-3814., 2002

[169] Davis DW, Shen Y, Mullani NA, et al: Quantitative Analysis of Biomarkers Defines an Optimal Biological Dose for Recombinant Human Endostatin in Primary Human Tumors. *Clin Cancer Res 10*:33-42, 2004

[170] Rosner GL, Stadler W, Ratain MJ: Randomized discontinuation design: application to cytostatic antineoplastic agents. *J Clin Oncol 20*:4478-84, 2002

[171] Kisker O, Becker CM, Prox D, et al: Continuous administration of endostatin by intraperitoneally implanted osmotic pump improves the efficacy and potency of therapy in a mouse xenograft tumor model. *Cancer Res 61*:7669-74., 2001

[172] van der Schaft DW, Seftor RE, Seftor EA, et al: Effects of angiogenesis inhibitors on vascular network formation by human endothelial and melanoma cells. *J Natl Cancer Inst 96*:1473-7, 2004

[173] Shi W, Teschendorf C, Muzyczka N, et al: Gene therapy delivery of endostatin enhances the treatment efficacy of radiation. *Radiother Oncol 66*:1-9, 2003

[174] Hanna NN, Seetharam S, Mauceri HJ, et al: Antitumor interaction of short-course endostatin and ionizing radiation. *Cancer J 6*:287-93., 2000

[175] Plum SM, Hanson AD, Volker KM, et al: Synergistic activity of recombinant human endostatin in combination with adriamycin: analysis of in vitro activity on endothelial cells and in vivo tumor progression in an orthotopic murine mammary carcinoma model. *Clin Cancer Res 9*:4619-26, 2003

[176] te Velde EA, Vogten JM, Gebbink MF, et al: Enhanced antitumour efficacy by combining conventional chemotherapy with angiostatin or endostatin in a liver metastasis model. *Br J Surg 89*:1302-9, 2002

[177] Ponnazhagan S, Mahendra G, Kumar S, et al: Adeno-Associated Virus 2-Mediated Antiangiogenic Cancer Gene Therapy: Long-Term Efficacy of a Vector Encoding Angiostatin and Endostatin over Vectors Encoding a Single Factor. *Cancer Res 64*:1781-7, 2004

[178] Abdollahi A, Lipson KE, Sckell A, et al: Combined therapy with direct and indirect angiogenesis inhibition results in enhanced antiangiogenic and antitumor effects. *Cancer Res 63*:8890-8, 2003

[179] Yokoyama Y, Ramakrishnan S: Improved biological activity of a mutant endostatin containing a single amino-acid substitution. *Br J Cancer 90*:1627-35, 2004

[180] Yokoyama Y, Ramakrishnan S: Addition of integrin binding sequence to a mutant human endostatin improves inhibition of tumor growth. *Int J Cancer 111*:839-48, 2004

[181] Cattaneo MG, Pola S, Francescato P, et al: Human endostatin-derived synthetic peptides possess potent antiangiogenic properties in vitro and in vivo. *Exp Cell Res 283*:230-6, 2003

[182] Beerepoot LV, Witteveen EO, Groenewegen G, et al: Recombinant human angiostatin by twice-daily subcutaneous injection in advanced cancer: a pharmacokinetic and long-term safety study. *Clin Cancer Res 9*:4025-33, 2003

[183] O'Reilly MS, Holmgren L, Chen C, et al: Angiostatin induces and sustains dormancy of human primary tumors in mice. *Nat Med 2*:689-92, 1996

[184] Lu H, Dhanabal M, Volk R, et al: Kringle 5 causes cell cycle arrest and apoptosis of endothelial cells. *Biochem Biophys Res Commun 258*:668-73, 1999

[185] Cao Y, Chen A, An SS, et al: Kringle 5 of plasminogen is a novel inhibitor of endothelial cell growth. *J Biol Chem 272*:22924-8, 1997

[186] Ji WR, Barrientos LG, Llinas M, et al: Selective inhibition by kringle 5 of human plasminogen on endothelial cell migration, an important process in angiogenesis. *Biochem Biophys Res Commun 247*:414-9, 1998

[187] Kim TH, Kim E, Yoon D, et al: Recombinant human prothrombin kringles have potent anti-angiogenic activities and inhibit Lewis lung carcinoma tumor growth and metastases. *Angiogenesis 5*:191-201, 2002

[188] Lee TH, Rhim T, Kim SS: Prothrombin kringle-2 domain has a growth inhibitory activity against basic fibroblast growth factor-stimulated capillary endothelial cells. *J Biol Chem 273:*28805-12, 1998

[189] O'Reilly MS, Pirie-Shepherd S, Lane WS, et al: Antiangiogenic activity of the cleaved conformation of the serpin antithrombin. *Science 285*:1926-8, 1999

[190] Bootle-Wilbraham CA, Tazzyman S, Marshall JM, et al: Fibrinogen E-fragment inhibits the migration and tubule formation of human dermal microvascular endothelial cells in vitro. *Cancer Res 60*:4719-24, 2000

[191] Brown NJ, Staton CA, Rodgers GR, et al: Fibrinogen E fragment selectively disrupts the vasculature and inhibits the growth of tumours in a syngeneic murine model. *Br J Cancer 86*:1813-6, 2002

[192] Colman RW, Jameson BA, Lin Y, et al: Domain 5 of high molecular weight kininogen (kininostatin) down-regulates endothelial cell proliferation and migration and inhibits angiogenesis. *Blood 95:*543-50, 2000

[193] Xu R, Yao ZY, Xin L, et al: NC1 domain of human type VIII collagen (alpha 1) inhibits bovine aortic endothelial cell proliferation and causes cell apoptosis. *Biochem Biophys Res Commun 289*:264-8, 2001

[194] Hata K, Dhar DK, Kanasaki H, et al: Serum endostatin levels in patients with epithelial ovarian cancer. *Anticancer Res 23*:1907-12, 2003

[195] Miyashita M, Tajiri T, Yanagi K, et al: Serum levels of vascular endothelial growth factor, basic fibroblast growth factor and endostatin in human metastatic liver tumors. *Hepatogastroenterology 50*:308-9, 2003

[196] Urbanska-Rys H, Robak T: High serum level of endostatin in multiple myeloma at diagnosis but not in the plateau phase after treatment. *Mediators Inflamm 12*:229-35, 2003

[197] Feldman AL, Alexander HR, Jr., Bartlett DL, et al: A prospective analysis of plasma endostatin levels in colorectal cancer patients with liver metastases. *Ann Surg Oncol 8*:741-5, 2001

[198] Shaarawy M, El-Sharkawy SA: Biomarkers of intrinsic angiogenic and anti-angiogenic activity in patients with endometrial hyperplasia and endometrial cancer. *Acta Oncol 40*:513-8, 2001

[199] Hefler L, Tempfer C, Kainz C, et al: Serum concentrations of endostatin in patients with vulvar cancer. *Gynecol Oncol 74*:151-2, 1999

[200] Yamagata M, Shiratori Y, Dan Y, et al: Serum endostatin levels in patients with hepatocellular carcinoma. *Ann Oncol 11*:761-2, 2000

In: Trends in Angiogenesis Research
Editor: Roberta V. Zubar, pp. 43-69
ISBN 1-59454-452-2

Chapter II

STUDIES OF THE ENDOTHELIAL CELL-SPECIFIC SIGNAL TRANSDUCTION PATHWAYS (NEW PARADIGM FOR THE DEVELOPMENT OF POTENT ANTI-ANGIOGENIC THERAPIES)

***Shigeru Kanda*[1,*], *Yasuyoshi Miyata*[2] *and Hiroshi Kanetake*[2]**
[1]Department of Molecular Microbiology and Immunology, Division of Endothelial Cell biology, and [2]Department of Urology, Nagasaki University Graduate School of Biomedical Science, Nagasaki, Japan

ABSTRACT

Angiogenesis plays pivotal roles in pathophysiological conditions, such as solid tumor growth, ischemic retinopathy, and collateral formation after the occlusion of arteries. Inhibition of angiogenesis is anticipated to control human advanced malignant tumors. In animal studies, various anti-angiogenic strategies significantly reduce the size of preexisting, transplanted tumors, or retard the growth of tumors, leading to the extension of survival of tumor-bearing animals. However, in humans, almost no anti-angiogenic agent has solely been reported to cause regression of advanced tumors and only a few clinical studies showed enhanced survival of patients. In this regard, we may have to re-evaluate the anti-angiogenic strategies for the remedy of patients with advanced malignant tumors. Assessment of anti-angiogenic agents against transplanted tumors in rodent may yield different results from those in humans. Furthermore, a positive effect for anti-angiogenic therapy in animal studies does not necessarily guarantee inhibition of tumor angiogenesis in humans. It is also possible that the dose of anti-angiogenic agents used in human may not be sufficient to cause regression of tumors. In this chapter, we

* Correspondence concerning this article should be addressed to Dr. Shigeru Kanda, Department of Molecular Microbiology and Immunology, Division of Endothelial Cell biology, Nagasaki University Graduate School of Biomedical Science, 1-7-1, Sakamoto, Nagasaki 852-8501, Japan. Phone: +81 95 849 7340; Fax: +81 95 849 7343; E-mail: shigeruk@net.nagasaki-u.ac.jp.

discuss the impact of attenuation of the anti-angiogenic actions by particular agents and the possible studies that could solve these problems.

Color graphics are presented at the end of the chapter.

Key words: Signal transduction,hypoxia, Ras, MAPK, Fes, molecular target

Introduction

Under normal conditions, endothelial cells do not proliferate but rather stay in a static state. Less than 0.1% of endothelial cells can be labeled as proliferating cells [1]. Once endothelial cells are activated, they produce proteases that can digest the basement membrane of blood vessels, and migrate into surrounding interstitial tissues from preexisting vessels by proangiogenic factors, where they proliferate to form lumen-containing tube-like structures. The final step in this process involves surrounding of the newly formed tubes by a layer of pericytes or smooth muscle cells [2]. These cellular responses are collectively known as angiogenesis. While these cellular responses are observed sequentially *in vivo*, each of the above cellular response steps can be examined separately when cultured endothelial cells are adopted.

Importantly, the behavior of tumor cells during invasion and metastasis is quite similar to the cellular responses of endothelial cells during angiogenesis [3, 4]. Local invasion is initiated by the proteolytic digestion of neighboring tissues by tumor cells, followed by the migration into surrounding interstitial tissues and proliferation. For metastasis, the tumor cells digest the basement membrane of blood or lymphatic vessels and migrate into the lumen. After translocation into the circulation and adhesion to particular sites, tumor cells settle in the surrounding tissues after digestion of the vessel wall, where they proliferate and form a distant metastatic site. The main feature of endothelial cells that is distinct from tumor cells is their ability to form lumen-containing tubes.

Vascular Endothelial Growth Factors and Tumor Angiogenesis

Vascular endothelial growth factor (VEGF) gene family is composed of several members including VEGF-A (a prototype VEGF), -B, -C, -D, -E, and placental growth factors (PlGFs) [5, 6]. Receptors for these growth factors are VEGF receptor-1 (VEGFR-1, also known as Flt-1), VEGFR-2 (KDR/Flk-1), and VEGFR-3 (Flt-4), all of which have a tyrosine kinase domain in the cytoplasmic region [7, 8]. VEGF-A binds to VEGFR-1 and –2, whereas VEGF-B and PlGFs bind only to VEGFR-1. VEGF-C and VEGF-D bind to VEGFR-2 and –3. Expression of VEGRFR-3 is highly specific for lymphatic endothelial cells [7, 9]. Both VEGF-C and –D are involved in lymphangiogenesis, which participates in the lymphatic metastasis of tumor cells [9]. VEGF-E only binds to VEGFR-2 [10].

Accumulating evidence suggests that VEGF-A plays central roles in tumor angiogenesis. VEGF-A promotes proliferation, migration, production of proteases, survival, and tube formation of cultured endothelial cells, all of which are critical responses in angiogenesis. Recent studies demonstrated the contribution of circulating endothelial precursor cells (EPCs) immobilized from bone marrow to the process of neovascularization in tumor tissue [11, 12]. Mobilization of EPCs is regulated by signaling via VEGFR-1 [11].

Neovascularization is required for the supply of oxygen to ischemic tissues. Hypoxic condition provides a feedback signal for the production of VEGF-A [13, 14]. Hypoxia inducible factor (HIF) family proteins transcriptionally regulate VEGF-A production. Although the β-subunit of HIF-1 and –2 is constitutively expressed in cells, their α-subunit is upregulated in hypoxic cells. The α-subunit of HIF heterodimerizes with β-subunit of HIF in nuclei, followed by binding to the specific DNA binding sites containing the core sequence 5'-RCGTG-3' and recruitment of co-activators such as p300 [13]. In oxygenated cells, von Hippel Lindau protein interacts with the α-subunit of HIF as the recognition component of an E3 ubiquitin ligase complex, resulting in degradation through proteasome [15, 16].

Recent studies have shown that VEGF-A-mediated signaling is involved in angiogenesis promoted by other proangiogenic factors, such as fibroblast growth factor (FGF)-2. The angiogenic activity of FGF-2 in endothelial cells was modulated by VEGF-A in an autocrine manner [17]. Antagonizing VEGFR-2 inhibited both VEGF-A- and FGF-2-promoted angiogenesis both *in vitro* and *in vivo* [18]. The blockade of VEGFR-3 signaling inhibited FGF-2-induced lymphangiogenesis [19]. FGF-2-promoted capillary morphogenesis of cultured endothelial cells requires c-Akt activity through endogenous VEGF-A/VEGFR-1 interaction [20]. Endogenous VEGF is also required for angiopoietin (Ang) 1-induced tube formation by endothelial cells in culture [21]. These studies suggest that the blockade of VEGF signaling may also inhibit angiogenesis induced by other proangiogenic factors. Thus, it seems that the inhibition of VEGF-A possess is a potentially suitable strategy to block tumor angiogenesis.

Compared to the normal microvessels, tumor vessels have a distinct structure [22]. Most endothelial cells with scanty perivascular cells exhibit tortuous and saccular morphology of vessels with disorganization and hyperpermeability. In animal models, VEGF blockade decreased the diameter of microvessels, vessel tortuosity, and permeability [23]. This improvement of microvasculature is called "normalization of vessels" [24]. These structural changes are often associated with functional changes such as reduction of interstitial fluid pressure in tumor tissues and increased oxygenation and blood flow [25, 26]. These alterations may support the penetration of chemotherapeutic agents into tumor tissue and enhance the cytotoxic effect of irradiation [25, 27].

Several inhibitors of VEGF signaling have been examined clinically. These inhibitors can be classified into four classes: 1) anti-VEGF blocking antibodies or soluble forms of extracellular domain of VEGF receptors, 2) anti-VEGF receptor blocking antibodies, 3) VEGFR or VEGF-directed ribozymes, and 4) small molecule VEGFR tyrosine kinase inhibitors [28]. Accumulating evidence suggests that anti-VEGF strategies might be useful when combined with cytotoxic chemotherapeutic agents. Especially in patients with metastatic colorectal cancers, significant prolongation of survival rate or time for tumor progression was observed. In addition, anti-VEGF monoclonal antibody exhibited antivascular effect in patients with rectal cancer, assessed by tumor blood perfusion, vascular volume, interstitial fluid pressure, and microvessel density [29]. However, the antibody had little effect on tumor regression in human when used alone. With regard to the toxic effects of these treatment modalities, headache, nausea, vomiting and increased risk of thromboembolic events may limit the dose of compounds used for VEGF blockade [28]. Thrombomodulin is an anti-thrombotic protein produced by endothelial cells, and VEGF-A upregulates its expression [30]. Anti-VEGF strategies may down-regulate the expression of this protein, resulting in thromboembolus formation.

Does Solid Tumor Growth Require Angiogenesis?

In ischemic retinopathy, such as diabetic retinopathy, neovascularization is required for proper oxygen supply to the retinal tissue. In diabetic retinopathy, leaky fragile vessels cause hemorrhage, which ultimately causes blindness if not treated [31]. In addition, loss of pericytes from microvessel wall leads to microaneurysm formation and edema, which worsen the loss of visual acuity [32]. The phenotype of such vasculature is observed in VEGF-promoted angiogenesis. Thus, the formation of mature new vessels covered with pericytes would be favorable for ischemic retinopathy than simple inhibition of angiogenesis itself. Efficient anti-VEGF strategies for the treatment of diabetic retinopathy should thus include blockade of immature neovascularization [32, 33].

Irradiation could cause tissue ischemia [34]. Radiotherapy has long been used for the treatment of many cancers, e.g., uterine cervical cancer. One of the complications of this therapy is radiation cystitis. Chronic ischemia induces angiogenesis with leaky fragile vessels in the mucosa of the urinary bladder, which could result in massive hemorrhage [35]. Interestingly, hyperbaric oxygenation improves such hemorrhagic state [36]. Hypoxia induces upregulation of VEGF-A, resulting in angiogenesis with leaky vessels. VEGF-A-induced vessels showed rapid regression upon downregulation of VEGF-A [37]. Based on our experience, microvessels in the mucosa of the irradiated bladder were markedly decreased after hyperbaric oxygenation (unpublished observations). It is likely that the hemorrhage seen in radiation-related cystitis may be the result of VEGF-A-induced angiogenesis. Therefore, in addition to inhibition of angiogenesis, it would be also preferable for radiation-induced ischemic complications to generate neovascularization in which the newly formed vessels are surrounded by pericytes.

Judah Folkman, a highly respected pioneer of tumor angiogenesis, reported a number of observations that suggest the requirement for angiogenesis for solid tumor growth [38]. In normal tissue, the percentage of labeled endothelial cells following a single injection of tritiated thymidine was around 0.1% [1]. Furthermore, the doubling time of the normal endothelium was 20-2,000 times longer than that of the endothelium of tumor tissues [39]. In fact, tumor cells could not grow more than 1 mm^3 upon inhibition of angiogenesis [40], and tumor growth was rapid after vascularization [41]. In addition, treatment with anti-angiogenic agents markedly repressed the growth of transplanted tumors in rodents. These results strongly support the idea that tumor growth is angiogenesis-dependent. When angiogenesis does not occur, tumor stays in a dormant state (tumor dormancy) [42], which may enable patients to live an entire life in the presence of quiescent malignant tumor. Transgenic mouse models carrying dominant oncogenes demonstrated that tumor cells became angiogenic just before they started to grow rapidly [43]. This phenomenon is called as "angiogenic switch". Tumor cells exhibit genetic instability and can change their characteristics as an adaptation to the surrounding conditions. Thus, tumor cells gain drug-resistance to survive during chemotherapies. Since anti-angiogenic strategies target normal endothelial cells, repeated treatments with anti-angiogenic agents do not induce resistance to the therapy [44]. Why does anti-angiogenic therapy fail to cause regression of malignant tumors in human? While the exact reason is unknown at present, several mechanisms could explain this finding.

1) Tumor cells transplanted into rodents may have different characteristics from cells of spontaneously grown tumors. Many studies on anti-angiogenesis have employed the transplanted tumor model into syngenic or immunodeficient rodents, in which tumor cells are usually cultured under normoxic condition (21% oxygen corresponds to O_2 partial pressure; pO_2 of 160 mmHg) [45]. Only a limited number of studies used spontaneous tumor models with specific genetic background [46, 47]. In the end-capillary blood, pO_2 is 45-50 mmHg, indicating that the pO_2 of normoxic culture condition is at least 3 times higher than physiological normoxia *in vivo* [48]. Thus, transplanted tumor cells into rodents are exposed to acute severe hypoxic environment. HIF target genes encode proteins that support energy metabolism of tumor cells and oxygen supply by inducing a multitude of angiogenic factors, such as VEGF-A, VEGFR-1, transforming growth factor-β (TGF- β), insulin-like growth factor (IGF)-II, epidermal growth factor (EGF) receptor, glucose transporters, and hexokinases [13]. In animal models of tumor angiogenesis, hypoxia and expression of HIF may strongly modulate angiogenesis. Since tissue pO_2 of around 10 mmHg reflects a borderline between well and poorly oxygenated tissue environment [49], many malignant tumors in human grow under chronic hypoxic condition. The oxygen dependency of many chemotherapies and radiotherapy has been documented [48]. Therefore, the efficacy of anti-angiogenic agents should be re-evaluated by using transplanted tumor models cultured under chronic hypoxic condition.

2) Increased expression of VEGF-A in tumor cells does not simply account for the requirement of VEGF-A-dependent angiogenesis for tumor growth. Many clinicopathological studies have suggested that high expression of VEGF-A in tumor cells is closely associated with tumor aggressiveness and enhanced angiogenesis. However, the expression of thymidine phosphorylase was significantly higher in high-grade (aggressive) urinary bladder tumors than in low-grade tumors, which correlated with microvessel density [50]. Conversely, the expression of VEGF-A was higher in low-grade tumors [51]. We have also obtained similar results (unpublished observations). Importantly, careful examination of low-grade bladder tumors in our study showed high expression of VEGF-A in tumors containing small numbers of apoptotic tumor cells and few microvessels. This result suggests that poorly vascularized tumor cells are resistant to hypoxia and overexpression of VEGF-A may simply reflect the presence of hypoxia. Several reports have demonstrated the lack of angiogenesis in aggressive non-small lung cancers [52]. It seems that these cancers depended on preexisting large vessels for the blood supply. Other studies also showed that tumor cells resistant to hypoxia showed diminished apoptotic potential [53]. Taken together, the angiogenesis-independent fraction of tumor cells may exhibit resistance to anti-angiogenic therapies.

3) The oxygenation status of endothelial cells may alter the signal transduction pathways or responsiveness to anti-angiogenic factors. Endothelial cells in tumor tissues are frequently exposed to hypoxia. The anti-angiogenic effects of particular molecules are often examined using endothelial cells cultured under 21% oxygen environment. Various growth factors play pivotal roles in the regulation of angiogenic responses of endothelial cells. At present, only a few studies have examined the effect of hypoxia on signal transduction pathways in endothelial cells. Under hypoxic condition, endothelial cells express VEGF-A, Ang 2, Ang 4, Tie 1, and Tie 2 [54]. However, the roles of these proteins in hypoxic endothelial cells are not clarified well. AMP-activated protein kinase is activated by hypoxia, and its inhibition attenuated VEGF-A-induced motility and tube formation in hypoxic, but not normoxic endothelial cells [55]. Mitogen-activated protein kinase-activated protein kinase is activated by hypoxia and regulates cytoskeletal changes through heat-shock protein 27 [56]. However, other important signaling pathways regulated by proangiogenic growth factors or cytokines remain to be elucidated. In addition, the response of hypoxic endothelial cells to anti-angiogenic molecules is totally unknown. These missing points should be extensively studied in the future.

4) The dose of anti-angiogenic agents may be insufficient to cause regression of tumors in human. The dose of each agent is usually determined by the balance between efficacy and toxicity. Anti-angiogenic agents are roughly divided into two categories; endothelial cell-specific growth inhibitors without better understanding of the mechanism of action, and agents that target previously identified molecules expressed in endothelial cells. The former group includes TNP 470, thalidomide, angiostatin, and endostatin, whereas the latter includes agents for VEGF blockade and anti-αvβ3 integrin. Although these anti-angiogenic agents inhibit angiogenesis and result in tumor regression in animal models, a few such cases have been reported in human. It is possible that spontaneous human malignant tumors are more resistant to anti-angiogenic therapies than transplanted tumor models in rodents. Based on this feature, it is conceivable that the dose of anti-angiogenic agents should be increased in the treatment of tumors in human. However, the use of high doses of agents with unidentified mechanism may cause unexpected toxicities. Thus, even when the mechanism of action is well understood, such as VEGF blockade, the use of high doses could result in thromboembolism. Since VEGF signaling promotes the recovery of damaged bone marrow induced by chemotherapeutic agents [57], the dose of anti-VEGF-A antibodies or VEGFR tyrosine kinase inhibitors cannot be increased when used in combination with chemotherapy or raditherapy. In this regard, blockade of downstream signaling molecules of VEGFR, of which pathways do not affect the anti-thrombotic activity of endothelial cells or reconstitution of bone marrow cells, would be favorable.

5) Tumors treated with VEGF blockade may change their characteristics from VEGF-dependent angiogenesis to other proangiogenic factor-dependent angiogenesis. Several reports described the efficacy of anti-angiogenic strategies that significantly inhibit tumor growth. However, the duration of experiments in these reports is not sufficiently long to see the effect of anti-angiogenesis by a single agent (usually less than 6-8 weeks). Furthermore, it is not clear whether blockade of VEGF-A by the antibody renders all tumors examined dormant during the entire life of the experimental animals. There may be re-growth of tumors, which may not respond to VEGF blockade. For example, more than 50% of breast

cancer cells express VEGF-A in the early phase of tumor development, but during tumor progression, tumor cells start to express other proangiogenic factors, such as FGF-2, thymidine phosphorylase, and pleiotropin [58]. It has also been reported that simultaneous blockade of VEGF and FGF produces a stronger anti-tumor effect than VEGF blockade alone [59]. Thus, it seems likely that blockade of a single proangiogenic factor promotes tumor cells to secrete other proangiogenic factors for survival. This could be viewed as resistance to prior therapy. Although normal cells (*i.e.,* endothelial cells) do not develop resistance to repeated therapy in mice, it is possible that alteration of angiogenic factor-dependency still causes resistance.

Endothelial Cell-Specific Signaling Molecules as Targets of Anti-Angiogenic Therapy

Various types of proteins are exclusively expressed on the surface of endothelial cells. Among these proteins, VEGFRs, platelet endothelial cell adhesion molecule-1 (PECAM-1) [60], vascular endothelial-cadherin [61], Endoglin [62], and Tie 2 [63] are considered key molecules in tumor angiogenesis. These cell surface proteins transduce extracellular signals into the cells. In addition, several growth factor receptors are involved in the regulation of tumor angiogenesis, such as FGF receptors, EGF receptor, hepatocyte growth factor (HGF) receptor, platelet-derived growth factor (PDGF) receptors, IGF receptor, and TGF-β receptors. Signals via cell surface receptors can be blocked with specific blocking antibodies against ligands and receptors, soluble receptors, ribozymes, and small molecule protein kinase inhibitors. The demerits of using these agents to control angiogenesis are; 1) inhibition of the target molecules is specific and does not exhibit broad-range inhibition, 2) blockade of all reactions regulated via targeted receptors though some are required for the maintenance of physiological functions of endothelial cells (*i.e.*, hematopoiesis and anti-thrombotic effect of VEGF-A), and 3) modulation of molecule-dependent angiogenesis of tumor cells (*e.g.*, from VEGF-A-dependent angiogenesis to FGF-2-dependent angiogenesis). To solve these problems, inhibition of intracellular signaling molecules would be favorable. Anti-angiogenic therapy should specifically target endothelial cells. Thus, one can suggest that improved anti-angiogenic strategies should result in block the signaling molecules that are exclusively expressed in endothelial cells and are commonly used as downstream signaling molecules via several kinds of cell surface receptors.

Hematopoietic cells and endothelial cells arise from the same origin; the hemangioblasts [64]. In addition, angiogenesis and hematopoiesis are to a large extent regulated by common growth factors and cytokines [65]. Thus, it is likely that endothelial cells and hematopoietic cells commonly express a large number of proteins. Hematopoietic cells can proliferate, migrate, and produce proteases [66, 67], which are all involved in angiogenic behaviors of endothelial cells. However, only endothelial cells can form lumen-containing tube-like structures. Therefore, to identify endothelial cell-specific signaling molecules, examination of signal transduction pathways that lead to tube formation is important for our understanding of the angiogenic process. This strategy may also be beneficial for avoiding of cells of non-endothelial cell origin and may allow the use of high doses of anti-angiogenic agents to efficiently inhibit tumor angiogenesis in human.

Targeted Deletion of Signaling Molecules Related to Ras/Mark Pathways and Vascular Development in Mice

Blood vessel development in the embryo and tumor angiogenesis in adult have distinct, but in part, similar features [68]. The yolk sac is the source of early embryonic blood. Development of the yolk sac vasculature begins with the formation of blood islands containing hematopoietic stem cells, surrounded by angioblasts. Then, the blood islands fuse together and form an organized, honeycombed array of endothelial cells. Between E8.5 and 9.5, the endothelial cells again alter their location and adherence patterns as they reorganize into a highly organized vascular network that feeds the embryo. The vascular network including heart and major blood vessels (vasculogenesis) are observed in the embryo. Subsequently, small blood vessels sprout from the large vascular network to form fine mesh-like capillaries (angiogenesis). In tumor tissues, endothelial cells of preexisting vessels digest the basement membrane of the vessel wall by proteases, migrate toward various proangiogenic factors secreted in the surrounding interstitial tissues by tumor cells, proliferate, and form new microvessels (angiogenesis). Furthermore, circulating endothelial precursor cells also accumulate in the tumor tissue and are incorporated into the tumor vasculature (vasculogenesis). To identify the functional signaling molecules that are preferentially expressed in endothelial cells, there is a need to examine the vascular development in transgenic or gene targeting mouse models. Targeted disruption of the genes of molecules involved in Ras/mitogen-activated protein kinase (MAPK) pathway and related pathways can cause vascular defect.

ShcA is an adaptor molecule that contains the Src-Homology (SH) 2 domain and the phosphotyrosine-binding domain [69]. Three splice variants have been identified, denoted p46, p52, and p66. ShcA forms complexes with tyrosine-phosphorylated proteins, such as growth factor receptor tyrosine kinases and the adopter protein, Grb 2. Subsequently, the Ras-specific guanine nucleotide exchanger factor, son of sevenless (Sos), is recruited to the plasma membrane, where GDP-bound Ras exist. Sos releases GDP from Ras, and causes conformational change of Ras to allow it to bind to GTP [70]. During early development, ShcA is most prominently expressed in endothelial cells and surrounding mesenchymal cells of the cardiovascular system [71]. In ShcA-homozygous ($shcA^{-/-}$) mutant embryos, no absolute block of early vasculogenesis and angiogenesis was observed. However, large and uniformly sized lumens were observed in the yolk sac vasculature and dilatation and reduced complexity of the primary head vessels were observed at E10.5, indicating perturbation in the later phase of angiogenesis. By using isolated cells from the mutant ($shcA^{-/-}$) and wild type embryos, it was shown that ShcA sensitized cells for MAPK activation [71]. ShcA is involved in FGF-2-promoted proliferation and differentiation of cultured endothelial cells [72]. ShcA also acts as a downstream signaling molecule of VEGF receptors [73, 74].

Sos activates Ras by removing GDP from the inactive form Ras. The closely related Sos1 and Sos2 are widely expressed, as is true of Ras. Targeted deletion of Sos1 is embryonically lethal due to poor development of placenta [75]. In the placenta, Sos1 is strongly expressed in the spongiotrophoblasts and labyrinth trophoblasts. Lack of Sos1 resulted in disorganization of the trophoblasts layers and incomplete vascularization of the placenta and embryo. Since the placenta is required for nutrient supply and waste exchange, deletion of Sos1-promoted fetal death may be a secondary effect of the poor development of the placenta. Sos1 acts as a Ras activator downstream of a number of cell surface receptors, including proangiogenic growth factor receptor tyrosine kinase and integrins.

Ras is activated following the release of GDP and its subsequent binding to GTP. Ras has an intrinsic weak GTPase activity, but its activity is enhanced by GTPase activating protein (GAP). It then hydrolyzes GTP to form GDP-bound inactive form [76]. Thus, Ras-GAP is a negative regulator of Ras signaling. Targeted disruption of Ras-GAP is embryonically lethal in homozygous mice (*ras-gap*$^{-/-}$) at E10.5 [77]. The remarkable phenotype is the vascular abnormality. At E9.5, the yolk sac of the mutant exhibits a roughened, wrinkled appearance and at E10.5, reorganization of endothelial cells is delayed. These findings suggest the involvement of Ras-GAP in the morphological maturation of the vasculature. In cultured endothelial cells, Ras-GAP acted as a downstream signaling molecule of VEGF receptor, Tie 2, and EphB receptors [78-80].

Raf was the first effecter identified downstream of Ras. Raf is a protein serine/threonine kinase, which is activated by the association of Ras binding domain with GTP-bound Ras, followed by changes in phosphorylation status due to conformational changes and recruitment to the plasma membrane [81]. There are three human Raf, A-Raf, B-Raf, and C-Raf (also known as Raf-1) [82]. Targeted disruption of B-Raf caused death of homozygous embryo (*B-raf*$^{-/-}$) *in utero* between E10.5 and E12.5 with evidence of vascular defects [83]. Early vasculogenesis and angiogenesis were intact. However, all vessels were incompletely lined with endothelial cells, resulting in vessel rupture and hemorrhage. The defect in suitable lining was due to abundant apoptosis of endothelial cells, suggesting the possible involvement of B-Raf in the survival of endothelial cells during development. Raf-mediated survival signals include the MAPK/Erk kinase (Mek)/extracellular signal-regulated kinase (Erk)/p92 ribosomal S6 kinase (p92 Rsk) pathway, Bcl-2 family proteins, and nuclear factor-κB (NF-κB) pathway [82].

Mek1 is activated by Raf kinases following extracellular stimulation. Activated Mek1 phosphorylates threonine and tyrosine residues in Erk1 and Erk2. Targeted deletion of Mek1 causes vascular defect in placenta and yolk sac [84]. Importantly, embryonic fibroblasts obtained from Mek1-deficient embryos failed to migrate by fibronectin, although Erk activation was intact, suggesting that Mek1 may utilize yet unknown signaling pathways other than Erk.

Mekk3 is a protein serine/threonine kinase implicated in the activation of c-Jun NH2-terminal kinases (JNK), p38 mitogen-activated protein kinases (MAPK), and Erk5 [85]. Mekk3-deficient mice die at E11.0 with vascular anomalies [86]. The phenotype is characterized by the absence of vessels in the yolk sac, few complex vessels in the embryo, and retarded development of the myocardium. Blood islands were observed in mutant mice, indicating that Mekk3 might be involved in the later phase of angiogenesis. In cultured endothelial cells, VEGF-A-induced activation of c-Akt resulted in enhanced phosphorylation of Mekk3, which decreased its activity, with subsequent inhibition of p38 MAPK-mediated apoptosis [87].

Erk5 is a member of the MAPK family, which contains three subfamilies: the Erks, the JNKs, and p38 MAPKs. Erk5 is activated through Mekk3/Mek5 pathway [81]. Three reports have shown that deletion of Erk5 in mice was embryonically lethal at around E10.5 with defective vascular development in the yolk sac and reduced complexity of the embryonic vascular network [88-90]. In cultured endothelial cells obtained from Erk5-deficient embryo, Erk5 negatively regulated hypoxia-induced expression of VEGF-A [89]. While it is known that Erk5 is activated by epidermal growth factor, serum, neurotropins, and oxidative or osmotic stress [91-94], its role in the regulation of angiogenic responses by cultured endothelial cells is not well defined.

p38 MAPK (α and β) is activated by cytokines and environmental stress through Mekk3/Mkk3&6 pathways [95]. Four studies reported that deletion of p38 MAPK α gene caused fetal death [96-99]. Two of these studies showed vascular defect in placenta and yolk sac [96, 97]. Another report described lack of erythropoietin expression, with resultant impairment of erythropoiesis [98]. The reason for the two different phenotypes is not clear. As has been described before, incomplete vascularization of the placenta may secondarily impede the development and survival of the embryo. p38 MAPK is involved in FGF-2- and Ang 1-induced apoptosis of cultured endothelial cells [100, 101].

Targeted deletion of proangiogenic factors and their receptors demonstrates two classes of vascular defects in the mouse embryo. Deletion of a single allele of VEGF-A gene (*vegf-A*$^{+/-}$) or homozygous mutant of VEGFR-2 (*vegfr-2*$^{-/-}$) resulted in defective early-stage vasculogenesis, i.e., severe impairment of blood island formation [102-104]. In contrast, disruption of genes encoding Ang 1 and Tie 2 results in vascular defect at a later phase, characterized by reduced complexity and disorganization of the vascular network [105, 106]. Thus, the phenotypes observed in Ang 1- and Tie 2-knockout mice seem to be highly specific for endothelial cells, because developmental defect including both endothelial cells and hematopoietic cells (blood island formation and early-stage vasculogenesis) is not affected. The knockout mice of Ras/MAPK-related signaling molecules, except Sos1 and p38 MAPK α, have quite similar phenotypes to Ang 1- and Tie 2-knockout mice, suggesting that these molecules may act downstream of Tie 2. Since the ShcA/Sos1/Ras/Raf/Mek pathway is essential for many physiological processes in all cell types, targeting these molecules for anti-angiogenesis may produce unexpected toxicities. At this stage, it is unknown whether Mekk3 and Erk5 are required for VEGF-, Ang 1-, or FGF-driven tumor angiogenesis.

Targeted Disruption of Genes Encoding Other Signaling Molecules and Vascular Development in Mice

Akt (1, 2, and 3)/protein kinase B (α, β, and γ) is a protein serine/threonine kinase that is activated through phosphoinositide-dependent kinase (PDK) and Ca^{2+}/calmodulin-dependent protein kinase kinase [107, 108]. Akt is involved in a number of cellular responses, especially apoptosis and motility of endothelial cells [109]. Deletion of Akt1 resulted in growth retardation of embryo and neonate [110]. Some mice died *in utero* probably due to hypotrophy of the placenta and reduced angiogenesis. Growth retardation was also noted in the neonates. Phosphorylation of endothelial nitric-oxide synthase (eNOS) at Ser^{1177} by Akt is required in VEGF-A-driven migration and this phosphorylation was decreased in the placenta of mutant mice. Akt is a downstream signaling molecule of many proangiogenic growth factor receptors, such as VEGF receptors, Tie 2, and EGF receptor [109].

Focal adhesion kinase (FAK) is a non-receptor protein tyrosine kinase, which plays pivotal roles in the assembly and disassembly of focal adhesion, and actin reorganization [111]. Targeted disruption of the gene encoding FAK resulted in embryonic lethality at E8.5 with severe impairment of vascular development [112]. Development of the heart and circulatory system was defective in FAK mutant embryos, similar to fibronectin-deficient mice [113]. FAK-deficient embryos did not form well-organized vascular network but no defect in differentiation to endothelial cells was noted in cultured cells, suggesting the involvement of FAK in late-stage vascular development. FAK is a downstream signaling molecule of FGF receptors, VEGF receptors, and Tie 2 [114-116]. Isolated endothelial cells from FAK mutant embryo demonstrated impaired motility and tubulogenesis.

WAVE2, a protein related to Wiskott-Aldrich syndrome protein, is important for Rac-induced actin reorganization and cell motility [117]. WAVE2 is expressed predominantly in vascular endothelial cells during embryogenesis [118]. Targeted deletion of WAVE2 caused embryonic death around E10 in association with decreased sprouting and branching of vessels [118]. WAVE2-deficient endothelial cells showed impaired lamellipodia formation and tubulogenesis in response to VEGF-A. As is true of FAK, actin remodeling by WAVE2 is also essential for vascular development. Endothelial cell-specific downstream signaling molecules of FAK and WAVE2 have not yet been identified.

Non-Receptor Protein Tyrosine Kinase c-Fes in Angiogenesis

c-Fes/Fps is a non-receptor protein tyrosine kinase and belongs to a family of tyrosine kinase c-Fer [119, 120]. Both kinases have an amino-terminal unique region, an SH2 domain, and a catalytic domain. Unlike c-Fer, expression of c-Fes is exclusively limited to hematopoietic cells, endothelial cells, and some neuronal cells [121]. c-Fes is activated by oligomerization of coiled-coil domain that exists in the N-terminal unique region, followed by autophosphorylation [122, 123]. Although targeted disruption of c-Fes gene did not cause any defect in vascular development [124-127], expression of the activated form of c-Fes, which was fused with myristylation signal of c-Src at the N-termini, in transgenic mice resulted in widespread hypervascularity [128]. Endothelial cells from this transgenic mouse showed increased response of c-Fes activation to treatment with VEGF-A or platelet-derived growth factor (PDGF) [129]. In addition, the activated c-Fes partially rescued the defective development of blood vessels in VEGFR-2 null mice [130]. These results indicate that c-Fes is involved in angiogenesis. By using cultured endothelial cells, overexpression of wild type c-Fes promoted proangiogenic factor-independent, spontaneous tube formation or capillary morphogenesis [131, 132]. Stromal cell-derived factor-1α and sonic hedgehog induced tube formation or capillary morphogenesis through c-Fes/phosphoinositide 3-kinase (PI3-kinase) pathway [133, 134]. Endothelial cell-specific signaling molecules may exist downstream of c-Fes.

Important Issues for the Study of Signal Transduction Pathways in Endothelial Cells

To identify endothelial cell-specific signaling molecules that act downstream of a variety of proangiogenic factor receptors, could potentially allow the development of novel anti-angiogenic therapies. Examination of signal transduction pathways that lead to cellular responses in endothelial cells should be examined using cultured endothelial cells. Upon ligand-binding, receptor tyrosine kinases are oligomerized followed by transphosphorylation to increase their intrinsic tyrosine kinase activity [135, 136]. Activation of receptor tyrosine kinases yields autophosphorylation sites in the intracellular domain of the receptor molecule, which creates binding sites for SH2-domain containing proteins [137]. Phospholipase C-γ (PLC-γ) is directly associated with activated receptor tyrosine kinases, followed by tyrosine phosphorylation and activation [138]. Tyrosine phosphorylation of PLC-γ was observed in VEGF-A-treated NIH3T3 cells expressing VEGFR-1 [139]. In overexpression of intracellular domain of VEGFR-1 in Baculovirus expression system or yeast two-hybrid system, autophosphorylation sites of VEGFR-1, which corresponded to the binding of PLC-γ, were identified [140-143]. However, in endothelial cells, no report demonstrated the tyrosine phosphorylation of PLC-γ downstream of VEGFR-1. Class Ia PI3-kinase is composed of p85 regulatory subunit and p110 catalytic subunit [144, 145]. The former subunit has two SH2 domains split by an inter SH2 domain, which constitutively associates with the p110 catalytic subunit. Activation of PI3-kinase requires the binding of p85 to tyrosine phosphorylated receptor tyrosine kinases or adaptor proteins, which recruit the kinase to plasma membranes. Another mechanism is the direct association of activated Ras with p110 subunit. The yeast two hybrid system and synthetic peptide from VEGFR-1 demonstrated the binding of p85 subunit to VEGFR-1 [146]. However, no activation and association with VEGFR-1 were observed in VEGF-A-treated endothelial cells. Furthermore, it has been shown that PI3-kinase was activated through Tie 2 by direct binding of p85 subunit to Tie 2 [147, 148]. These studies used the yeast two-hybrid system, GST-fusion protein pull-down method, or co-transfection of p85 and Tie 2 in non-endothelial, 293T cells. In murine brain capillary endothelial cells, activation of Tie 2 by high concentration of Ang 2 failed to induce the association of PI3-kinase activity with Tie 2 [149]. In this study, activated PI3-kinase was associated with c-Fes. In murine brain capillary endothelial cells and human umbilical vein endothelial cells, recombinant Ang 1 activated PI3-kinase, which was associated with endogenous c-Fes, but not with Tie 2 [150]. These results emphasize the need to examine the signal transduction pathways leading to angiogenesis in endothelial cells.

Activation of endothelial cells, which can allow quiescent endothelial cells to respond to proangiogenic factors, may also endothelial cell-specific feature. The expression of VEGFR-2 and Ang 2 was observed in endothelial cells at the beginning of tumor angiogenesis [151], and transcriptional upregulation of these molecules may be the molecular marker of endothelial cell activation. It has been shown that the basic helix-loop-helix transcription factor HESR1 downregulated the expression of VEGFR-2 [152]. Ets-1 upregulates the expression of VEGFR-2 and Ang 2 [153, 154]. Signal transduction pathways leading to activation of these transcription factors may also allow the design of novel anti-angiogenic therapies.

Conclusion

Employment of anti-angiogenic strategy is an attractive option for the treatment of malignant tumors in human. Several evidences suggest that blockade of angiogenesis is effective in reducing tumor tissue volume and induction of dormancy in animal models. However, as described above, more detailed basic examination of endothelial cell biology and identification of anti-angiogenic molecules with defined molecular mechanisms is necessary to reveal the effectiveness of anti-angiogenic tumor therapy in human.

In addition, verifying the effects of current therapies may be also valuable for improving the overall effect of anti-angiogenic therapies. For example, arterial embolization to shut out the feeding artery is frequently used for the reduction of solid tumors, such as renal cell carcinomas and hepatocellular carcinomas [155, 156]. After embolization, a large proportion of tumor tissue becomes necrotic, however, surviving tumor cells frequently grow again in association with the development of new collateral vessels. This phenomenon can be characterized by the hypoxic response, in which angiogenesis and upregulation of metabolic enzymes are involved [13]. The use of anti-angiogenic therapy immediately after embolization may achieve a more potent blockade of feeding blood vessels.

We can also try anti-angiogenic gene therapies by intra-arterial infusion. Recent reports have shown that combination of genes of interest with Tie 2 promotor allowed the expression of gene products specifically in endothelial cells [157]. In addition, adeno-associated virus vector utilizing the heparan sulfate proteoglycan and FGFR-1 for the entry and FGF-2 enhanced the transport of genes [158]. Endothelial cells express FGFR-1, and expression of FGF-2 is frequently upregulated in endothelial cells as well as tumor cells. Combination of these technologies and intra-arterial infusion may potently block angiogenesis without dilution of vectors by circulated blood.

Acknowledgements

We are grateful to the members of the Department of Urology, Nagasaki University Graduate School of Biomedical Science for sharing important clinical findings in the preparation of this review. This work was partly supported by a grant from the Japan Society for the Promotion of Science.

REFERENCES

[1] Engerman, R. L,, Pfaffenbach, D., and Davis, M. D. (1967). Cell turnover of capillaries. *Lab Invest. 17*, 738-743.

[2] Beck, L. Jr,, and D'Amore, P. A. (1997). Vascular development: cellular and molecular regulation. *FASEB J. 11*, 365-373.

[3] Fidler, I. J., and Ellis, L. M. (1994). The implications of angiogenesis for the biology and therapy of cancer metastasis. *Cell. 79*, 185-188.

[4] Liotta, L. A., and Stetler-Stevenson, W. G. (1991). Tumor invasion and metastasis: an imbalance of positive and negative regulation. *Cancer Res. 51*, 5054s-5059s.

[5] Ferrara, N., Gerber, H. P., and LeCouter, J. (2003). The biology of VEGF and its receptors. *Nat Med. 9*, 669-676.

[6] Dvorak, H. F. (2002). Vascular permeability factor/vascular endothelial growth factor: a critical cytokine in tumor angiogenesis and a potential target for diagnosis and therapy. *J Clin Oncol. 20*, 4368-4380.

[7] Veikkola, T., Karkkainen, M., Claesson-Welsh, L., and Alitalo, K. (2000). Regulation of angiogenesis via vascular endothelial growth factor receptors. *Cancer Res. 60*, 203-212.

[8] Cross, M.J., Dixelius, J., Matsumoto, T., and Claesson-Welsh, L. (2003). VEGF-receptor signal transduction. *Trends Biochem Sci. 28*, 488-494.

[9] Lohela, M., Saaristo, A., Veikkola, T., and Alitalo, K. (2003). Lymphangiogenic growth factors, receptors and therapies. *Thromb Haemost. 90*, 167-184.

[10] Shibuya, M. (2003). Vascular endothelial growth factor receptor-2: its unique signaling and specific ligand, VEGF-E. *Cancer Sci. 94*, 751-756.

[11] Lyden, D., Hattori, K., Dias, S., Costa, C., Blaikie, P., Butros, L., Chadburn, A., Heissig, B., Marks, W., Witte, L., Wu, Y., Hicklin, D., Zhu, Z., Hackett, N. R., Crystal, R. G., Moore, M. A., Hajjar, K. A., Manova, K., Benezra, R., and Rafii, S. (2001). Impaired recruitment of bone-marrow-derived endothelial and hematopoietic precursor cells blocks tumor angiogenesis and growth. *Nat Med. 7*, 1194-1201.

[12] Bagley, R. G., Walter-Yohrling, J., Cao, X., Weber, W., Simons, B., Cook, B. P., Chartrand, S. D., Wang, C., Madden, S. L., and Teicher, B. A. (2003). Endothelial precursor cells as a model of tumor endothelium: characterization and comparison with mature endothelial cells. *Cancer Res. 63*, 5866-5873.

[13] Semenza, G. L. (2001). Hypoxia-inducible factor 1: oxygen homeostasis and disease pathophysiology. *Trends Mol Med. 7*, 345-350.

[14] Semenza, G. L. (2003). Targeting HIF-1 for cancer therapy. *Nat Rev Cancer. 3,* 721-32.

[15] Maxwell, P.H., Wiesener, M. S., Chang, G. W., Clifford, S. C., Vaux, E. C., Cockman, M. E., Wykoff, C. C., Pugh, C. W., Maher, E. R., and Ratcliffe, P. J. (1999). The tumour suppressor protein VHL targets hypoxia-inducible factors for oxygen-dependent proteolysis. *Nature. 399*, 271-275.

[16] Ivan, M., Kondo, K., Yang, H., Kim, W., Valiando, J., Ohh, M., Salic, A., Asara, J. M., Lane, W. S., and Kaelin, W. G. Jr. (2001). HIFalpha targeted for VHL-mediated

destruction by proline hydroxylation: implications for O2 sensing. *Science*. 292, 464-468.

[17] Seghezzi, G., Patel, S., Ren, C. J., Gualandris, A., Pintucci, G., Robbins, E. S., Shapiro, R. L., Galloway, A. C., Rifkin, D. B., and Mignatti, P. (1998). Fibroblast growth factor-2 (FGF-2) induces vascular endothelial growth factor (VEGF) expression in the endothelial cells of forming capillaries: an autocrine mechanism contributing to angiogenesis. *J Cell Biol. 141*,1659-1673.

[18] Tille, J. C., Wood, J., Mandriota, S. J., Schnell, C., Ferrari, S., Mestan, J., Zhu, Z., Witte, L., and Pepper, M. S. (2001). Vascular endothelial growth factor (VEGF) receptor-2 antagonists inhibit VEGF- and basic fibroblast growth factor-induced angiogenesis in vivo and in vitro. *J. Pharmacol. Exp. Ther. 299*, 1073-1085.

[19] Kubo, H., Cao, R., Brakenhielm, E., Makinen, T., Cao, Y., and Alitalo, K. (2002). Blockade of vascular endothelial growth factor receptor-3 signaling inhibits fibroblast growth factor-2-induced lymphangiogenesis in mouse cornea. *Proc Natl Acad Sci U S A. 99*, 8868-8873.

[20] Kanda, S., Miyata, Y., and Kanetake, H. (2004). Fibroblast growth factor-2-mediated capillary morphogenesis of endothelial cells requires signals via Flt-1/vascular endothelial growth factor receptor-1: possible involvement of c-Akt. *J Biol Chem. 279*, 4007-4016.

[21] Saito, M., Hamasaki, M., and Shibuya, M. (2003). Induction of tube formation by angiopoietin-1 in endothelial cell/fibroblast co-culture is dependent on endogenous VEGF. *Cancer Sci. 94*, 782-790.

[22] Hashizume, H., Baluk, P., Morikawa, S., McLean, J. W., Thurston, G., Roberge, S., Jain, R. K., and McDonald, D. M. (2000). Openings between defective endothelial cells explain tumor vessel leakiness. *Am J Pathol. 156*, 1363-1380.

[23] Yuan, F., Chen, Y., Dellian, M., Safabakhsh, N., Ferrara, N., and Jain, R. K. (1996). Time-dependent vascular regression and permeability changes in established human tumor xenografts induced by an anti-vascular endothelial growth factor/vascular permeability factor antibody. *Proc Natl Acad Sci U S A. 93*, 14765-14770.

[24] Jain, R. K. (2001). Normalizing tumor vasculature with anti-angiogenic therapy: a new paradigm for combination therapy. *Nat Med. 7*, 987-989.

[25] Hansen-Algenstaedt, N., Stoll, B. R., Padera, T. P., Dolmans, D. E., Hicklin, D. J., Fukumura, D., and Jain, R. K. (2000). Tumor oxygenation in hormone-dependent tumors during vascular endothelial growth factor receptor-2 blockade, hormone ablation, and chemotherapy. *Cancer Res. 60*, 4556-4560.

[26] Tong, R. T., Boucher, Y., Kozin, S. V., Winkler, F., Hicklin, D. J., and Jain, R. K. (2004). Vascular normalization by vascular endothelial growth factor receptor 2 blockade induces a pressure gradient across the vasculature and improves drug penetration in tumors. *Cancer Res. 64*, 3731-3736.

[27] Lee, C. G., Heijn, M., di Tomaso, E., Griffon-Etienne, G., Ancukiewicz, M., Koike, C., Park, K. R., Ferrara, N., Jain, R. K., Suit, H. D., and Boucher, Y. (2000). Anti-Vascular endothelial growth factor treatment augments tumor radiation response under normoxic or hypoxic conditions. *Cancer Res. 60*, 5565-5570.

[28] Manley, P. W., Bold, G., Bruggen, J., Fendrich, G., Furet, P., Mestan, J., Schnell, C., Stolz, B., Meyer, T., Meyhack, B., Stark, W., Strauss, A., and Wood, J. (2004) Advances in the structural biology, design and clinical development of VEGF-R kinase inhibitors for the treatment of angiogenesis. *Biochim Biophys Acta. 1697*, 17-27.

[29] Willett, C. G., Boucher, Y., di Tomaso, E., Duda, D. G., Munn, L. L., Tong, R. T., Chung, D. C., Sahani, D. V., Kalva, S. P., Kozin, S. V., Mino, M., Cohen, K. S., Scadden, D. T., Hartford, A. C., Fischman, A. J., Clark, J. W., Ryan, D. P., Zhu, A. X., Blaszkowsky, L. S., Chen, H. X., Shellito, P. C., Lauwers, G. Y., and Jain, R. K. (2004). Direct evidence that the VEGF-specific antibody bevacizumab has antivascular effects in human rectal cancer. *Nat Med. 10*, 145-147.

[30] Calnek, D. S., and Grinnell, B. W. (1998). Thrombomodulin-dependent anticoagulant activity is regulated by vascular endothelial growth factor. *Exp Cell Res. 238*, 294-298.

[31] Spranger, J., and Pfeiffer, A. F. H. (2001). New concepts in pathogenesis and treatment of diabetic retinopathy. *Exp Clin Endocrinol Diabetes. 109*, S438-450.

[32] Das, A., and McGuire, P. G. (2003). Retinal and choroidal angiogenesis: pathophysiology and strategies for inhibition. *Prog Retin Eye Res. 22*, 721-748.

[33] Hammes, H. P., Lin, J., Renner, O., Shani, M., Lundqvist, A., Betsholtz, C., Brownlee, M., and Deutsch, U. (2002). Pericytes and the pathogenesis of diabetic retinopathy. *Diabetes. 51*, 3107-3112.

[34] Marx, R. E., and Johnson, R. P. (1987). Studies in the radiobiology of osteoradionecrosis and their clinical significance. *Oral Surg Oral Med Oral Pathol. 64*, 379-390.

[35] Ennis, R. D. (2002). Hyperbaric oxygen for the treatment of radiation cystitis and proctitis. *Curr Urol Rep. 3*, 229-231.

[36] Corman, J. M., McClure, D., Pritchett, R., Kozlowski, P., and Hampson, N. B. (2003). Treatment of radiation induced hemorrhagic cystitis with hyperbaric oxygen. *J Urol. 169*, 2200-2202.

[37] Benjamin, L. E., Golijanin, D., Itin, A., Pode, D., and Keshet, E. (1999). Selective ablation of immature blood vessels in established human tumors follows vascular endothelial growth factor withdrawal. *J Clin Invest. 103*, 159-165.

[38] Folkman, J. (1971). Tumor angiogenesis: therapeutic implications. *N Engl J Med. 285*, 1182-1186.

[39] Hobson, B., and Denekamp, J. (1984). Endothelial proliferation in tumours and normal tissues: continuous labelling studies. *Br J Cancer. 49*, 405-413.

[40] Folkman, J., Cole, P., and Zimmerman, S. (1966). Tumor behavior in isolated perfused organs: in vitro growth and metastases of biopsy material in rabbit thyroid and canine intestinal segment. *Ann Surg. 164*, 491-502.

[41] Algire, G. H., and Chalkley, H. W. (1945). Vascular reactions of normal and malignant tissues *in vivo*: vascular reactions of mice to wounds and to normal and neoplastic transplants. *J. Natl. Cancer Inst. 6*, 73-85.

[42] Gimbrone, M. A. Jr,, Leapman, S. B., Cotran, R. S., and Folkman, J. (1972). Tumor dormancy in vivo by prevention of neovascularization. *J Exp Med. 136*, 261-276.

[43] Hanahan, D., and Folkman, J. (1996). Patterns and emerging mechanisms of the angiogenic switch during tumorigenesis. *Cell. 86*, 353-364.

[44] Boehm, T., Folkman, J., Browder, T., and O'Reilly, M. S. (1997). Antiangiogenic therapy of experimental cancer does not induce acquired drug resistance. *Nature. 390*, 404-407.

[45] Blagosklonny, M. V. (2004). Antiangiogenic therapy and tumor progression. *Cancer Cell. 5*, 13-17.

[46] Yokoyama, Y., Green, J. E., Sukhatme, V. P., and Ramakrishnan, S. (2000). Effect of endostatin on spontaneous tumorigenesis of mammary adenocarcinoma in a transgenic mouse model. *Cancer Res. 60*, 4362-4365.

[47] Ruzinova, M. B., Schoer, R. A., Gerald, W., Egan, J. E., Pandolfi, P. P., Rafii, S., Manova, K., Mittal, V., and Benezra, R. (2003). Effect of angiogenesis inhibition by Id loss and the contribution of bone-marrow-derived endothelial cells in spontaneous murine tumors. *Cancer Cell. 4*, 277-289.

[48] Hockel, M., and Vaupel, P. (2001). Tumor hypoxia: definitions and current clinical, biologic, and molecular aspects. *J Natl Cancer Inst. 93*, 266-276.

[49] Hockel, M., Schlenger, K., Hockel, S., and Vaupel, P. (1999). Hypoxic cervical cancers with low apoptotic index are highly aggressive. *Cancer Res. 59*, 4525-4528.

[50] O'Brien, T. S., Fox, S. B., Dickinson, A. J., Turley, H., Westwood, M., Moghaddam, A., Gatter, K. C., Bicknell, R., and Harris, A. L. (1996). Expression of the angiogenic factor thymidine phosphorylase/platelet-derived endothelial cell growth factor in primary bladder cancers. *Cancer Res. 56*, 4799-4804.

[51] Crew, J. P., O'Brien, T., Bradburn, M., Fuggle, S., Bicknell, R., Cranston, D., and Harris, A. L. (1997). Vascular endothelial growth factor is a predictor of relapse and stage progression in superficial bladder cancer. *Cancer Res. 57*, 5281-5285.

[52] Pezzella, F., Pastorino, U., Tagliabue, E., Andreola, S., Sozzi, G., Gasparini, G., Menard, S., Gatter, K. C., Harris, A. L., Fox, S., Buyse, M., Pilotti, S., Pierotti, M., and Rilke, F. (1997). Non-small-cell lung carcinoma tumor growth without morphological evidence of neo-angiogenesis. *Am J Pathol. 151*, 1417-1423.

[53] Graeber, T. G., Osmanian, C., Jacks, T., Housman, D. E., Koch, C. J., Lowe, S. W., and Giaccia, A. J. (1996). Hypoxia-mediated selection of cells with diminished apoptotic potential in solid tumours. *Nature. 379*, 88-91.

[54] Yamakawa, M., Liu, L. X., Date, T., Belanger, A. J., Vincent, K. A., Akita, G. Y., Kuriyama, T., Cheng, S. H., Gregory, R. J., and Jiang, C. (2003). Hypoxia-inducible factor-1 mediates activation of cultured vascular endothelial cells by inducing multiple angiogenic factors. *Circ Res. 93*, 664-673.

[55] Nagata, D., Mogi, M., and Walsh, K. (2003). AMP-activated protein kinase (AMPK) signaling in endothelial cells is essential for angiogenesis in response to hypoxic stress. *J Biol Chem. 278*, 31000-31006.

[56] Kayyali, U. S., Pennella, C. M., Trujillo, C., Villa, O., Gaestel, M., and Hassoun, P. M. (2002). Cytoskeletal changes in hypoxic pulmonary endothelial cells are dependent on MAPK-activated protein kinase MK2. *J Biol Chem. 277*, 42596-42602.

[57] Rafii, S., Avecilla, S., Shmelkov, S., Shido, K., Tejada, R., Moore, M. A., Heissig, B., and Hattori, K. (2003). Angiogenic factors reconstitute hematopoiesis by recruiting stem cells from bone marrow microenvironment. *Ann N Y Acad Sci. 996*, 49-60.

[58] Relf, M., LeJeune, S., Scott, P. A., Fox, S., Smith, K., Leek, R., Moghaddam, A., Whitehouse, R., Bicknell, R., and Harris, A. L. (1997). Expression of the angiogenic factors vascular endothelial cell growth factor, acidic and basic fibroblast growth factor, tumor growth factor beta-1, platelet-derived endothelial cell growth factor, placenta growth factor, and pleiotrophin in human primary breast cancer and its relation to angiogenesis. *Cancer Res. 57*, 963-969.

[59] Ogawa, T., Takayama, K., Takakura, N., Kitano, S., and Ueno, H. (2002). Anti-tumor angiogenesis therapy using soluble receptors: enhanced inhibition of tumor growth when soluble fibroblast growth factor receptor-1 is used with soluble vascular endothelial growth factor receptor. *Cancer Gene Ther. 9*, 633-640.

[60] Zhou, Z., Christofidou-Solomidou, M., Garlanda, C., and DeLisser, H. M. (1999). Antibody against murine PECAM-1 inhibits tumor angiogenesis in mice. *Angiogenesis. 3*, 181-188.

[61] Corada, M., Zanetta, L., Orsenigo, F., Breviario, F., Lampugnani, M. G., Bernasconi, S., Liao, F., Hicklin, D. J., Bohlen, P., and Dejana, E. (2002). A monoclonal antibody to vascular endothelial-cadherin inhibits tumor angiogenesis without side effects on endothelial permeability. *Blood. 100*, 905-911.

[62] Takahashi, N., Haba, A., Matsuno, F., and Seon. B. K. (2001). Antiangiogenic therapy of established tumors in human skin/severe combined immunodeficiency mouse chimeras by anti-endoglin (CD105) monoclonal antibodies, and synergy between anti-endoglin antibody and cyclophosphamide. *Cancer Res. 61*, 7846-7854.

[63] Lin, P., Polverini, P., Dewhirst, M., Shan, S., Rao, P. S., and Peters, K. (1997). Inhibition of tumor angiogenesis using a soluble receptor establishes a role for Tie2 in pathologic vascular growth. *J Clin Invest. 100*, 2072-2078.

[64] Traver, D., and Zon, L. I. (2002). Walking the walk: migration and other common themes in blood and vascular development. *Cell. 108*, 731-734.

[65] Bikfalvi, A., and Han, Z. C. (1994). Angiogenic factors are hematopoietic growth factors and vice versa. *Leukemia. 8*, 523-529.

[66] Steinman, R. A. (2002). Cell cycle regulators and hematopoiesis. *Oncogene. 21*, 3403-3413.

[67] Bene, M. C., Castoldi, G., Knapp, W., Rigolin, G. M., Escribano, L., Lemez, P., Ludwig, W. D., Matutes, E., Orfao, A., Lanza, F., and van't Veer, M; EGIL, European Group on Immunological Classification of Leukemias. (2004). CD87 (urokinase-type plasminogen activator receptor), function and pathology in hematological disorders: a review. *Leukemia. 18*, 394-400.

[68] Risau, W. (1997). Mechanisms of angiogenesis. *Nature. 386*, 671-674.

[69] Pawson, T., and Scott, J. D. (1997). Signaling through scaffold, anchoring, and adaptor proteins. *Science. 278*, 2075-2080.

[70] Boriack-Sjodin, P. A., Margarit, S. M., Bar-Sagi, D., and Kuriyan, J. (1998). The structural basis of the activation of Ras by Sos. *Nature. 394*, 337-343.

[71] Lai, K. M., and Pawson T. (2000). The ShcA phosphotyrosine docking protein sensitizes cardiovascular signaling in the mouse embryo. *Genes Dev. 14*, 1132-1145.

[72] Klint, P., Kanda, S., Kloog, Y., and Claesson-Welsh, L. (1999). Contribution of Src and Ras pathways in FGF-2 induced endothelial cell differentiation. *Oncogene. 18*, 3354-3364.

[73] Kroll, J., and Waltenberger, J. (1997). The vascular endothelial growth factor receptor KDR activates multiple signal transduction pathways in porcine aortic endothelial cells. *J Biol Chem. 272*, 32521-32527.

[74] Fournier, E., Blaikie, P., Rosnet, O., Margolis, B., Birnbaum, D., and Borg, J. P. (1999). Role of tyrosine residues and protein interaction domains of SHC adaptor in VEGF receptor 3 signaling. *Oncogene. 18*, 507-514.

[75] Qian, X., Esteban, L., Vass, W. C., Upadhyaya, C., Papageorge, A. G., Yienger, K., Ward, J. M., Lowy, D. R., and Santos, E. (2000). The Sos1 and Sos2 Ras-specific exchange factors: differences in placental expression and signaling properties. *EMBO J. 19*, 642-654.

[76] Boguski, M. S., and McCormick, F. (1993). Proteins regulating Ras and its relatives. *Nature. 366*, 643-654.

[77] Henkemeyer, M., Rossi, D. J., Holmyard, D. P., Puri, M. C., Mbamalu, G., Harpal, K., Shih, T. S., Jacks, T., and Pawson, T. (1995). Vascular system defects and neuronal apoptosis in mice lacking ras GTPase-activating protein. *Nature. 377*, 695-701.

[78] Guo, D., Jia, Q., Song, H. Y., Warren, R. S., and Donner, D. B. (1995). Vascular endothelial cell growth factor promotes tyrosine phosphorylation of mediators of signal transduction that contain SH2 domains. Association with endothelial cell proliferation. *J Biol Chem. 270*, 6729-6733.

[79] Jones, N, and Dumont, D. J. (1998). The Tek/Tie2 receptor signals through a novel Dok-related docking protein, Dok-R. *Oncogene. 17*, 1097-1108.

[80] Kim, I., Ryu, Y. S., Kwak, H. J., Ahn, S. Y., Oh, J. L., Yancopoulos, G. D., Gale, N. W., and Koh, G. Y. (2002). EphB ligand, ephrinB2, suppresses the VEGF- and angiopoietin 1-induced Ras/mitogen-activated protein kinase pathway in venous endothelial cells. *FASEB J. 16*, 1126-1128.

[81] Chong, H., Vikis, H. G., and Guan, K. L. (2003). Mechanisms of regulating the Raf kinase family. *Cell Signal. 15*, 463-469.

[82] Herrera, R., and Sebolt-Leopold, J. S. (2002). Unraveling the complexities of the Raf/MAP kinase pathway for pharmacological intervention. *Trends Mol Med. 8*, S27-31.

[83] Wojnowski, L., Zimmer, A. M., Beck, T. W., Hahn, H., Bernal, R., Rapp, U. R., and Zimmer, A. (1997). Endothelial apoptosis in Braf-deficient mice. *Nat Genet. 16*, 293-297.

[84] Giroux, S., Tremblay, M., Bernard, D., Cardin-Girard, J. F., Aubry, S., Larouche, L., Rousseau, S., Huot, J., Landry, J., Jeannotte, L., and Charron, J. (1999). Embryonic death of Mek1-deficient mice reveals a role for this kinase in angiogenesis in the labyrinthine region of the placenta. *Curr Biol. 9*, 369-372.

[85] Hagemann, C., and Blank, J. L. (2001). The ups and downs of MEK kinase interactions. *Cell Signal. 13*, 863-875.

[86] Yang, J., Boerm, M., McCarty, M., Bucana, C., Fidler, I. J., Zhuang, Y., and Su, B. (2000). Mekk3 is essential for early embryonic cardiovascular development. *Nat Genet. 24*, 309-313.

[87] Gratton, J. P., Morales-Ruiz, M., Kureishi, Y., Fulton, D., Walsh, K., and Sessa, W. C. (2001). Akt down-regulation of p38 signaling provides a novel mechanism of vascular endothelial growth factor-mediated cytoprotection in endothelial cells. *J Biol Chem. 276*, 30359-30365.

[88] Regan, C. P., Li, W., Boucher, D. M., Spatz, S., Su, M. S., and Kuida, K. (2002). Erk5 null mice display multiple extraembryonic vascular and embryonic cardiovascular defects. *Proc Natl Acad Sci U S A. 99*, 9248-9253.

[89] Sohn, S. J., Sarvis, B. K., Cado, D., and Winoto, A. (2002). ERK5 MAPK regulates embryonic angiogenesis and acts as a hypoxia-sensitive repressor of vascular endothelial growth factor expression. *J Biol Chem. 277*, 43344-43351.

[90] Yan, L., Carr, J., Ashby, P. R., Murry-Tait, V., Thompson, C., and Arthur, J. S. (2003). Knockout of ERK5 causes multiple defects in placental and embryonic development. *BMC Dev Biol. 3*, 11.

[91] Abe, J., Kusuhara, M., Ulevitch, R. J., Berk, B. C., and Lee, J. D. (1996). Big mitogen-activated protein kinase 1 (BMK1) is a redox-sensitive kinase. *J Biol Chem. 271*, 16586-16590.

[92] Abe, J., Takahashi, M., Ishida, M., Lee, J. D., and Berk, B. C. (1997). c-Src is required for oxidative stress-mediated activation of big mitogen-activated protein kinase 1. *J Biol Chem. 272*, 20389-20394.

[93] Kato, Y., Kravchenko, V. V., Tapping, R. I., Han, J., Ulevitch, R. J., and Lee, J. D. (1997). BMK1/ERK5 regulates serum-induced early gene expression through transcription factor MEF2C. *EMBO J. 16*, 7054-7066.

[94] Kato, Y., Tapping, R. I., Huang, S., Watson, M. H., Ulevitch, R. J., and Lee, J. D. (1998). Bmk1/Erk5 is required for cell proliferation induced by epidermal growth factor. *Nature. 395*, 713-716.

[95] Ono, K., and Han, J. (2000). The p38 signal transduction pathway: activation and function. *Cell Signal. 12*, 1-13.

[96] Mudgett, J. S., Ding, J., Guh-Siesel, L., Chartrain, N. A., Yang, L., Gopal, S., and Shen, M. M. (2000). Essential role for p38alpha mitogen-activated protein kinase in placental angiogenesis. *Proc Natl Acad Sci U S A. 97*, 10454-10459.

[97] Adams, R. H., Porras, A., Alonso, G., Jones, M., Vintersten, K., Panelli, S., Valladares, A., Perez, L., Klein, R., and Nebreda, A. R. (2000). Essential role of p38alpha MAP kinase in placental but not embryonic cardiovascular development. *Mol Cell. 6*, 109-116.

[98] Tamura, K., Sudo, T., Senftleben, U., Dadak, A. M., Johnson, R., and Karin, M. (2000). Requirement for p38alpha in erythropoietin expression: a role for stress kinases in erythropoiesis. *Cell. 102*, 221-231.

[99] Allen, M., Svensson, L., Roach, M., Hambor, J., McNeish, J., and Gabel, C. A. (2000). Deficiency of the stress kinase p38alpha results in embryonic lethality: characterization of the kinase dependence of stress responses of enzyme-deficient embryonic stem cells. *J Exp Med. 191*, 859-870.

[100] Matsumoto, T., Turesson, I., Book, M., Gerwins, P., and Claesson-Welsh, L. (2002). p38 MAP kinase negatively regulates endothelial cell survival, proliferation, and differentiation in FGF-2-stimulated angiogenesis. *J Cell Biol. 156*, 149-160.

[101] Harfouche, R., Gratton, J. P., Yancopoulos, G. D., Noseda, M., Karsan, A., Hussain, S. N. (2003). Angiopoietin-1 activates both anti- and proapoptotic mitogen-activated protein kinases. *FASEB J. 17*, 1523-1525.

[102] Shalaby, F., Rossant, J., Yamaguchi, T. P., Gertsenstein, M., Wu, X. F., Breitman, M. L., and Schuh, A. C. (1995). Failure of blood-island formation and vasculogenesis in Flk-1-deficient mice. *Nature. 376*, 62-66.

[103] Carmeliet, P., Ferreira, V., Breier, G., Pollefeyt, S., Kieckens, L., Gertsenstein, M., Fahrig, M., Vandenhoeck, A., Harpal, K., Eberhardt, C., Declercq, C., Pawling, J., Moons, L., Collen, D., Risau, W., and Nagy, A. (1996). Abnormal blood vessel development and lethality in embryos lacking a single VEGF allele. *Nature. 380*, 435-439.

[104] Ferrara, N., Carver-Moore, K., Chen, H., Dowd, M., Lu, L., O'Shea, K. S., Powell-Braxton, L., Hillan, K. J., and Moore, M. W. (1996). Heterozygous embryonic lethality induced by targeted inactivation of the VEGF gene. *Nature. 380*, 439-442.

[105] Sato, T. N., Tozawa, Y., Deutsch, U., Wolburg-Buchholz, K., Fujiwara, Y., Gendron-Maguire, M., Gridley, T., Wolburg, H., Risau, W., and Qin, Y. (1995). Distinct roles of the receptor tyrosine kinases Tie-1 and Tie-2 in blood vessel formation. *Nature. 376*, 70-74.

[106] Suri, C., Jones, P. F., Patan, S., Bartunkova, S., Maisonpierre, P. C., Davis, S., Sato, T. N., and Yancopoulos, G. D. (1996). Requisite role of angiopoietin-1, a ligand for the TIE2 receptor, during embryonic angiogenesis. *Cell. 87*, 1171-1180.

[107] Chan, T. O., Rittenhouse, S. E., and Tsichlis, P. N. (1999). AKT/PKB and other D3 phosphoinositide-regulated kinases: kinase activation by phosphoinositide-dependent phosphorylation. *Annu Rev Biochem. 68*, 965-1014.

[108] Nicholson, K. M., and Anderson, N. G. (2002). The protein kinase B/Akt signalling pathway in human malignancy. *Cell Signal. 14*, 381-395.

[109] Shiojima, I., and Walsh, K. (2002). Role of Akt signaling in vascular homeostasis and angiogenesis. *Circ Res. 90*, 1243-1250.

[110] Yang, Z. Z., Tschopp, O., Hemmings-Mieszczak, M., Feng, J., Brodbeck, D., Perentes, E., and Hemmings, B. A. (2003). Protein kinase B alpha/Akt1 regulates placental development and fetal growth. *J Biol Chem. 278*, 32124-32131.

[111] Carragher, N. O., and Frame, M.,C. (2004). Focal adhesion and actin dynamics: a place where kinases and proteases meet to promote invasion. *Trends Cell Biol. 14*, 241-249.

[112] Ilic, D., Kovacic, B., McDonagh, S., Jin, F., Baumbusch, C., Gardner, D. G., and Damsky, C. H. (2003). Focal adhesion kinase is required for blood vessel morphogenesis. *Circ Res. 92*, 300-307.

[113] George, E. L., Georges-Labouesse, E. N., Patel-King, R.S., Rayburn, H., and Hynes, R. O. (1993). Defects in mesoderm, neural tube and vascular development in mouse embryos lacking fibronectin. *Development. 119*, 1079-1091.

[114] Rousseau, S., Houle, F., Kotanides, H., Witte, L., Waltenberger, J., Landry, J., and Huot, J. (2000). Vascular endothelial growth factor (VEGF)-driven actin-based

motility is mediated by VEGFR2 and requires concerted activation of stress-activated protein kinase 2 (SAPK2/p38) and geldanamycin-sensitive phosphorylation of focal adhesion kinase. *J Biol Chem. 275*, 10661-10672.

[115] Holmqvist, K., Cross, M., Riley, D., and Welsh, M. (2003). The Shb adaptor protein causes Src-dependent cell spreading and activation of focal adhesion kinase in murine brain endothelial cells. *Cell Signal. 15*, 171-179.

[116] Kim, I., Kim, H. G., Moon, S. O., Chae, S. W., So, J. N., Koh, K. N., Ahn, B. C., and Koh, G. Y. (2000). Angiopoietin-1 induces endothelial cell sprouting through the activation of focal adhesion kinase and plasmin secretion. *Circ Res. 86*, 952-959.

[117] Miki, H., Suetsugu, S., and Takenawa, T. (1998). WAVE, a novel WASP-family protein involved in actin reorganization induced by Rac. *EMBO J. 17*, 6932-6941.

[118] Yamazaki, D., Suetsugu, S., Miki, H., Kataoka, Y., Nishikawa, S., Fujiwara, T., Yoshida, N., and Takenawa, T. (2003). WAVE2 is required for directed cell migration and cardiovascular development. *Nature. 424*, 452-456.

[119] Greer, P. (2002). Closing in on the biological functions of Fps/Fes and Fer. *Nat Rev Mol Cell Biol. 3*, 278-289.

[120] Smithgall, T. E., Rogers, J. A., Peters, K. L., Li, J., Briggs, S. D., Lionberger, J. M., Cheng, H., Shibata, A., Scholtz, B., Schreiner, S., and Dunham, N. (1998). The c-Fes family of protein-tyrosine kinases. *Crit Rev Oncog. 9*, 43-62.

[121] Haigh, J., McVeigh, J., and Greer, P. (1996). The fps/fes tyrosine kinase is expressed in myeloid, vascular endothelial, epithelial, and neuronal cells and is localized in the trans-golgi network. *Cell Growth Differ. 7*, 931-944.

[122] Read, R. D., Lionberger, J. M., and Smithgall, T. E. (1997). Oligomerization of the Fes tyrosine kinase. Evidence for a coiled-coil domain in the unique N-terminal region. *J Biol Chem. 272*, 18498-18503.

[123] Rogers, J. A., Read, R. D, Li, J., Peters, K. L., and Smithgall, T. E. (1996). Autophosphorylation of the Fes tyrosine kinase. Evidence for an intermolecular mechanism involving two kinase domain tyrosine residues. *J Biol Chem. 271*, 17519-17525.

[124] Senis, Y., Zirngibl, R., McVeigh, J., Haman, A., Hoang, T., and Greer, P. A. (1999). Targeted disruption of the murine fps/fes proto-oncogene reveals that Fps/Fes kinase activity is dispensable for hematopoiesis. *Mol Cell Biol. 19*, 7436-7446.

[125] Hackenmiller, R., Kim, J., Feldman, R. A., and Simon, M. C. (2000). Abnormal Stat activation, hematopoietic homeostasis, and innate immunity in c-fes-/- mice. *Immunity. 13*, 397-407.

[126] Zirngibl, R. A., Senis, Y., and Greer, P. A. (2002). Enhanced endotoxin sensitivity in fps/fes-null mice with minimal defects in hematopoietic homeostasis. *Mol Cell Biol. 22*, 2472-2486.

[127] Hackenmiller, R., and Simon, M. C. (2002). Truncation of c-fes via gene targeting results in embryonic lethality and hyperproliferation of hematopoietic cells. *Dev Biol. 245*, 255-269.

[128] Greer, P., Haigh, J., Mbamalu, G., Khoo, W., Bernstein, A., and Pawson, T. (1994). The Fps/Fes protein-tyrosine kinase promotes angiogenesis in transgenic mice. *Mol Cell Biol. 14*, 6755-6763.

[129] Sangrar, W., Mewburn, J. D., Vincent, S. G., Fisher, J. T., and Greer, P. A. (2004). Vascular defects in gain-of-function fps/fes transgenic mice correlate with PDGF- and VEGF-induced activation of mutant Fps/Fes kinase in endothelial cells. *J Thromb Haemost. 2*, 820-832.

[130] Haigh, J. J., Ema, M., Haigh, K., Gertsenstein, M., Greer, P., Rossant, J., Nagy, A., and Wagner, E. F. (2004). Activated Fps/Fes partially rescues the in vivo developmental potential of Flk1-deficient vascular progenitor cells. *Blood. 103*, 912-920.

[131] Kanda, S., Lerner, E. C., Tsuda, S., Shono, T., Kanetake, H., Smithgall, T. E. (2000). The nonreceptor protein-tyrosine kinase c-Fes is involved in fibroblast growth factor-2-induced chemotaxis of murine brain capillary endothelial cells. *J Biol Chem. 275*, 10105-10111.

[132] Kanda, S., Mochizuki, Y., Miyata, Y., and Kanetake, H. (2003). The role of c-Fes in vascular endothelial growth factor-A-mediated signaling by endothelial cells. *Biochem Biophys Res Commun. 306*, 1056-1063.

[133] Kanda, S., Mochizuki, Y., and Kanetake, H. (2003). Stromal cell-derived factor-1alpha induces tube-like structure formation of endothelial cells through phosphoinositide 3-kinase. *J Biol Chem. 278*, 257-262.

[134] Kanda, S., Mochizuki, Y., Suematsu, T., Miyata, Y., Nomata, K., and Kanetake, H. (2003). Sonic hedgehog induces capillary morphogenesis by endothelial cells through phosphoinositide 3-kinase. *J Biol Chem. 278*, 8244-8249.

[135] Ullrich, A., and Schlessinger, J. (1990). Signal transduction by receptors with tyrosine kinase activity. *Cell. 61*, 203-212.

[136] Heldin,C.-H. (1995). Dimerization of cell surface receptors in signal transduction. *Cell. 80*, 213-223.

[137] Pawson, T. (1995). Protein modules and signalling networks. *Nature. 373*, 573-580.

[138] Kamat, A., and Carpenter G. (1997). Phospholipase C-γ1: regulation of enzyme function and role in growth factor-dependent signal transduction. *Cytokine Growth Factor Rev. 8*, 109-117.

[139] Seetharam, L., Gotoh, N., Maru, Y., Neufeld, G., Yamaguchi, S., and Shibuya, M. (1995). A unique signal transduction from FLT tyrosine kinase, a receptor for vascular endothelial growth factor VEGF. *Oncogene. 10*, 135-147.

[140] Sawano, A., Takahashi, T., Yamaguchi, S., and Shibuya, M. (1997). The phosphorylated 1169-tyrosine containing region of flt-1 kinase (VEGFR-1) is a major binding site for PLCγ. *Biochem Biophys Res Commun. 238*, 487-491.

[141] Cunningham, S. A., Arrate, M. P., Brock, T. A., and Waxham, M. N. (1997). Interactions of FLT-1 and KDR with phospholipase Cγ: identification of the phosphotyrosine binding sites. *Biochem Biophys Res Commun. 240*, 635-639.

[142] Igarashi, K., Isohara, T., Kato, T., Shigeta, K., Yamano, T., and Uno, I. (1998). Tyrosine 1213 of Flt-1 is a major binding site of Nck and SHP-2. *Biochem Biophys Res Commun. 246*, 95-99.

[143] Ito, N., Wernstedt, C., Engstrom, U., and Claesson-Welsh, L. (1998). Identification of vascular endothelial growth factor receptor-1 tyrosine phosphorylation sites and binding of SH2 domain-containing molecules. *J Biol Chem. 273*, 23410-23418.

[144] Vanhaesebroeck, B., Leevers, S. J., Panayotou, G., and Waterfield, M. D. (1997). Phosphoinositide 3-kinases: a conserved family of signal transducers. *Trends Biochem Sci. 22*, 267-272.

[145] Fruman, D. A., Meyers, R. E., and Cantley, L. C. (1998). Phosphoinositide kinases. *Annu Rev Biochem. 67*, 481-507.

[146] Cunningham, S. A., Waxham, M. N., Arrate, P. M., and Brock, T. A. (1995). Interaction of the Flt-1 tyrosine kinase receptor with the p85 subunit of phosphatidylinositol 3-kinase. Mapping of a novel site involved in binding. *J Biol Chem. 270*, 20254-20257.

[147] Kontos, C. D., Stauffer, T. P., Yang, W. P., York, J. D., Huang, L., Blanar, M. A., Meyer, T., and Peters, K. G. (1998). Tyrosine 1101 of Tie2 is the major site of association of p85 and is required for activation of phosphatidylinositol 3-kinase and Akt. *Mol Cell Biol. 18*, 4131-4140.

[148] Jones, N., Master, Z., Jones, J., Bouchard, D., Gunji, Y., Sasaki, H., Daly, R., Alitalo, K., and Dumont, D. J. (1999). Identification of Tek/Tie2 binding partners. Binding to a multifunctional docking site mediates cell survival and migration. *J Biol Chem. 274*, 30896-30905.

[149] Mochizuki, Y., Nakamura, T., Kanetake, H., and Kanda, S. (2002). Angiopoietin 2 stimulates migration and tube-like structure formation of murine brain capillary endothelial cells through c-Fes and c-Fyn. *J Cell Sci. 115*, 175-183.

[150] Kanda, S., Miyata, Y., Mochizuki, Y., Matsuyama, T., and Kanetake, H. (2005). Angiopoietin 1 is mitogenic for cultured endothelial cells. *Cancer Res*. In press.

[151] Vajkoczy, P., Farhadi, M., Gaumann, A., Heidenreich, R., Erber, R., Wunder, A., Tonn, J. C., Menger, M. D., and Breier, G. (2002). Microtumor growth initiates angiogenic sprouting with simultaneous expression of VEGF, VEGF receptor-2, and angiopoietin-2. *J Clin Invest. 109*, 777-785.

[152] Henderson, A. M., Wang, S. J., Taylor, A. C., Aitkenhead, M., and Hughes, C. C. (2001). The basic helix-loop-helix transcription factor HESR1 regulates endothelial cell tube formation. *J Biol Chem. 276*, 6169-6176.

[153] Elvert, G., Kappel, A., Heidenreich, R., Englmeier, U., Lanz, S., Acker, T., Rauter, M., Plate, K., Sieweke, M., Breier, G., and Flamme, I. (2003). Cooperative interaction of hypoxia-inducible factor-2α (HIF-2α) and Ets-1 in the transcriptional activation of vascular endothelial growth factor receptor-2 (Flk-1). *J Biol Chem. 278*, 7520-7530.

[154] Hasegawa, Y., Abe, M., Yamazaki, T., Niizeki, O., Shiiba, K., Sasaki, I., and Sato, Y. (2004). Transcriptional regulation of human angiopoietin-2 by transcription factor Ets-1. Biochem Biophys Res Commun. 316, 52-58.

[155] Munro, N. P., Woodhams, S., Nawrocki, J. D., Fletcher, M. S., and Thomas, P. J. (2003). The role of transarterial embolization in the treatment of renal cell carcinoma. *BJU Int. 92*, 240-244.

[156] Chang, J. M., Tzeng, W. S., Pan, H. B., Yang, C. F., and Lai, K. H. (1994). Transcatheter arterial embolization with or without cisplatin treatment of hepatocellular carcinoma. A randomized controlled study. *Cancer. 74*, 2449-2453.

[157] De Palma, M., Venneri, M. A., and Naldini, L. (2003). In vivo targeting of tumor endothelial cells by systemic delivery of lentiviral vectors. *Hum Gene Ther. 14*, 1193-1206.

[158] Hadaczek, P., Mirek, H., Bringas, J., Cunningham, J., and Bankiewicz, K. (2004). Basic fibroblast growth factor enhances transduction, distribution, and axonal transport of adeno-associated virus type 2 vector in rat brain. *Hum Gene Ther. 15*, 469-479.

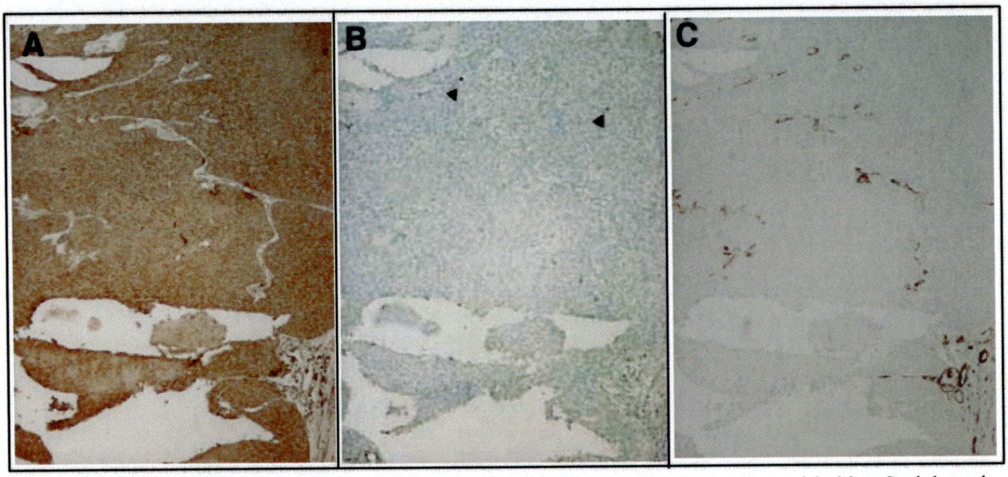

Fig. 1. Expression of VEGF-A in low-grade transitional cell carcinoma of the urinary bladder. Serial sections of papillary transitional cell carcinoma of the urinary bladder were examined. VEGF-A was stained by a specific antibody against VEGF-A (**A**) and vessels were visualized by endothelial cell staining by anti-CD31 antibody (**C**). Apoptotic cells (arrow heads) were examined by the TUNEL method (**B**). Note the expression of VEGF-A in tumor cells and the presence of few microvessels and apoptotic tumor cells. In papillary carcinoma of the urinary bladder, blood vessels are usually observed at the narrow base of the tumor. When the size of the tumor is more than 2 cm, vessels in the tumor tissue are still vacant.

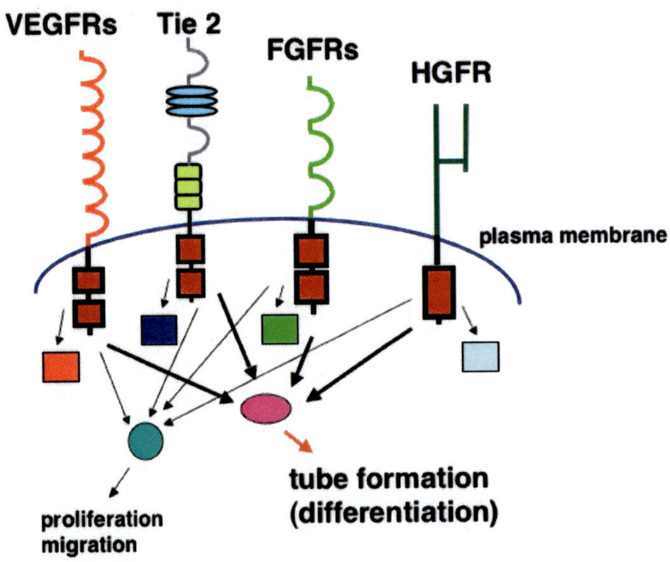

Fig. 2. Strategy to identify novel targets of ant-angiogenic therapy. Growth factors play pivotal roles in the regulation of angiogenic cellular responses by endothelial cells and their signals are transduced into the cells via specific receptor tyrosine kinases, such as VEGF receptors, FGF receptors, hepatocyte growth factor receptor and Tie 2. Downstream of these receptors, signaling molecules specific for each receptor (rectangle) and common molecules (blue circle) leading to proliferation and migration of endothelial cells, may exist. Cellular proliferation and migration are not unique for endothelial cells (also observed in hematopoietic cells and tumor cells). Tube formation (differentiation) is rather distinctive of endothelial cells. Targeted inhibition of signaling molecule(s) involved in the regulation of endothelial cell differentiation, which commonly acts downstream of receptor tyrosine kinases (red oval), could be potentially useful specific anti-angiogenic therapy.

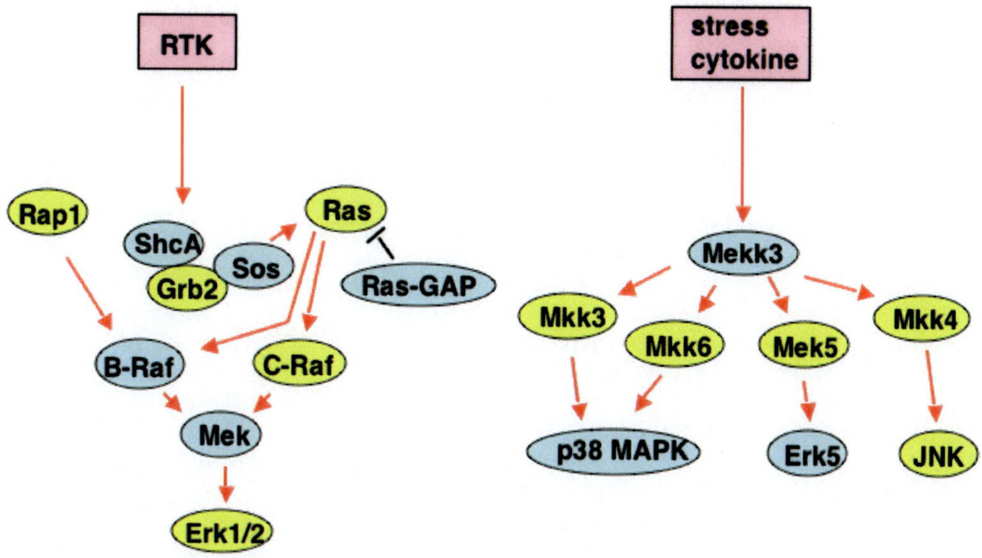

Fig. 3. Targeted disruption of genes encoding signaling molecules of Ras/MAPK and related pathways (blue oval) causes defect in vascular development in mice. Deletion of genes encoding the molecules encircled by blue oval causes vascular defects. Activated receptor tyrosine kinases (RTK) phosphorylate ShcA and Grb2 at tyrosine residues, which in turn form complexes with Ras-specific guanine nucleotide exchanger factor, Sos. Sos activates Ras and the activated Ras (GTP-bound form) further activates Raf kinases, followed by subsequent activation of Mek and Erk kinases. GTP-bound Ras is inactivated by hydrolyzing GTP by Ras-GTPase activating protein (Ras-GAP)-promoted increased intrinsic GTPase activity. Stress and cytokines activate Mekk3, resulting in the activation of signaling cascades leading to the activation of MAPKs, such as p38 MAPK, Erk5, and JNK.

In: Trends in Angiogenesis Research
Editor: Roberta V. Zubar, pp. 71-102

ISBN 1-59454-452-2

Chapter III

HORMONAL EFFECTS ON ENDOMETRIAL ANGIOGENESIS

Gareth C. Weston**, Jane E. Girling, Caroline E. Gargett and Peter A. W. Rogers

Centre for Women's Health Research, Department of Obstetrics and Gynaecology, Monash University, Melbourne, Australia

ABSTRACT

Angiogenesis in the endometrium occurs in a cyclic manner under the influence of the steroid hormones estrogen and progesterone. Whether effects by these hormones on the endothelial cells are direct, indirect, or a combination of both, is unclear. In addition, little is known of the mechanisms by which estrogen and progesterone influence angiogenesis in the endometrium.

Here, we describe our work examining possible direct and indirect effects of these hormones on endometrial angiogenesis. Overall effects of estrogen and progesterone on vessel proliferation were examined in a mouse model. The same mouse model was then used to demonstrate the modulation of vascular endothelial growth factor by estrogen. An in vitro model of microvascular endothelial cell cultures derived from the myometrium were used to demonstrate estrogen and progesterone receptors, and screening with gene expression microarrays performed to investigate direct transcriptional effects of estrogen and progesterone stimulation of the endothelial cells.

Finally, a possible role of circulating neutrophils in endometrial angiogenesis is postulated based upon an immunohistochemical study of human endometrium. The possibility of direct modulation of this interaction by progesterone is investigated using flow cytometry and gene expression microarrays on our in vitro myometrial microvascular endothelial cell model.

* Correspondence concerning this article should be addressed to Dr Gareth C Weston, Department of Obstetrics & Gynaecology, Level 5 Monash Medical Centre, 246 Clayton Rd, Clayton VIC 3168, Australia. Email: gareth.weston@med.monash.edu.au

Color graphics are presented at the end of the chapter.

Key words: Endometrium; Angiogenesis; Estrogen; Progesterone; Neutrophils

1. INTRODUCTION

The ovarian steroid hormones, estrogen and progesterone, vary cyclically with, and are key regulators of, endometrial remodeling during the menstrual cycle. It is likely that the cyclical changes in the endometrial vasculature are influenced, either directly or indirectly, by the actions of one or both of these hormones.

There is considerable evidence that estrogen regulates physiological angiogenesis in the endometrium. In the ERα knockout mouse, uterine angiogenesis is impaired (Johns *et.al.*, 1996), and antiestrogenic compounds have angiogenesis inhibitory activity (Gagliardi and Collins, 1993). However, the precise mechanism by which estrogen affects the endometrial vasculature in the human is unclear.

The literature on progesterone effects on angiogenesis is scant when compared with estrogen. Nonetheless, there are important clinical implications of progesterone effects on angiogenesis in the endometrium. The systemic delivery of progesterone is part of several contraceptive regimes, as well as post-menopausal hormone replacement therapy. In up to forty percent of women commencing continuous progesterone in hormone replacement therapy regimes, irregular endometrial bleeding will occur within the first six months of treatment, often leading to cessation of therapy (Odmark *et.al.*, 2001).

The endometrium of women taking progesterone continuously as a contraceptive is thin, with an increased microvessel density (Rogers *et.al.*, 1993). However, the vessels show evidence of increased fragility (Hickey *et.al.*, 2000), and suppression of angiogenic activity as evidenced by a reduced endothelial cell proliferation (Goodger *et.al.*, 1994) and migratory activity (Subakir *et.al.*, 1995). The progestin medroxyprogesterone acetate was one of the first compounds found to have angiogenic inhibitory activity in tumors (Gross *et.al.*, 1981). Although the effects of long-term progestins on the endometrial vasculature continue to be investigated, the role of progesterone in physiological angiogenesis in the endometrium has yet to be determined.

A key issue is whether estrogen and progesterone act directly or indirectly on endometrial vessels. Both estrogen and progesterone upregulate production of a potent angiogenic promoter, vascular endothelial growth factor (VEGF), by the endometrial stroma (Shifren *et.al.*, 1996). However, progesterone also upregulates angiogenesis inhibitors, such as thrombospondin-1 (TSP-1) (Iruela-Arispe *et.al.*, 1996). The net effect, if any, of these kinds of indirect effects on the endometrial vasculature is unknown.

If the effects of estrogen on angiogenesis are mediated directly, then they may be via the endothelial cells, the vascular smooth muscle cells, or a combination of the two cell types. Both endothelial cells (Venkov *et.al.*, 1996) and vascular smooth muscle cells (Karas *et.al.*, 1994) have been shown to express estrogen receptors. There have now been several studies examining ER expression in the uterine microvasculature (Iruela-Arispe *et.al.*, 1999; Wu *et.al.*, 2000; Critchley *et.al.*, 2001; Lecce *et.al.*, 2001; Gargett *et.al.*, 2002). Expression of estrogen receptor has been shown in all of these studies in both the smooth muscle cell and endothelial cell components of the vessels.

There are an increasing number of direct effects reported for estrogen on endothelial cells. Many of the studies of estrogen effects on endothelial cells use endothelial cells from non-human species, or from large vessels, making extrapolation of results to the uterine microvasculature problematic. It has been shown that effects of estrogen on one endothelial cell type do not necessarily translate to effects on other cell types, even within the same species (Seli *et.al.*, 2002). There are few studies looking specifically at the direct effects of estrogen on uterine microvascular endothelial cells. Our in vitro work has used microvascular endothelial cells from the myometrium as a model for the endometrial vasculature, as, unlike our experience with endometrium, the cells can be isolated in sufficient quantities from the myometrium to be experimented on at an early passage. We postulate that myometrial microvascular endothelial cells are far more likely to be similar to endometrial microvascular endothelial cells than those of different organs, or large vessel endothelial cells.

In contrast to estrogen, there have been very few studies examining direct effects of progesterone on endothelial cells, and the literature that exists is contradictory. A need for in-vitro genomic studies addressing the regulation of the uterine vasculature by progesterone has been recognized (Smith, 2000), owing to the lack of studies in the literature.

In this chapter, we present some of the work of the past few years in our department investigating the role of estrogen and progesterone in angiogenesis in the endometrium. In particular, this chapter describes work examining indirect effects of steroid hormones on endometrial angiogenesis via production of vascular endothelial growth factor (VEGF), or manipulation of contact between endothelial cells and intravascular neutrophil sources of VEGF. Further, we describe attempts to investigate possible direct effects of steroid hormones on angiogenesis via direct effects on endothelial cells.

2. Effects of Estrogen on Vessel Proliferation in the Endometrium

In recent years, there has been some disagreement about the role that estrogen plays in stimulating endometrial angiogenesis. Using recently developed stereological methods to measure anisotropic structures, we have been able to demonstrate that vessel elongation, the lengthways growth of the vessel without formation of new vascular junctions, is a major angiogenic mechanism during the mid-late estrogen-driven proliferative phase of the human menstrual cycle (Gambino et al., 2002). This work suggests, but does not prove a role for estrogen in this process.

More convincing evidence is provided by experimental work using ovariectomised mice in which endometrial endothelial cell proliferation increases significantly within 24 hours of estrogen treatment (Heryanto and Rogers, 2002). In this experiment, ovariectomised mice (25-30 g, C57BL/6J x CBA) were treated with daily steroid injections for seven days: days 1-3 – 100 ng estradiol in 0.1 ml peanut oil (denoted E1-E3), days 4-5 – 10 ng estradiol plus 500 µg progesterone in 1 ml peanut oil (denoted P1-P3), and day 7: 100 ng estradiol plus 500 µg progesterone (denoted PE). Groups of mice (n=5) were dissected 24 h after each day of treatment. Four hours prior to dissection, mice received an injection of bromodeoxyuridine (BrdU, 40 mg/kg) to label proliferating cells (thymidine analogue that is incorporated into DNA during the S phase of the cell cycle). A sample of one uterine horn was snap frozen in OCT medium before the mouse was perfusion fixed and the remaining uterine tissue fixed in 10 % formalin before embedding in paraffin. Immunohistochemistry was used to identify proliferating cells on sections from paraffin-embedded tissues (5 µm sections; primary antibody = sheep anti-BrdU [10 µg/ml, BioDesign, Saco, ME]) and vascular profiles on frozen tissues (5 µm; monoclonal primary antibody = rat anti-mouse CD31 [10 µg/ml, PharMingen, Los Angeles, CA]). The number of proliferating endothelial cells on a section from each mouse was counted and expressed as a percentage of the total number of endothelial cells. Vascular density was quantified by counting the number of capillary profiles immunostained with CD31 per mm^2. Stromal cell density was quantified by counting the number of stromal cells per mm^2. A ratio of vascular density: stromal cell density was calculated for each stage with the ratio in untreated, ovariectomised mice made to equal one.

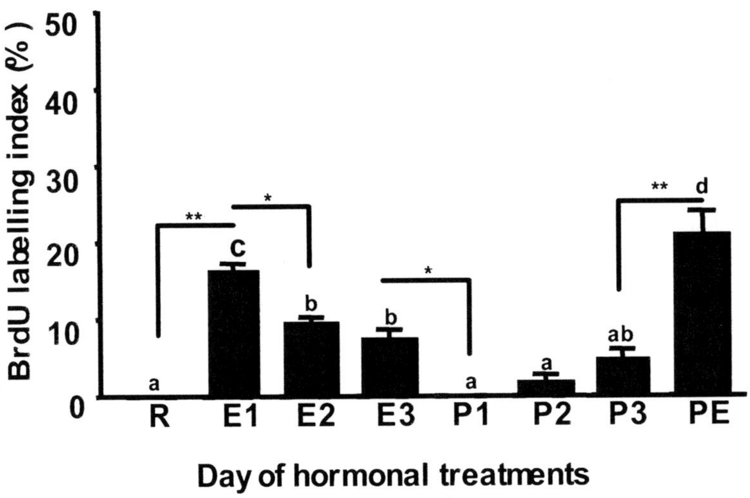

Fig. 1. Bromodeoxyuridine labeling index (%) in the endothelium of mouse endometrium. Values are means ± SE (n=5 per group). Columns with different superscripts are significantly different ($^{a\text{-}d}p < 0.05$, $*p < 0.01$, $**p < 0.001$). R: untreated, ovariectomised mice; E1, E2 and E3: days 1-3 of treatment with estradiol (100 ng/mouse/day); P1, P2 and P3: days 4-6 of treatment with progesterone (500 µg/mouse/day) and estradiol (10 ng/mouse/day); PE: day 7 of treatment with progesterone (500 µg/mouse/day) and estradiol (100 ng/mouse/day). (Reproduced from Heryanto and Rogers, 2002 with permission).

BrdU labeling was undetectable in endothelial cells in untreated ovariectomised mice (Heryanto and Rogers, 2002; Fig. 1). After one day of estradiol treatment (E1), endothelial cell proliferation increased significantly (p<0.05). Endothelial cell proliferation was also observed at E2, E3, P2 and P3, although the percentage was lower than at E1. The highest amount of endothelial cell proliferation was observed at PE; however, the design of this experiment does not allow us to determine the relative roles of oestrogen and progesterone at this stage. Differing patterns of glandular epithelial, luminal epithelial and stromal cell proliferation were also observed (data not shown).

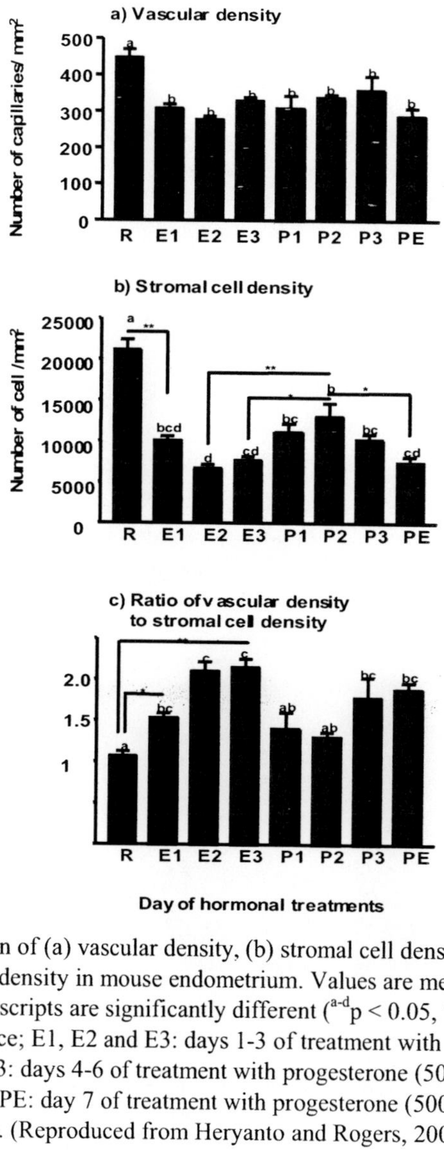

Fig. 2. Quantitative evaluation of (a) vascular density, (b) stromal cell density and (c) the ratio of vascular density:stromal cell density in mouse endometrium. Values are means ± SE (n=5 per group). Columns with different superscripts are significantly different ($^{a-d}p < 0.05$, $*p < 0.01$, $**p < 0.001$). R: untreated, ovariectomised mice; E1, E2 and E3: days 1-3 of treatment with estradiol (100 ng/mouse/day); P1, P2 and P3: days 4-6 of treatment with progesterone (500 μg/mouse/day) and estradiol (10 ng/mouse/day); PE: day 7 of treatment with progesterone (500 μg/mouse/day) and estradiol (100 ng/mouse/day). (Reproduced from Heryanto and Rogers, 2002 with permission).

There was a significant decrease in both vascular density and stromal cell density at all treatment stages in contrast to untreated, ovariectomised mice; this reflected the increased tissue oedema caused by steroid treatment (Fig. 2). Despite this, however, there was a significant increase in the ratio of vessel density: stromal cell density at all stages. We hypothesized that the increase in this ratio at E1 reflected estrogen-induced endometrial angiogenesis. In ovariectomised sheep also, estrogen treatment caused an almost 2-fold increase in endometrial microvascular volume density (percentage of tissue volume occupied by microvessels) within 24 hours; this reflected an approximately 5-fold increase in total endometrial microvascular volume (Reynolds et al., 1998a). In contrast, uterine tissue weight only increased approximately 3-fold. Reynolds et al. (1998a) hypothesized that the increase in microvascular volume reflected an increase in both microvascular vasodilation and growth.

In contrast, Ma et al. (2001) have hypothesized that estrogen promotes vascular permeability, but 'profoundly inhibits' angiogenesis. Ma's hypothesis was based on a lack of stromal VEGF mRNA (and Flk-1) after 24 h of estrogen treatment and a reduction in the stromal area occupied by blood vessels after two days in ovariectomised mice (although no account was taken for tissue oedema in this study). Ma et al. (2001) also found an increase in stromal VEGF mRNA at 2 h (and Flk1 mRNA at 6 h) after estrogen treatment, which they considered to be responsible for the increased vascular permeability only. However, this observation could also be consistent with endothelial cell proliferation, such as that observed in our 24 h estrogen-treated mice (Heryanto et al., 2002, 2003). In a similar study to our own, Hasting's et al. (2003) found there was no increase in volume fraction occupied by endothelial cells following 24 hours of estrogen treatment. Many of the discrepancies between these studies are likely to be due to methodological differences. Calculating changes in blood vessel density, for instance, is a relatively crude method and does not necessarily take into account changes in oedema and tissue expansion. In addition, unless carefully validated double-immunostaining techniques identifying vessels and proliferating cells are used, it is difficult to identify proliferating endothelial cells present within the stroma. Many vessels do not have an obvious vessel lumen to aid identification.

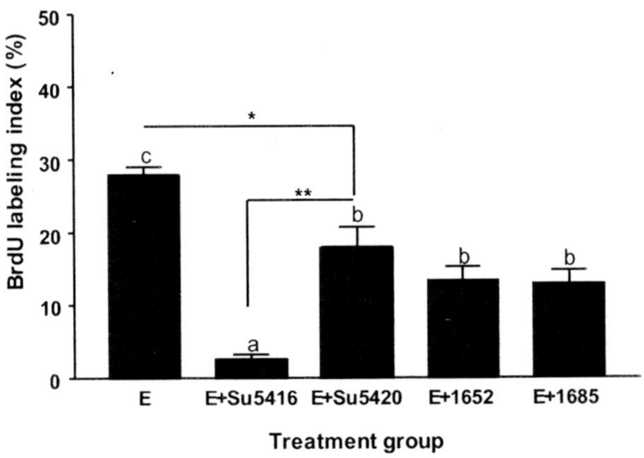

Fig. 3. Bromodeoxyuridine labeling index (%) in the endometrial endothelium of ovariectomised mice treated with a single injection of estradiol (100 ng/mouse) plus one of four angiogenesis inhibitor compounds: SU5416, SU5420, SU11652 or SU11685. Values are means ± SE (n=6 per group). Columns with different superscripts are significantly different ($^{a\text{-}c}p < 0.05$, $^{*}p < 0.01$, $^{**}p < 0.001$). (Reproduced from Heryanto et al., 2003 with permission).

The estrogen-induced endothelial cell proliferation observed in our experiment outlined above (Heryanto and Rogers 2002) was found to be dependent on vascular endothelial growth factor (VEGF). In an ensuing experiment (Heryanto et al., 2003), in conjunction with the steroid hormone treatment regime discussed above, mice were treated with one of four SUGEN pyrrole indolinone angiogenesis inhibitor compounds: SU5416, SU5402, SU11682 and SU11685. SU5416 and SU5402 are inhibitors of VEGF receptor 2 (Flk-1/KDR) and fibroblast growth factor receptor 1 (FGFR-1), respectively. Su11652 exhibits nM potencies for inhibition of platelet-derived growth factor receptor (PDGFR), Flk-1/KDR and FGFR-1, whereas SU11685 exhibits comparable nM potency for inhibition of PDGFR and Flk-1/KDR, but is about tenfold less potent than SU11652 at inhibiting the kinase activity of FGFR-1. The effects of these various inhibitors were tested after the first day of estradiol treatment (E1) and after the last day of steroid treatment (PE). Groups of six mice were injected (100 mg/kg/day s.c.) with one of the four SUGEN angiogenesis inhibitors for three days prior to and at the same time as the first estradiol injection, or at the same time as daily steroid injections on days 4-7 (P1-P3, PE). A further group of mice (n=6) were also treated with a VEGF antiserum raised in rabbits against mouse $VEGF_{164}$ to further investigate the role of VEGF in endothelial cell proliferation at E1 (0.2 ml antiserum injected one day prior to and at the same time as the estradiol injection). Mice were injected with BrdU four hours prior to their dissection 24 h after their last hormone injection. Uterine tissues were processed for immunohistochemistry as described above.

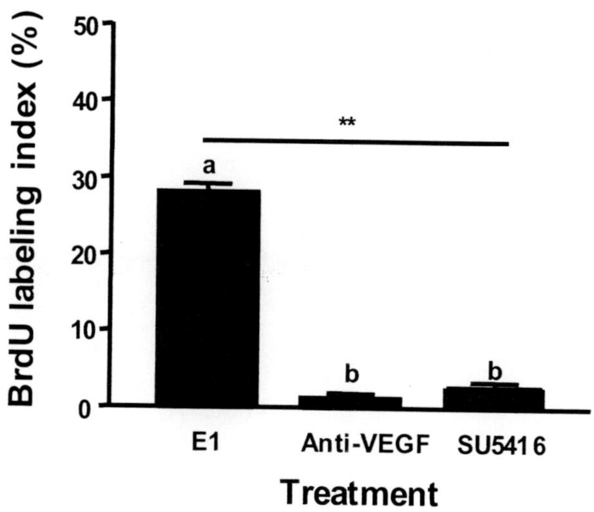

Fig. 4. Bromodeoxyuridine labeling index (%) in the endometrial endothelium of ovariectomised mice treated with a single injection of estradiol (100 ng/mouse) plus the angiogenesis inhibitor SU5416, or an anti-VEGF serum. Values are means ± SE (n=6 per group). Columns with different superscripts are significantly different ($^{a\text{-}c}p < 0.05$, $*p < 0.01$, $**p < 0.001$). (Reproduced from Heryanto et al., 2003 with permission).

The endothelial cell proliferation induced by the single injection of estradiol (E1) was significantly reduced by all four SUGEN angiogenesis inhibitors (Heryanto et al., 2003); the greatest reduction was observed following treatment with SU5416 ($p < 0.001$; Fig. 3). Oestradiol-induced endometrial endothelial cell proliferation was also significantly reduced by the anti-VEGF serum (Fig. 4). All four angiogenesis inhibitor compounds significantly reduced (but only partially) endothelial cell proliferation at the PE stage ($P < 0.01$; Fig. 5). In contrast to the results at E1, there were no differences in the extent of reduction among the four different inhibitors. These results demonstrate that endometrial angiogenesis after acute estrogen treatment is primarily due to VEGF; additional research is required to determine which cell(s) type provide the source of this growth factor.

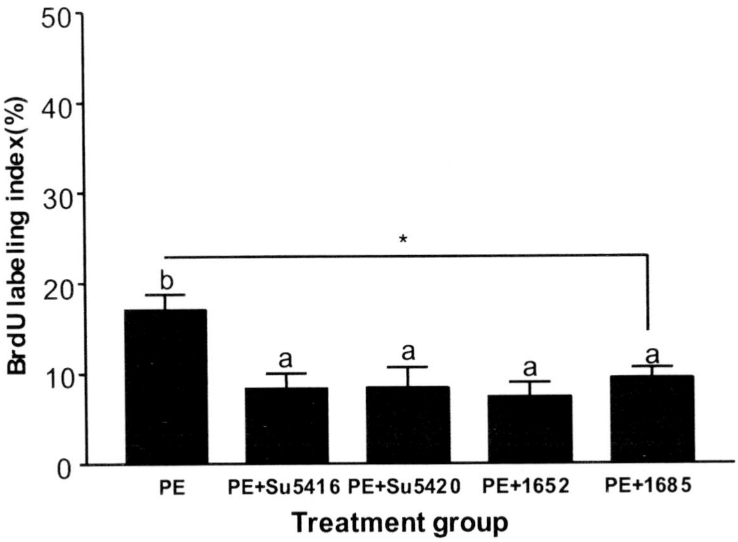

Fig. 5. Bromodeoxyuridine labeling index (%) in the endometrial endothelium of ovariectomised mice treated with a seven day steroid hormone regime (see text for details) plus one of four angiogenesis inhibitor compounds: SU5416, SU5420, SU11652 or SU11685. Values are means ± SE (n=6 per group). Columns with different superscripts are significantly different ($^{a,b}p < 0.05$, $^{*}p < 0.01$). (Reproduced from Heryanto et al, 2003 with permission).

3. Effects of Progesterone on Vessel Proliferation in the Endometrium

There is considerably less data available concerning the role of progesterone in endometrial angiogenesis. Functional nuclear progesterone receptors have been identified on approximately 25-30 % of endothelial cells from a wide variety of tissue types, including endometrium (Vázquez et al., 1999). Progesterone was found to promote cell cycle arrest in the G_0/G_1 phase, thereby inhibiting proliferation of endothelial cells. Despite these *in vitro* results, however, endometrial angiogenesis is observed in response to progesterone. During the secretory phase of the human menstrual cycle, our morphometric studies suggest some form of branching angiogenesis is occurring (Gambino et al., 2002). As with the observations in the proliferative stage of the cycle, however, these observations suggest, but do not prove, a role for progesterone in endometrial angiogenesis. In the rat, considerable endothelial cell proliferation is observed during early pregnancy, correlating with increasing progesterone production by the developing corpora luteum (Goodger and Rogers, 1993). In ovariectomised mice also, there is an increase in vascular density following progesterone treatment (Ma et al., 2001). Unlike the response to estrogen, in which VEGF mRNA was upregulated in the endometrial stroma of rats only transiently shortly after treatment was initiated, progesterone stimulated prominent stromal VEGF mRNA accumulation which was still present after two days of treatment (Ma et al., 2001). There is currently minimal data to suggest how progesterone may elicit endometrial angiogenesis or capillary remodelling. In our experiments (outlined in the section above), treatment of ovariectomised mice with oestradiol and progesterone caused endometrial endothelial cell proliferation; this proliferation was partially blocked using inhibitors against each of VEGF, FGF and PDGF (Fig. 5; Heryanto et al., 2003). Although this model does implicate these growth factors in progesterone-induced endometrial angiogenesis, it does not exclude the effects of concurrent oestrogen administration.

4. Direct Effects of Estrogen and Progesterone on Endothelian Cells

We have demonstrated, in the mouse model, that steroid hormones have indirect effects on endometrial endothelial cell function, and hence on angiogenesis, as they are dependent on VEGF. What is less certain is whether steroid hormones have direct effects on endothelial cells in the endometrium.

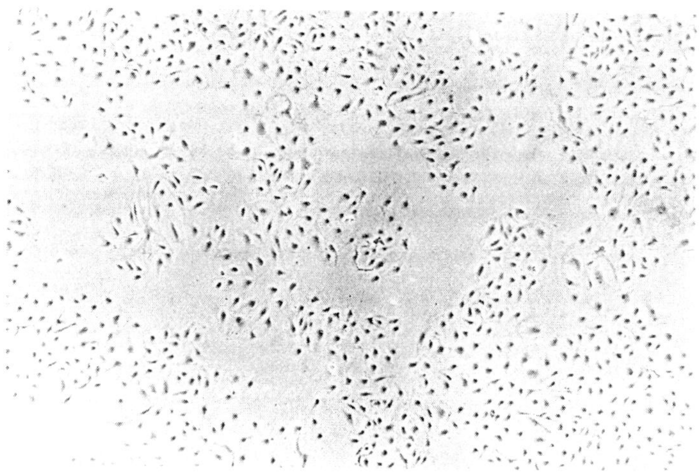

Fig. 6. Myometrial microvascular endothelial cells (MMECs) in vitro.

A key issue in examining direct effects of estrogen and progesterone on endometrial angiogenesis is the presence or absence of estrogen and progesterone receptors in endothelial cells. Both endothelial cells (Venkov *et.al.*, 1996) and vascular smooth muscle cells (Karas *et.al.*, 1994) have been shown to express estrogen receptors. There have now been several studies examining ER expression in the uterine microvasculature (Iruela-Arispe *et.al.*, 1999; Wu *et.al.*, 2000; Critchley *et.al.*, 2001; Lecce *et.al.*, 2001; Gargett *et.al.*, 2002). Expression of estrogen receptor has been shown in all of these studies in both the smooth muscle cell and endothelial cell components of the vessels. While ERβ is invariably present in microvascular endothelial cells in both endometrial and myometrial microvessels, the expression of ERα appears to be variable. In one study of cultured myometrial microvascular endothelial cells, only about 50% of the isolates expressed ERα, but all expressed ERβ (Gargett *et.al.*, 2002). This has functional implications for the individual variablility in estrogen effects on the vasculature, due to the different, and often opposing, transcriptional effects of the two receptor isoforms.

Functional progesterone receptors in microvascular endothelial cells isolated from the endometrium, dermis, and coronary vessels have been reported (Vazquez *et al.*, 1999). In human umbilical vein endothelial cells, functional progesterone receptors have been reported by one group (Otsuki *et al.*, 2001), but were absent in another study (Rodriguez-Manzaneque *et al.*, 2000). Progesterone has been reported to have antiproliferative (Vazquez *et al.*, 1999) and anti-inflammatory (Otsuki *et al.*, 2001) effects on endothelial cells.

The in vitro endothelial cell model used for the experiments described in this chapter has been described in detail elsewhere (Gargett *et.al.*, 2000). Myometrial microvascular endothelial cells (MMECs) were isolated from hysterectomy specimens, purified and cultured (see Figure 6). The purity of the cultures was confirmed by flow cytometry using the endothelial cell marker CD31, with experiments performed only on early passage (< 4) cultures >97% pure.

Expression of ER Isoform mRNA in MMECs in Vitro

One microgram of total RNA isolated from MMEC cultures was reverse transcribed for 90 minutes at 42 C in a total volume of 20µL using AMV-RT (Roche). First strand synthesis was performed with 30pmol of antisense primer (universal for both ERα and ERβ: sense primer 5'-CCGGAATTCTTC/TGACATGCTC/GCTGG-3'; antisense primer 5'-GATGC/TTCCATGCCC/TTTGTTACTC-3'). Two microliters of each RT reaction were amplified in a single stage PCR for 30 cycles with 10pmol of the universal primers for ERα and ERβ, and 2.5 U *Taq* polymerase (Roche) in a total volume of 50µL. Products were visualized on a 1.8% agarose gel, stained with ethidium bromide, and photographed under UV transillumination. For Southern blot analysis, ^{32}P-labeled probes specific for ERα or ERβ were used (ERα probe 5'-GGTTGTGTGCCTCAAATCTATTATTT-3'; ERβ probe 5'-ATATCTCTGTGTCAAGGCCATGA-3'), after PCR products were transferred to Hybond N^+ membranes (Amersham, Little Chaltfont, Buckinghamshire, UK).

Fifteen separate biological isolates of MMECs were assessed for their expression of the two ER isoforms: ERα and ERβ. All of the isolates expressed ERβ mRNA (Figure 7), but only 7/15 (46.7%) of the isolates tested expressed ERα. Therefore, roughly half of the MMEC isolates were ERα +ve ERβ +ve, while the other half were ERα –ve ERβ +ve.

Progesterone Receptor Expression in MMECs

The presence of progesterone receptor mRNA and protein investigated in the following manner:

First, MMEC were grown on 13mm gelatin-coated Thermanox coverslips (Nunc, Roskilde, Denmark) and when confluent were rinsed in PBS and fixed in cold 2% paraformaldehyde for 2 min. Subsequently, the cells were washed with glycine 0.1mol/L in PBS, and incubated for 5 min in 1% TritonX (MERCK, Kilsyth, Australia) /PBS to permeabilise the cells. After a PBS wash, a protein blocking reagent (DAKO Ltd, High Wycombe, UK) was added for 10 min at room temperature. Progesterone receptor was detected using 1mg/L rabbit anti-human polyclonal progesterone receptor IgG (cat#sc-538; Santa Cruz Biotech, Santa Cruz, CA, USA). As a negative control, 1mg/L rabbit IgG (Sigma, Saint Louis, Missouri, USA) was used. Cells were incubated with primary antibody or negative control at 4°C overnight, followed by secondary antibody and horseradish-peroxidase steps at RT for 15 min each, using reagents of the LSAB+ Kit (DAKO, Carpinteria, CA, USA). AEC chromogen (Zymed, San Francisco, CA, USA), was applied for 5 min at RT prior to a distilled water wash and mounting with Faramount (DAKO).

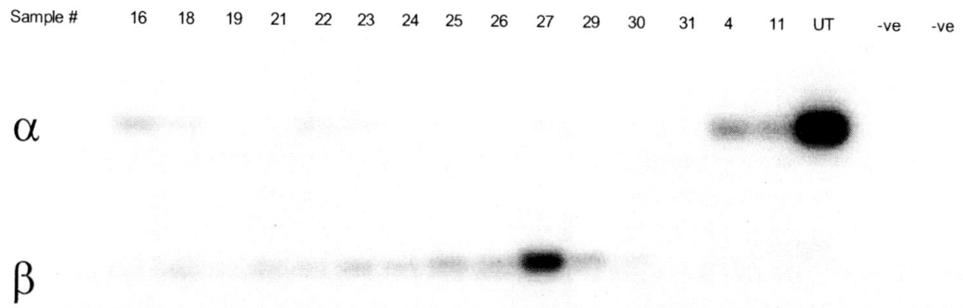

Fig. 7. RT-PCR Southern blot for ERα (top) and ERβ (bottom). A total of 15 separate biological MMEC isolates were assessed for expression of the two ER isoforms: UT=uterus positive control, with predominant expression of ERα; -ve = no RT negative controls.

Second, 1 µg total RNA from MMEC samples was DNase treated using the DNA-free kit (Ambion, Austin, Texas, USA) according to the manufacturers protocol, then reverse transcribed at 42°C for 1 hour in a total volume of 20µl (2.5µl anchor primer (oligodT$_{15}$;Roche), 2µl 10mmol/L dNTPs (Roche), 4µl 5 times RT buffer (Roche), 0.5µl RNasin (Promega), 2µl dithiothreitol (Promega), 0.2µl AMV-reverse transcriptase (Roche), total RNA and sterile H_2O to make up the volume). Amplification of cDNA was performed using 5µl RT product using primers for both a common fragment of progesterone receptor (PR) A/B (sense primer 5'-AGCCCACAATACAGCTTCGAG; antisense primer 5'-TTTCGACCTCCAAGGACCAT) and a PR-B specific fragment (sense primer 5'-CCTGAAGTTTCGGCCATACCT; antisense primer 5'-AGCAGTCCGCTGTCCTTTTCT) in a single stage PCR for 30 cycles. PCR was carried out in a total volume of 50µl (5µl RT product, 4.5µl 10 times PCR buffer (Roche), 0.9µl 10mmol/L dNTPs (Roche), 0.5µl Taq polymerase (Roche) and 0.15µmol/L concentration of primers, made up in H_2O). The cycling conditions were 95°C 3min; 30 cycles (95°C 1 min, 63°C 1min30sec), then 72°C for 7 min, using a GeneAmp Perkin Elmer PCR machine (Applied Biosystems). 10µl PCR product was run on a 2% agarose / TBE gel at 90V. After electrophoresis, PCR products were denatured by two 15 min washes in 0.5mol/L NaOH / 1.5mol/L NaCl, rinsed in H_2O, neutralized in 0.5mol/L Tris / 3mol/L NaCl, and transferred overnight at RT onto Hybond-N+ nylon membranes (Amersham) in 20 times SSC. Transferred PCR products were fixed onto the membrane by UV-crosslinking for 3 min. DIG wash and block kit and DIG easy hyb (Roche) were used according to the manufacturer's protocol. Oligonucleotide probes were labeled with DIG using the DIG Oligonucleotide 3'-End Labeling Kit (Roche) (PR-A/B probe 5'-AAGTAGTTGTGCTGCCCTTCCATTGCCCTC; PR-B probe 5'-TTGTAGCTTCAGCTCTGGAATATGCGCCCTCCACG) according to the manufacturer's protocol. Expected sizes of PCR products were 250bp (PR-A/B) and 198bp (PR-B), and amplicons were verified by sequencing using the dideoxy chain termination method.

Weak, but consistently positive nuclear staining for progesterone receptor protein was detected in MMECs by immunohistochemistry (Figure 8a). The cells used for the immunohistochemistry were of the same passage as those used for all subsequent experiments (ie. passages 2-4). T47D breast cancer cell line cells were used as a positive control and showed considerably stronger staining than the MMECs (data not shown). RT-PCR for PR-A/B and PR-B was performed on T47D cells, both to optimize the reaction, and to confirm the presence of progesterone receptors in the positive control cells. DNase treatment of the RNA was found to be necessary to prevent genomic amplification. Both PR-A/B and PR-B mRNA were confirmed in the T47D cells (Figure 8b). Next, progesterone receptor mRNA was detected both for a PR-A/B common fragment and for a PR-B-specific fragment in four different isolates of myometrial microvascular endothelial cells by RT-PCR (Figure 8b), again, at passage 2-4. The amplicons were verified by sequencing to correspond with PR-A/B and PR-B respectively. Although formal quantification was not carried out, the expression of PR A and B appeared to be less than in T47D cells, but definitely present (see no RT controls in Figure 8b).

Direct Effects of Estrogen on Endothelial Cells in Vitro

Confluent MMECs were incubated for 48 hours in hormone-free medium (PRF-M199 with 5% ch-FCS, 0.005mg/L VEGF (R&D, Minneapolis, MN, USA), 100mg/L heparin(Gibco-BRL)) in order to achieve quiescence. Following this, the medium was replaced with fresh medium containing either 10nmol/L 17β-estradiol or 100% ethanol vehicle control (both 1:1000 dilution into media). After 8 hours of stimulation with 17β-estradiol or control, cells were harvested for total RNA extraction.

The total RNA samples were used to prepare fluorescent-labelled cDNA for probing with glass microarray slides spotted with 10500 human cDNA sequences (prepared in-house at the PeterMacCallum Cancer Institute Microarray Facility, Melbourne, Australia). 60-90μg of experiment total RNA (from estrogen-stimulated MMEC) was used for each microarray, with an equal amount of reference total RNA (vehicle-stimulated MMEC) used as the control. A direct-labelling procedure was used for creating fluorescent-labelled cDNA. The labeling, hybridization, and scanning of the slides has been described previously (Weston *et.al.*, 2002).

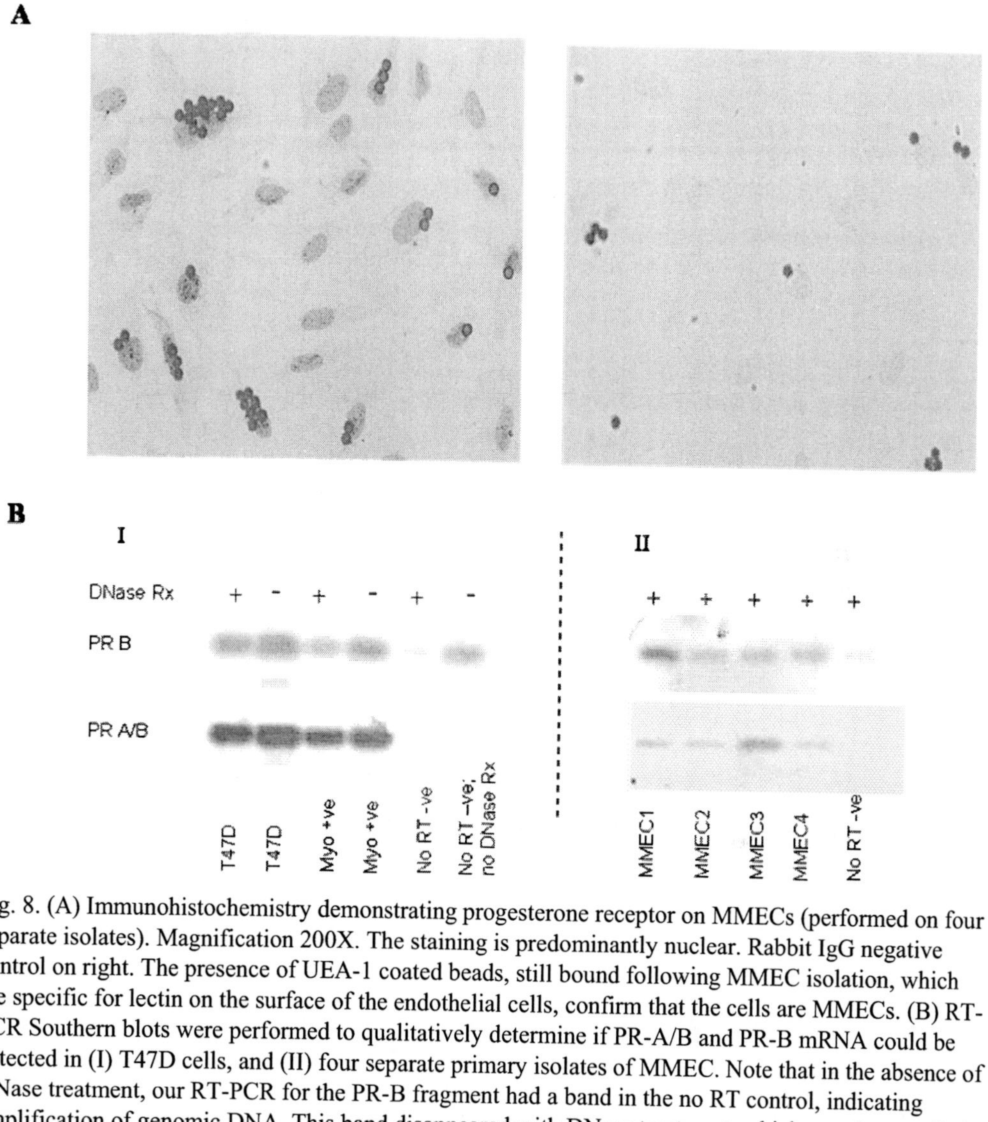

Fig. 8. (A) Immunohistochemistry demonstrating progesterone receptor on MMECs (performed on four separate isolates). Magnification 200X. The staining is predominantly nuclear. Rabbit IgG negative control on right. The presence of UEA-1 coated beads, still bound following MMEC isolation, which are specific for lectin on the surface of the endothelial cells, confirm that the cells are MMECs. (B) RT-PCR Southern blots were performed to qualitatively determine if PR-A/B and PR-B mRNA could be detected in (I) T47D cells, and (II) four separate primary isolates of MMEC. Note that in the absence of DNase treatment, our RT-PCR for the PR-B fragment had a band in the no RT control, indicating amplification of genomic DNA. This band disappeared with DNase treatment, which was then applied to the MMEC RNA samples. Both PR-A/B and PR-B were present in all four MMEC isolates. (Myo +ve = whole myometrium positive control; MMEC = myometrial microvascular endothelial cells).

The raw expression data was analysed using Genespring (Silicon Genetics, USA). The relative gene expression was obtained as a ratio by dividing the experimental value (estrogen-stimulated MMECs) by the control value (vehicle-stimulated MMECs). Genespring normalized each gene to itself by dividing all of the values for a gene by the median of the gene's expression values over all the samples. Normalized values less than zero were set to zero, and data was rejected if the background-subtracted control value was below 10.0. All data underwent, in addition, intensity-dependent normalization by use of a LOWESS fit. Data could then be analysed on the basis of both expression ratio and p value (by t-testing). Genes were to be considered if they were up or down regulated at least 1.5-fold in at least half of the isolates.

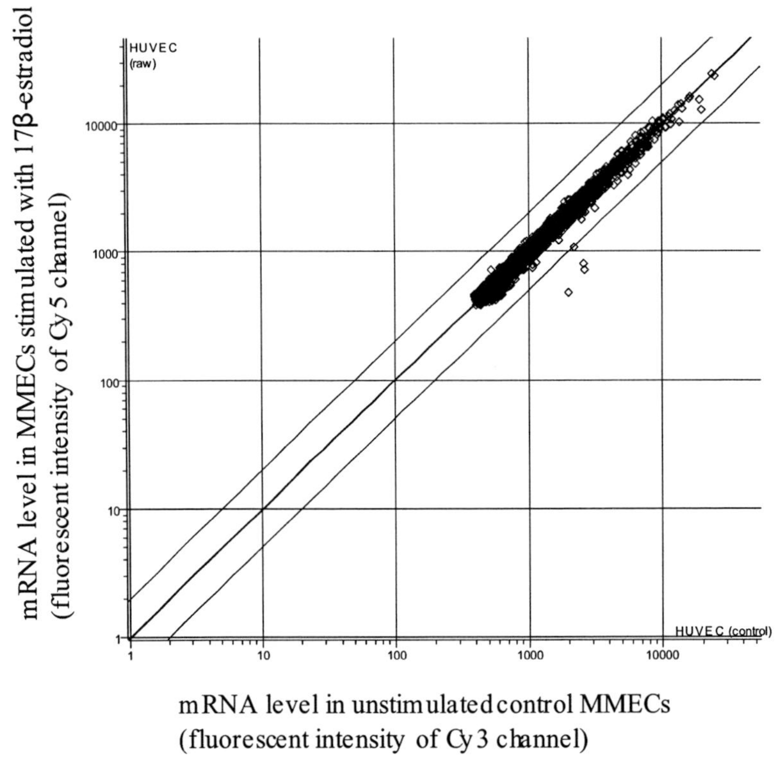

Fig. 9. A scatterplot representing gene expression ratios in one of nine experiments on different biological replicates. Gene expression in MMECs after 8 hours stimulation with 10nmol/L 17β-estradiol (Y-axis) or vehicle control (X-axis). Genes above and below the upper and lower lines on the graph would represent genes up or down-regulated, respectively, by at least two-fold. No genes were consistently up or down-regulated by estrogen (the few genes seen below the lower line were not downregulated in any of the other 8 experiments).

Of the nine biological isolates tested under identical conditions, four were positive for ERα, and five were negative for ERα. All of the isolates expressed ERβ. However, none of the cultures showed any consistent gene expression changes following stimulation with estrogen (see Figure 9). Given that some isolates expressed ERα, and some did not, the isolates were analysed separately depending upon their ERα expression. In neither the ERα +ve nor the ERα –ve cultures were there any gene expression changes of 1.5-fold or more up or down-regulation.

Direct Effects of Progesterone on Endothelial Cells in Vitro

Having demonstrated PR A and B in MMEC, we used a 10,500 gene cDNA glass slide microarray to examine gene expression in MMECs in response to 24hr stimulation with 100nmol/L progesterone. To verify our technique would identify genes with PR regulated expression, a positive control microarray was performed with the same conditions on T47D cells. Following 24 hours progesterone stimulation, the T47D cells showed 83 genes upregulated two-fold or more, and 25 genes down-regulated two-fold (Figure 10). No tests for statistical significance could be applied, as only one array was performed. In the three microarrays performed on progesterone stimulation of MMECs, none of the genes showed upregulation of more than 1.5-fold over control in at least 2 experiments, nor a downregulation of more than 0.7-fold in at least 2 experiments. None of the genes showed a statistically significant difference in expression after progesterone stimulation, as measured by t-tests. Thus, direct stimulation with progesterone had no detectable effect on gene expression in MMECs in any of the 10,500 genes studied (Figure 10). The concentration of progesterone in the media, and the absence of progesterone from the unstimulated control media, was verified by standard radio-immunoassay.

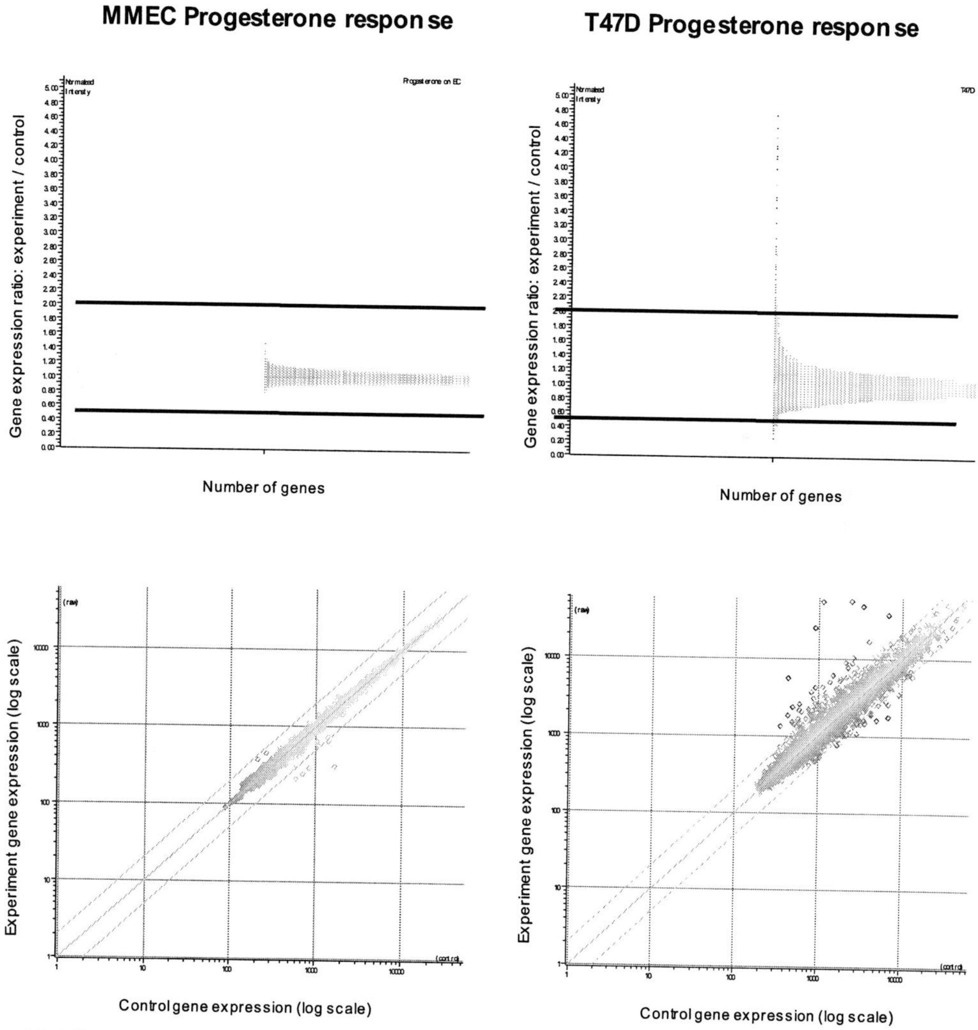

Fig. 10. Histograms (top) of the normalized ratio of gene expression in microarray experiments relative to controls (10,500 genes). The Y-axis indicates the ratio of gene expression relative to the control for each of the genes on the array, while the X-axis indicates the number of genes with the indicated ratio of gene expression. Changes are seen in gene expression relative to unstimulated controls in T47D (right) but not in MMEC (left – average of three repeats). Horizontal lines run at the level of two-fold up and down-regulation of gene expression. Genes above and below these lines are seen in T47D (top

right) but not in MMEC (top left). Scatterplots (bottom) of intensity of hybridized probe detected for each gene in the control channel (X axis) versus the progesterone treated channel (Y axis). The upper and lower diagonal lines on the scatterplots correspond to two-fold up and down-regulation respectively in gene expression in progesterone treated experiments relative to untreated controls.

Having shown no detectable alteration in gene expression by progesterone, we examined the effect of progesterone on MMEC proliferation rate. The CellTitre 96 MTS tetrazolium-based bioassay (Promega, Madison, WT, USA), was used as previously described (Gargett *et al.*, 2000) to measure cell number after incubation of MMECs with $VEGF_{165}$ (R&D Systems, Minneapolis, MN, USA) and bFGF (Gibco BRL, Gaithersburg, MD, USA) in the presence of a variety of different concentrations of progesterone (0.1nmol/L-1000nmol/L) (cat#P-0130; Sigma, St Louis, MO, USA). MMEC were seeded in hormone-free quiescent media with phenol red-free (PRF) M199 (Gibco-BRL) containing 5% charcoal-stripped (ch) FCS, and allowed to quiesce for 24 hrs. The medium was then replaced with a growth medium containing 5% ch-human serum (HS; pooled and heat inactivated from male staff volunteers and the Red Cross Blood Service), 15% ch-FCS, 0.01mg/L $VEGF_{165}$, 0.005mg/L bFGF, and 100mg/L heparin (Gibco-BRL). To examine the effects of progesterone on MMEC growth, progesterone (1:1000) at 0.1, 1, 10, 100, 1000nmol/L, or vehicle control (100% ethanol, final concentration 0.1%) was added to the growth medium starting from day 0. Cells were incubated at 37°C in 5% CO_2/air for 6 days, with culture medium changes every 2 days.

At a range of 0.1-1000 nmol/L, progesterone had no significant effect on MMEC proliferation compared with vehicle control in growth media with VEGF (0.01mg/L) and bFGF (0.005mg/L) added (Fig 11).

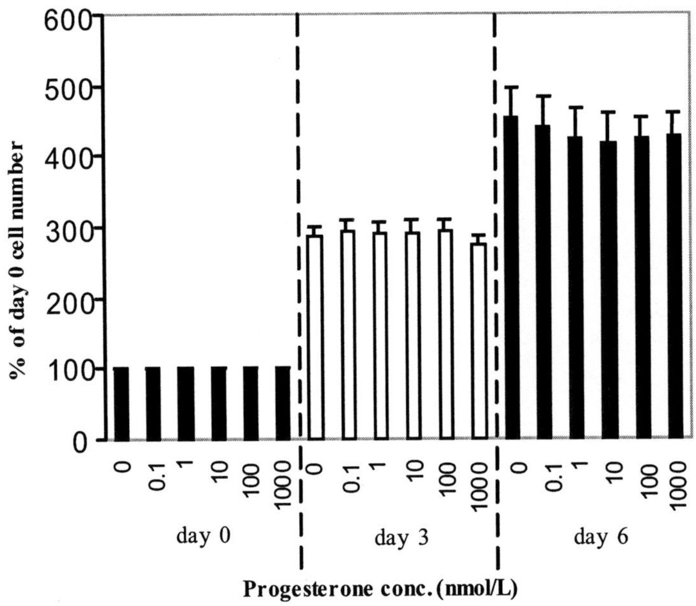

Fig. 11. Effect of progesterone on growth factor-induced MMEC proliferation using the MTS bioassay. MMEC were seeded into wells at 2000/cm2 in duplicates and stimulated with 0.01 mg/L VEGF and 0.005 mg/L bFGF in the presence or absence (vehicle control) of progesterone (0.1-1000 nmol/L). There was no difference in MMEC proliferation between vehicle control-treated cells and progesterone-treated cells at any of the concentrations or time points examined. Results are mean +/- SEM of 6 experiments on 3 different MMEC isolates.

Discussion of Experiments of Direct Effects of Estrogen and Progesterone on MMECs

a. Estrogen

No gene transcription was evident in MMECs by gene expression microarray after 8 hours of a physiological dose of estrogen. This was regardless of the presence or absence of ERα. . In the only study of cultured myometrial microvascular endothelial cells to accurately quantitate ERα expression in vessels from different individuals, only about 50% of the isolates expressed ERα (Gargett *et.al.*, 2002). However, all of the isolates expressed ERβ. The work reported in this chapter confirms the findings by Gargett *et.al.* (2002), with 46.7% of the isolates tested here being ERα +ve.

Various transcriptional events which have been reported in endothelial cells following an estrogen stimulus. Genes reported to be transcriptionally activated by an estrogen stimulus in endothelial cells include endothelial nitric oxide synthase (eNOS) (MacRitchie *et.al.*, 1997), cyclooxygenase-1 (COX-1) (Jun *et.al.*, 1998), plasminogen activator inhibitor (PAI-1) (Villablanca *et.al.*, 2002), and VEGFR-2 (Suzuma *et.al.*, 1999). Genes with suppressed transcription following an estrogen stimulus include thrombomodulin (Richardson *et.al.*, 2000), monocyte chemotactic protein-1 (MCP-1) (Seli *et.al.*, 2002), and endothelin-1 (ET-1) (Bilsel *et.al.*, 2000). There are several possibilities to consider when interpreting the negative result of this study.

Although ER mRNA expression was demonstrated by RT-PCR in this study, the technique used was not quantitative. Although ER was present in the cultures, it is not possible to tell if the levels of ER were sufficient to result in transcriptional effects following ligand-activation. Sex steroid hormone receptors have been shown to down-regulate rapidly in *in vitro* culture conditions, and in some studies (Sampath *et.al.*, 2001), transfection of the cells with ER was required to demonstrate an estrogen response. However, in the only study published to date on myometrial MECs (under similar growth conditions), estrogen was shown to upregulate the VEGFR-2 protein evident at the cell surface of the MMECs by flow cytometry (Gargett *et.al.*, 2002).

In this study, only an 8 hr time-point after estrogen stimulation was examined. Many of the transcriptional events which have been reported in endothelial cells following an estrogen stimulus have required 24-48 hrs. It is possible that the duration of estrogen stimulus in this study was insufficient to elicit a response.

There is evidence to suggest that endothelial cells display considerable heterogeneity, both between tissue beds of different organs and between normal and pathological tissue (Garlanda *et al.*, 1997). Thus, it is possible that direct estrogen effects on endothelial cells from the myometrium are not reflected in previously reported effects in endothelial cells from other tissues. Many studies utilize endothelial cells from large veins or arteries, rather than from the microvasculature as in this study.

Microarrays have been reported to be less sensitive than Northern blots in detecting changes in mRNA, with 9% of genes detected by Northern missed by gene expression microarray in one study (Taniguchi *et.al.*, 2001). It is possible that the gene expression microarrays were not sensitive enough to pick up the gene expression changes, or that the genes were not present on the array. Studies of mRNA changes do not rule out changes in protein levels in the absence of alteration of transcription, opening up the possibility of non-genomic effects of estrogen on MMECs (Gerdes *et.al.*, 2000).

The data here is the first to be reported of gene expression profiling of MMECs following an estrogen stimulus using a cDNA microarray. This work suggests that estrogen has no direct transcriptional effects on these cells. Further work should focus on longer time-points and higher doses of estrogen, as well as quantification of estrogen receptors in culture over time, to confirm this result, and ensure it is not due to down-regulation of estrogen receptor in culture.

b. Progesterone

The work in this chapter is the first to demonstrate the presence of progesterone receptors in isolated human myometrial microvascular endothelial cells, and to examine broad-scale transcriptional effects of progesterone stimulation on these cells. However, progesterone did not show anti-proliferative effects on isolated MMEC, and no transcriptional effects could be demonstrated by gene microarray following direct progesterone stimulation.

The presence of progesterone receptors within endothelial cells has previously been reported for human umbilical vein endothelial cells (HUVECs) (Otsuki *et al.*, 2001) and microvascular endothelial cells from human dermis and endometrium (Rodriguez-Manzaneque *et al.*, 2000). The work presented in this chapter confirms and extends these findings by showing progesterone receptor mRNA and protein within human myometrial MECs for the first time.

The limited literature on progesterone effects on endothelial cells has primarily been confined to functional effects, and has focused almost exclusively on changes in protein levels. The one exception to this is a study showing reduction of VCAM-1 mRNA by progesterone following stimulation with TNFα (Otsuki *et al.*, 2001). This study was performed on HUVEC's, not microvascular EC, which may explain the difference in results to our study (VCAM-1 was not altered on our arrays). Quantitative changes in protein levels reported to date following progesterone stimulation of endothelial cells are increased matrix-metalloprotease 9 and changed matrix protein components (Rodriguez-Manzaneque *et al.*, 2000).

Many of the same possibilities exist as for estrogen to explain the lack of transcriptional effects of progesterone despite demonstration of the receptor in our cultures: inadequate sensitivity of the microarrays, wrong time-point, lack of appropriate genes on the array, and effects being non-genomic rather than transcriptional. Although clearly present, the levels of progesterone receptor expression are low in MMECs when compared with T47D cells. It is also possible that in vitro culture in hormone-free media may result in the down-regulation of the receptor when compared to the in vivo situation. Estrogen has been shown to upregulate the expression of progesterone receptor in endometrial stromal cells (Kurita *et al.*, 2001). Both estrogen receptor subtypes (alpha and beta) have been demonstrated in endothelial cells (Andersson *et al.*, 2001; Gargett *et al.*, 2002), raising the possibility that estrogen stimulation is required to maintain progesterone receptor expression in culture. It is also possible that an essential progesterone-receptor co-factor is lost during in-vitro culture.

From the work presented here in this chapter, we must conclude that, although mRNA and protein for the progesterone receptor is present in MMECs, they are not transcriptionally active on direct hormonal stimulation.

5. Circulating Neutrophils and Endometrial Endothelial Cell Proliferation

Various investigators have endeavored to correlate levels of VEGF mRNA and protein with phases of the human menstrual cycle (Torry and Torry, 1997; Rogers and Gargett, 1999). Although there have been conflicting results, it appears the majority of endometrial VEGF is glandular in origin (Shifren *et al.*, 1996; Zhang *et al.*, 1998; Gargett *et al.*, 1999). More importantly, it is hypothesised that the glandular VEGF is secreted apically into the uterine lumen and is unlikely to have a role in endometrial angiogenesis (Hornung *et al.*, 1998). In a study in our laboratory, although epithelial, stromal or total VEGF expression did not correlate with endometrial endothelial cell proliferation (Gargett *et al.*, 1999), foci of intense VEGF immunostaining were observed within the human endometrium; many of these foci were within blood vessels.

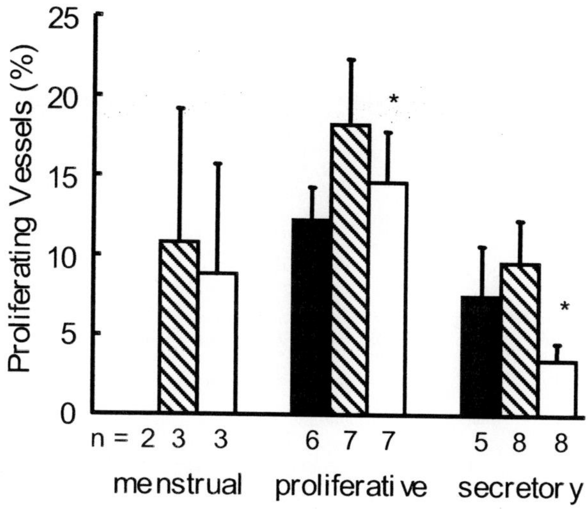

Fig. 12. Proliferating vessels in the subepithelial capillary plexus (black columns), functionalis (hatched columns) and basalis (white bars) layers of the human endometrium during three stages of the menstrual cycle. The number of samples examined is indicated under each bar. *Significantly more proliferative vessels in proliferative than secretory basalis ($p = 0.004$, Mann-Whitney U-Wilcoxon Rank Sum W). (Reproduced from Gargett et al., 2001 with permission).

An experiment was undertaken to identify these VEGF-positive foci and determine how they related to endometrial endothelial cell proliferation in the three layers of human endometrium (subepithelial capillary plexus, functionalis and basalis; Gargett *et al.*, 2001). Full-thickness human endometrial samples were obtained from 18 normal ovulating women following informed consent. The tissue was formalin-fixed and processed for routine paraffin embedding. Sections stained with haematoxylin and eosin were used for dating samples into three stages of the menstrual cycle (menstrual, proliferative or secretory). Serial sections (3 or 5 μm) were immunostained for VEGF (polyclonal primary antibody = rabbit anti-human VEGF; Santa Cruz Biotechnology Inc, Santa Cruz, CA, USA) and one of several markers for various leucocytes (monocytes and macrophages: monoclonal mouse anti-human CD68 IgG1 [7 μg/ml, clone KP1, Dako Ltd, High Wycombe, UK], neutrophils: monoclonal mouse anti-human neutrophil elastase IgG1 [1 μg/ml, clone NP57, Dako Ltd, High Wycombe, UK], T-lymphocytes: rabbit polyclonal anti-human CD3 IgG [3.3 μg/ml, Dako Ltd, High Wycombe, UK], NK cells and large granulated lymphocytes: monoclonal mouse anti-human N-CAM IgG1 [clone 123C3; Zymed, San Francisco, CA, USA], basophils and mast cells: monoclonal mouse anti-human tryptase IgG1 [clone AA1, Dako Ltd, High Wycombe, UK], circulating monocytes: monoclonal mouse anti-human CD14 [RPA-M1, Zymed, San Francisco, CA, USA]). Double immunostaining protocols combining antibodies against proliferating cell nuclear antigen (PCNA, clone PC10, Novacastra, Newcastle, UK) and CD34 (labels endothelial cells, clone QBEND/10, Serotc, oxford, UK), and antibodies against VEGF and CD34 were used to determine the percentage of proliferating vessels and the percentage of VEGF expressing vessels respectively.

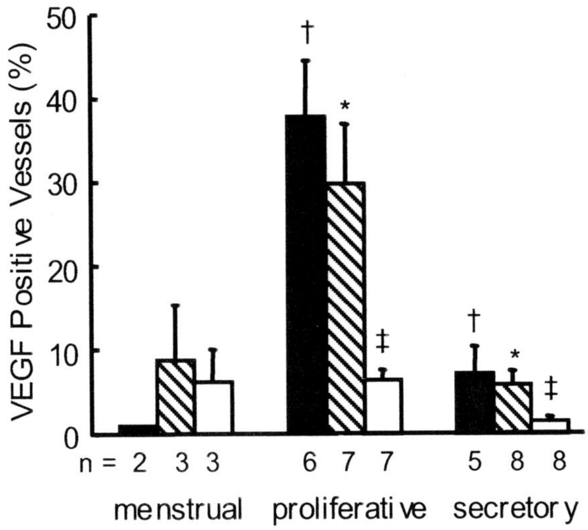

Fig. 13. Microvessels containing focal VEGF in the subepithelial capillary plexus (black columns), functionalis (hatched columns) and basalis (white bars) layers of the human endometrium during three stages of the menstrual cycle. The number of samples examined is indicated under each bar. For each layer, the number of VEGF positive vessels was significantly differently between cycle stages ($p < 0.01$ for the subepithelial capillary plexus, $p < 0.01$ for the functionalis and $p < 0.02$ for the basalis). Significantly more VEGF positive vessels were found in the proliferative than secretory phase in the subepithelial capillary plexus (†$p < 0.01$), the functionalis (*$p < 0.002$) and basalis (‡$p < 0.01$) by Mann-Whitney U-Wilcoxon Rank Sum W. (Reproduced from Gargett et al., 2001 with permission).

Proliferating vessels were observed in samples from all three stages of the menstrual cycle. The percentage of proliferating vessels was higher in proliferative compared to secretory endometrium, although this only reached significance in the basalis ($p = 0.004$, Fig. 12, Gargett et al., 2001). The focal VEGF was found to correlate both temporally and spatially with endometrial endothelial cell proliferation. A significantly greater percentage of focal VEGF-expressing microvessels were found during the proliferative phase in comparison to the secretory phase ($p < 0.05$), with the greatest numbers of VEGF-immunopositive vessels within the subepithelial capillary plexus (Fig. 13). A large proportion of proliferating vessels contained VEGF immunostained cells closely associated with vessel walls, particularly in the subepithelial capillary plexus during the proliferative stage (Fig. 14). There was also a significant correlation between focal VEGF-expressing microvessels and proliferating vessels in the subepithelial capillary plexus ($R = 0.70$, $p < 0.008$), functionalis ($R = 0.70$, $p < 0.001$) and basalis ($R = 0.76$, $p < 0.001$; Fig. 15). The focal VEGF associated with microvessels was found to best correspond with marginating and adherent neutrophils; the distribution of other leucocytes did not correlate with the distribution of VEGF-positive foci (Fig. 16). Based on these results, it was hypothesized that neutrophils provide a source of VEGF for the endometrial vessels undergoing proliferation.

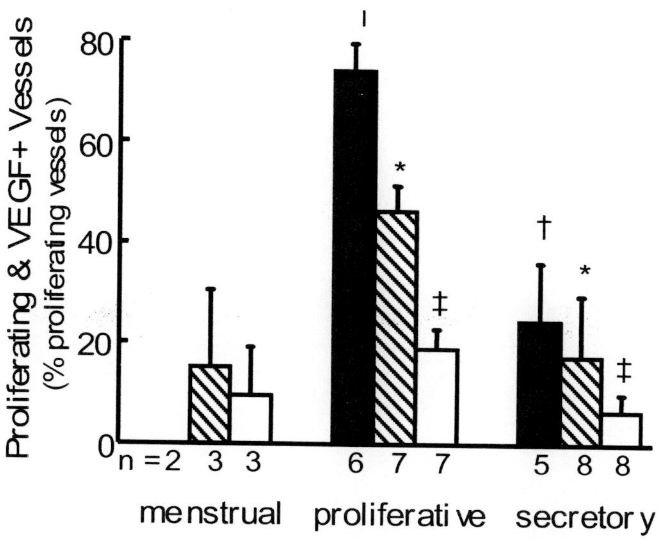

Fig. 14. Microvessels containing both focal VEGF and proliferating endothelial cells in the subepithelial capillary plexus (black columns), functionalis (hatched columns) and basalis (white bars) layers of the human endometrium during three stages of the menstrual cycle. The number of samples examined is indicated under each bar. The percentage of proliferating vessels containing focal VEGF was significantly greater in the proliferative than the secretory phase of the menstrual cycle for each of the three layers of human endometrium (†$p < 0.02$ for the subepithelial capillary plexus, *$p < 0.05$ for the functionalis and ‡$p < 0.02$ for the basalis) by Mann-Whitney U-Wilcoxon Rank Sum W. (Reproduced from Gargett et al., 2001 with permission).

Neutrophils are known to constitutively express VEGF, as well as other pro- and anti-angiogenic factors, within their specific (secondary) granules (Gaudry *et al.*, 1997; Cassatella, 1999). Current data also suggest that VEGF secreted by neutrophils may be essential for control of angiogenesis and vascular permeability during inflammatory processes (Cassatella, 1999) and in other models of angiogenesis (eg. angiogenesis induced in the normally avascular cornea, Taichman *et al.*, 1997; Edelman *et al.*, 1999). No studies, however, have directly addressed whether neutrophils play a role in endometrial angiogenesis. We have recently begun to address the role that neutrophils play in estrogen-induced endometrial angiogenesis using estrogen-treated ovariectomised mice (Heryanto et al., in press). Results to date suggest a role for neutrophils and further investigation is in progress.

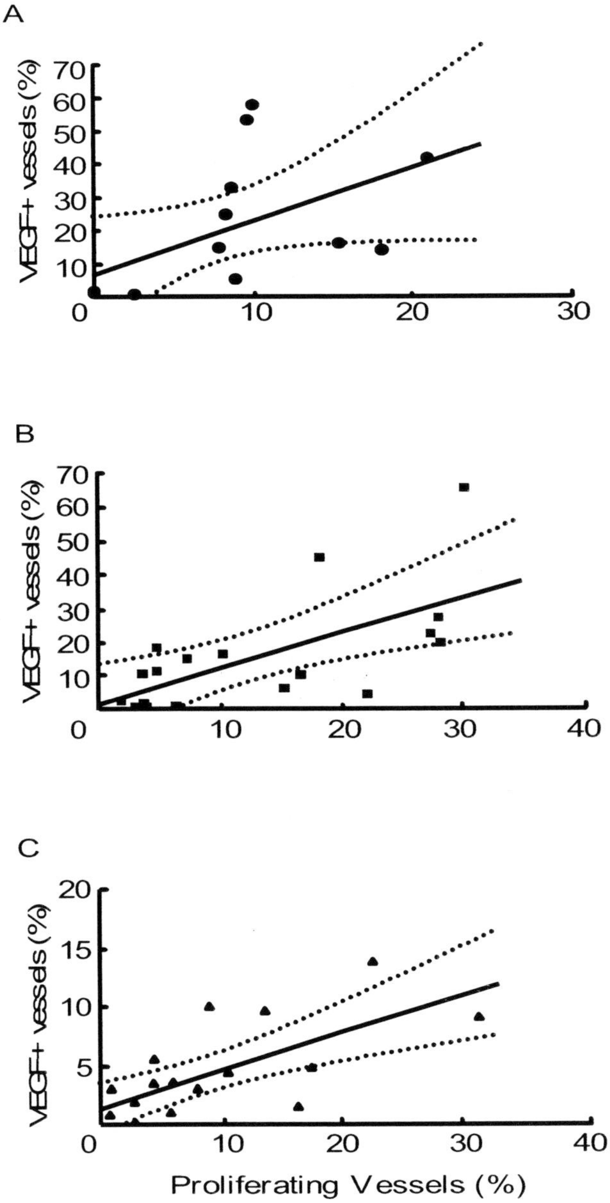

Fig. 15. Significant correlation between focal microvessel VEGF and proliferating vessels in the (A) subepithelial capillary plexus ($R = 0.70$, $p = 0.008$), (B) functionalis ($R = 0.70$, $p = 0.001$) and (C) basalis (R _ 0.76, $p < 0.001$) layers of human endometrium when combined for all stages of the menstrual cycle. Regression analysis showing line of best fit with 95 % confidence intervals are shown. (Reproduced from Gargett et al., 2001 with permission).

6. Progesterone Effects on Endothelial Cell-Inflammatory Cell Interactions

The work described above demonstrates an association between circulating neutrophil-sources of the angiogenic promoter VEGF, and endometrial endothelial cell proliferation. We decided to explore further possible modulation of this interaction by progesterone, again using our in vitro model of the endometrial vasculature.

Effects of Progesterone on MMECs with an Inflammatory Stimulus

We investigated the ability of progesterone to modulate the inflammation-induced expression of adhesion molecules on the surface of the endothelial cells. TNFα (0.1-25mg/L) increased E-selectin protein expression in a dose dependent manner in MMECs detected by flow cytometry (data not shown). Progesterone incubation for 48 hours prior to, and during, a 4 hour TNFα 400ng/L stimulus decreased the E-selectin protein expression relative to vehicle control. There was up to a 40% reduction in E-selectin protein which was statistically significant, and maximal at a concentration of 1nmol/L progesterone (Figure 17). Incubation with estrogen as well as progesterone (100nmol/L) negated this effect, and incubation with estrogen alone (0.1-100nmol/L) had no effect on TNFα-induced E-selectin protein expression (Figure 17).

Microarray experiments were then performed to examine the effect of progesterone on gene expression in response to TNFα 400ng/L, due to the effect demonstrated on E-selectin protein expression. The same conditions as for the flow experiment were repeated on two separate primary isolates of MMECs to generate RNA for the microarray experiments. Comparing gene expression in response to TNFα plus vehicle, with gene expression in response to TNFα plus progesterone (100nmol/L), there were no genes showing either greater than 1.5-fold or less than 0.6-fold in both of the microarrays (Figure 18). E-selectin gene expression as measured in the microarrays was 1.05 after normalization without a statistically significant difference by t-test ($p=0.71$) from control gene expression.

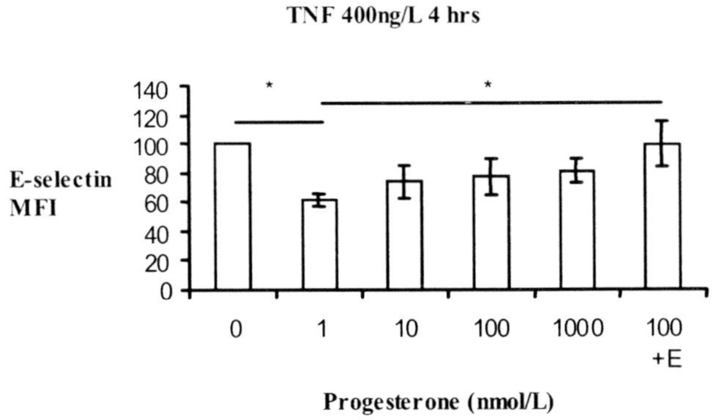

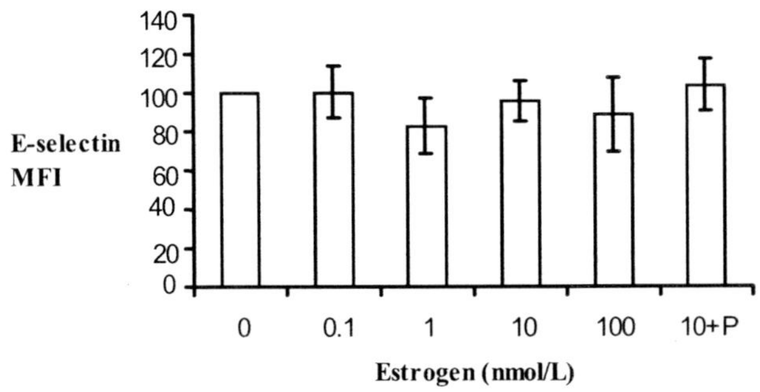

Fig. 17. Effect of TNFα on E-selectin expression in the presence of various concentrations of progesterone (top) and estrogen (bottom) measured by flow-cytometry. Means +/- SEM of n=6 experiments are shown (*$p<0.05$). MFI=mean fluorescent intensity, expressed as a percentage of the E-selectin expression in the absence of hormone treatment. There is a significant reduction in E-selectin expression in response to TNFα when incubated with 1nmol/L progesterone. There were non-statistically significant reductions with 10nmol/L, 100nmol/L, and 1000nmol/L progesterone added to TNFα. The effect by progesterone on TNF-regulated E-selectin expression was negated by incubation with 10nmol/L estrogen added to 100nmol/L progesterone.

Confirmation of Lack of Change in E-Selectin Gene Expression by Northern Blot

Northern blots were performed on RNA from the experiments above to confirm that progesterone did not alter mRNA abundance for E-selectin despite the alteration in protein detected (Figure 19). TNFα at 400pg/ml for 4 hrs resulted in an upregulation of E-selectin expression on MMEC which was less than the positive control (24 hours IL1β 10ng/ml; Montgomery *et al.*, 1991). However, the addition of progesterone did not alter the TNFα induced E selectin mRNA expression, as shown by the lack of significant difference between vehicle and progesterone co-stimulated cultures.

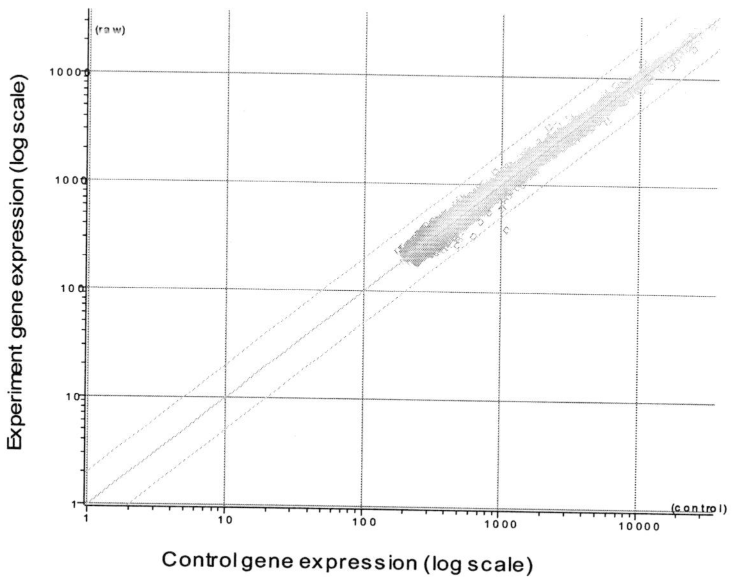

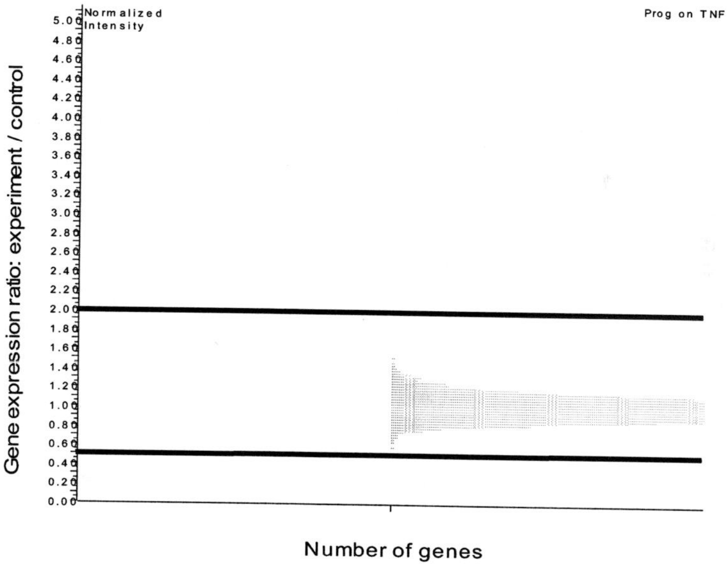

Fig. 18. A scatterplot (top) and histogram (bottom) representing gene expression ratios in one of two repeats of a microarray experiment. In the scatterplot (top) gene expression in MMECs after 4hrs with 400ng/L TNFα and progesterone 100nmol/L on the X axis is compared with gene expression in the same isolate after 4hrs with 400ng/L TNFα and vehicle on the Y axis. The upper and lower lines on the graph represent a two-fold difference in gene expression in TNFα-stimulated MMECs with the addition of progesterone. No gene expression changes could be seen, indicating that progesterone does not alter TNFα-mediated gene transcriprion. The histogram shows the normalized ratio of gene expression in MMEC treated with TNFα plus vehicle over the gene expression in MMEC treated with TNFα plus progesterone. Horizontal lines pass through the level at which genes vary by two-fold in either direction with the addition of progesterone. Again, no genes fall outside these lines, illustrating that no gene expression changes were detected in the inflammatory cytokine-stimulated cells with the addition of progesterone.

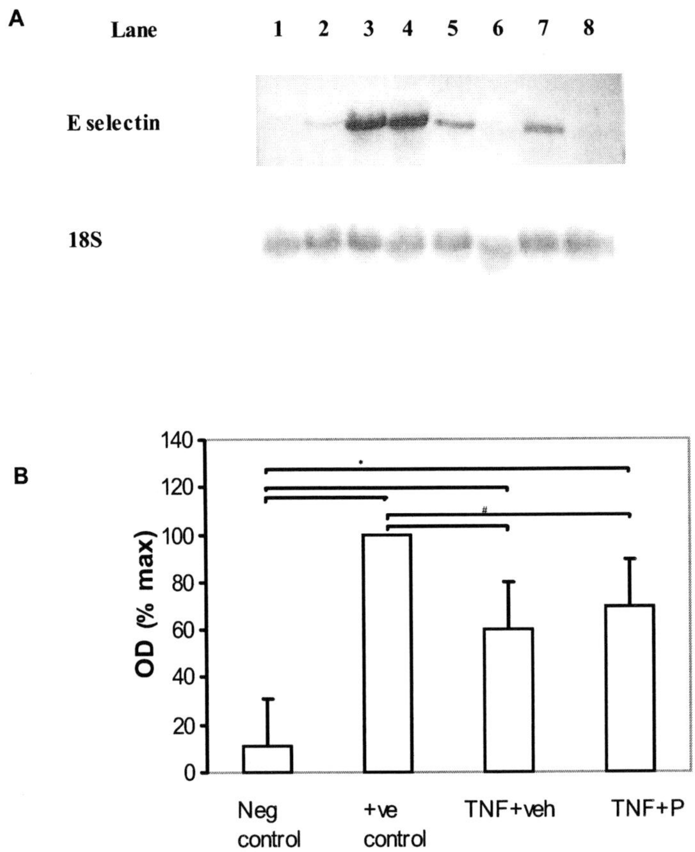

Fig. 19. A Northern blot analysis examining the effect of TNFα on E selectin mRNA expression in the presence and absence of progesterone 100nmol/L. Representative of three northern blots, on four biological replicates. In the northern blot shown, lanes 1-2 = negative control (no IL or TNFα); lanes 3-4 = positive control (10mg/L IL-1β for 24 hrs); lane 5 = TNFα 400ng/L plus vehicle for 4hrs; lane 7 = TNFα 400ng/L plus 100nmol/L progesterone for 4hrs. Lanes 6 and 8 show one MMEC isolate which did not respond to TNFα 400ng/L with an upregulation of E-selectin mRNA. Only one of the four MMEC isolates failed to respond to TNFα.**B** Summary of densitometry analysis of all Northern blots performed examining E-selectin expression. There were no significant differences between TNFα plus vehicle and TNFα plus progesterone following one way ANOVA and Tukey's multiple comparison test. (*, $P<0.001$; #, $P<0.05$).

Discussion

The addition of progesterone to TNFα-treated MMEC significantly altered the expression of E selectin protein detected by flow cytometry. However, it had no detectable effect on mRNA levels by Northern blot analysis. Given the Northern blot and microarray findings, it appears that if there is a transcriptional effect by progesterone causing the reduction in E-selectin response, it is not directly on the E selectin gene. Progesterone may have an indirect effect on E-selectin protein expression by affecting genes not on the 10.5K array. Another possibility is that progesterone has a non-genomic effect on translation.

It is emerging that progesterone and its metabolites have the ability to exert non-genomic effects, independent of changes in transcription via their nuclear receptors (Wehling, 1997). Progesterone has been shown to suppress the activity of G-protein coupled receptors, such as oxytocin receptors on uterine smooth muscle cells (Grazzini *et al.*, 1998), by acting at the cell surface. Vasodilatory effects by progesterone in coronary arteries have also been postulated to be via a non-genomic mechanism (Minshall *et al.*, 2002). It is possible that progesterone acts on the E-selectin adhesion molecule by altering the rate of internalization so as to reduce expression of E-selectin protein at the cell surface, without alteration of transcript abundance.

The effect of progesterone on E-selectin protein expression demonstrates the ability of progesterone to modulate leucocyte-endothelial cell interactions. Given the large number of cytokines and growth factors that can potentially be released by intravascular neutrophils, it is possible that progesterone could have profound effects on blood vessel pathology by affecting endothelial-leucocyte interactions. In the endometrium, focal sources of VEGF in intravascular neutrophils have been associated with angiogenesis (Gargett *et al.,* 2001). If long-term progestin administration alters the normal VEGF-stimulus received by endometrial endothelial cells, it might partially explain the disordered angiogenesis and vessel fragility associated with progestin-induced breakthrough bleeding.

REFERENCES

Andersson, C., Lydrup, M.L., Ferno, M., Idvall, I., Gustafsson, J.A., and Nilsson, B.O. (2001) Immunocytochemical demonstration of oestrogen receptor β in blood vessels of the female rat. *Journal of Endocrinology., 169,* 241-247.

Bilsel, A.S., Moini, H., Tetik, E., Aksunager, F., Kaynak, B., and Ozer, A. (2000) 17β-estradiol modulates endothelin-1 expression and release in human endothelial cells. *Cardiovasc Res., 46,* 579-84.

Cassatella, M.A. (1999) Neutrophil-derived proteins: selling cytokines by the pound. *Advances in Immunology, 73,* 369-509.

Critchley, H.O.D., Brenner, R.M., Henderson, T.A., Williams, K., Nayak, N.R., Slayden, O.D., Millar, M.R., and Saunders, P.T.K. (2001) Estrogen receptor β, but not estrogen receptor α, is present in the vascular endothelium of the human and nonhuman primate endometrium. *J Clin Endocrinol Metab., 86*, 1370-8.

Edelman, J.L., Castro, M.R., and Wen, Y. (1999) Correlation of VEGF expression by leukocytes with the growth and regression of blood vessels in the rat cornea. *Investigative Ophthalmology and Visual Science, 40*, 1112-1123.

Gagliardi, A., and Collins, D.C. (1993) Inhibition of angiogenesis by antiestrogens. *Cancer Res.*, 53, 533-5.

Gambino, L.S., Wreford, N.G., Bertram, J.F., Dockery, P., Lederman, F., and Rogers, P.A.W. (2002) Angiogenesis occurs by vessel elongation in proliferative phase human endometrium. *Hum Reprod., 17*, 1199-1206.

Gargett, C.E., Lederman, F.L., Lau, T.M., Taylor, N.H., and Rogers, P.A.W. (1999) Lack of correlation between vascular endothelial growth factor production and endothelial cell proliferation in the human endometrium. *Hum Reprod., 14*, 2080-2088.

Gargett, C.E., Bucak, K., and Rogers, P.A. (2000) Isolation, characterization, and long-term culture of human myometrial microvascular endothelial cells. *Hum Reprod., 15,* 293-301.

Gargett, C.E., Lederman, F., Heryanto, B., Gambino, L.S., and Rogers, P.A. (2001) Focal vascular endothelial growth factor correlates with angiogenesis in human endometrium. Role of intravascular neutrophils. *Hum Reprod., 16,* 1065-75.

Gargett, C.E., Zaitseva, M, Bucak, K., Chu, S., Fuller, P.J., and Rogers, P.A.W. (2002) 17β-Estradiol up-regulates vascular endothelial growth factor receptor-2 expression in human myometrial microvascular endothelial cells: role of estrogen receptors-α and –β. *J Clin Endocrinol Metab., 87,* 4341-9.

Garlanda, C., and Dejana, E. (1997) Heterogeneity of endothelial cells. *Arterioscler Thromb Vasc Biol., 17,* 1193-1202.

Gaudry, M., Bregerie, O., Andrieu, V., Benna, J.E., Pocidalo, M-A., and Hakim, J. (1997) Intracellular pool of vascular endothelial growth factor in human neutrophils. *Blood, 90,* 4153-4161.

Gerdes, D., Christ, M., Haseroth, K., Notzon, A., Falkenstein, E., and Wehling, M. (2000) Nongenomic actions of steroids – from the laboratory to clinical implications. *J Pediatr Endocrinol Metab., 13,* 853-78.

Goodger, A.M., and Rogers, P.A.W. (1993) Uterine endothelial cell proliferation before and after embryo implantation in rats. *Journal of Reproduction and Fertility 99,* 451-457.

Goodger, A.M., Rogers, P.A., and Affandi, B. (1994) Endometrial endothelial cell proliferation in long-term users of subdermal levonorgestrel. *Hum Reprod., 9,* 1647-51.

Grazzini, E., Guillon, G., Mouillac, B., and Zingg, H.H. (1998) Inhibition of oxytocin receptor function by direct binding of progesterone. *Nature, 392,* 509-12.

Gross, J., Azizkhan, R.G., Biswas, C., Bruns, R.R., Hsieh, D.S., and Folkman, J. (1981) Inhibition of tumor growth, vascularization, and collagenolysis in the rabbit cornea by medroxyprogesterone acetate. *PNAS., 78,* 1176-80.

Hastings, J.M., Licence, D.R., Burton, G.J., Charnock-Jones, D.S., and Smith, S.K. (2003) Soluble vascular endothelial growth factor receptor 1 inhbits edema and epithelial proliferation induced by 17β-estradiol in the mouse uterus. *Endocrinology, 144(1),* 326-334.

Heryanto, B., and Rogers, P.A.W. (2002) Regulation of endometrial endothelial cell proliferation by estrogen and progesterone in the ovariectomised mouse. *Reproduction, 123,* 107-113.

Heryanto, B., Lipson, K., and Rogers, P.A.W. (2003) Effect of angiogenesis inhibitors on oestrogen mediated endometrial endothelial cell proliferation in the ovariectomised mouse. *Reproduction, 125,* 1-10.

Heryanto, B., Girling, J.E., and Rogers, P.A.W. Intravascular neutrophils partially mediate the endometrial endothelial cell proliferative response to oestrogen in ovariectomised mice. *Reproduction,* in press.

Hickey, M., Dwarte, D., and Fraser, I.S. (2000) Superficial endometrial vascular fragility in Norplant user and in women with ovulatory dysfunctional uterine bleeding. *Hum Reprod., 15,* 1509-14.

Hornung, D., Lebovic, D.I., Shifren, J.L., Vigne, J-L., Taylor, R.N. (1998) Vectorial secretion of vascular endothelial growth factor by polarized human endometrial epithelial cells. *Fertil Steril.*, *69*, 909-915.

Iruela-Arispe, M.L., Porter, P., Bornstein, P., and Sage, E.H. (1996) Thrombospondin-1, an inhibitor of angiogenesis, is regulated by progesterone in the human endometrium. *J Clin Invest.*, *97*, 403-12.

Iruela-Arispe, M.L., Rodriguez-Manzaneque, J.C., and Abu-Jawdeh, G. (1999) Endometrial endothelial cells express estrogen and progesterone receptors and exhibit a tissue specific response to angiogenic growth factors. *Microcirculation, 6,* 127-40.

Johns, A., Freay, A.D., Fraser, W., Korach, K.S., and Rubanyi, G.M. (1996) Disruption of estrogen receptor gene prevents 17 beta estradiol-induced angiogenesis in transgenic mice. *Endocrinology*, *137*, 4511-3.

Jun, S.S., Chen, Z., Pace, M.C., and Shaul, P.W. (1998) Estrogen upregulates cyclooxygenase-1 gene expression in ovine fetal pulmonary artery endothelium. *J Clin Invest.*, *102*, 176-83.

Karas, R.H., Patterson, B.L., and Mendelsohn, M.E. (1994) Human vascular smooth muscle cells contain functional estrogen receptor. *Circulation*, *89*, 1943-1950.

Kurita, T., Lee, K., Saunders, P.T., Cooke, P.S., Taylor, J.A., Lubahn, D.B., Zhao, C., Makela, S., Gustafsson, J.A., Dahiya, R., and Cunha, G.R. (2001) Regulation of progesterone receptors and decidualization in uterine stroma of the estrogen receptor-alpha knockout mouse. *Biol Reprod.*, *64*, 272-283.

Lecce, G., Meduri, G., Ancelin, M., Bergeron, C., and Perrot-Applanat, M. (2001) Presence of estrogen receptor β in the human endometrium through the cycle: expression in glandular, stromal and vascular cells. *J Clin Endocrinol Metab.*, *86*, 1379-1386.

Ma, W., Tan, J., Matsumoto, H., Robert, B., Abrahamson, D.R., Das, S.K., and Dey, S.K. (2001) Adult tissue angiogenesis: evidence of negative regulation by estrogen in the uterus. *Molecular Endocrinology*, *15(11),* 1983-1992.

MacRitchie, A.N., Jun, S.S., Chen, Z., German, Z., Yuhanna, I.S., Sherman, T.S., and Shaul, P.W. (1997) Estrogen upregulates endothelial nitric oxide synthase gene expression in fetal pulmonary artery endothelium. *Circ Res., 81*, 355-62.

Minshall, R.D., Pavcnik, D., Browne, D.L., and Hermsmeyer, K. (2002) Nongenomic vasodilator action of progesterone on primate coronary arteries. *J Appl Physiol., 92,* 701-708.

Montgomery, K.F., Osborn, L., Hession, C., Tizard, R., Goff, D., Vassallo, C., Tarr, P.I., Bomsztyk, K., Lobb, R., Harlan, J.M., and Pohlman, T.H. (1991) Activation of endothelial-leukocyte adhesion molecule 1 (ELAM-1) gene transcription. *Proc Natl Acad Sci USA.*, *88,* 6523-6527.

Odmark, I., Jonsson, B., and Backstrom, T. (2001) Bleeding patterns in postmenopausal women using continuous combination hormone replacement therapy with conjugated estrogen and medroxyprogesterone acetate or with 17 beta estradiol and norethindrone acetate. *Am J Obstet Gynecol.*, *184,* 1131-1138.

Otsuki, M., Saito, H., Xu, X., Sumitani, S., Kouhara, H., Kishimoto, T., and Kasayama, S. (2001) Progesterone, but not medroxyprogesterone, inhibits vascular cell adhesion molecule-1 expression in human vascular endothelial cells. *Arterioscler Thromb Vasc Biol.*, 21, 243-248.

Reynolds, L.P., Kirsch, J.D., Kraft, K.C., Knutson, D.L., McClaflin, W.J., and Redmer, D.A. (1998) Time-course of the uterine response to estradiol-17beta in ovariectomised ewes: uterine growth and microvascular development. *Biol Reprod., 59,* 606-12.

Richardson, M.A., Berg, D.T., Calnek, D.S., Ciaccia, A.V., Joyce, D.E., and Grinnell, B.W. (2000) 17β-estradiol, but not raloxifene, decreases thrombomodulin in the antithrombotic protein C pathway. *Endocrinology, 141*, 3908-11.

Rodriguez-Manzaneque, J.C., Graubert, M., and Iruela-Arispe, M.L. (2000) Endothelial cell dysfunction following prolonged activation of progesterone receptor. *Hum Reprod., 15(suppl 3),* 39-47.

Rogers, P.A., Au, C.L., and Affandi, B. (1993) Endometrial microvascular density during the normal menstrual cycle and following exposure to long-term levonorgestrel. *Hum Reprod., 8*, 1396-404.

Rogers, P.A.W., and Gargett, C.E. (1999) Endometrial angiogenesis. *Angiogenesis, 2,* 287-294.

Sampath, D., Zhu, Y., Winneker, R.C., and Zhang, Z. (2001) Aberrant expression of Cyr61, a member of the CCN (CTGF/Cyr61/Cef10/NOVH) family, and dysregulation by 17 beta-estrdaiol and basic fibroblast growth factor in human uterine leiomyomas. *J Clin endocrinol Metab., 86,* 1707-15.

Seli, E., Pehlivan, T., Selam, B., Garcia-Velasco, J.A., and Arici, A. (2002) Estradiol down-regulates MCP-1 expression in human coronary artery endothelial cells. *Fertil Steril., 77,* 542-7.

Shifren, J.L., Tseng, J.F., Zaloudek, C.J., Ryan, I.P., Meng, Y.G., Ferrarra, N., Jaffe, R.., and Taylor, R.N. (1996) Ovarian steroid regulation of vascular endothelial growth factor in the human endometrium: implications for angiogenesis during the menstrual cycle and in the pathogenesis of endometriosis. *J Clin Endocrinol Metab., 81,* 3112-8.

Smith, S.K. (2000) Steroids and endometrial breakthrough bleeding: future directions for research. *Hum Reprod., 15(suppl 3),* 197-201.

Subakir, S.B., Hadisaputra, W., Siregar, B., Irawati, D., Santoso, D.I., Cornain, S., and Affandi, B. (1995) Reduced endothelial cell migratory signal production by endometrial explants from women using Norplant contraception. *Hum Reprod., 10,* 2579-83.

Suzuma, I., Mandai, M., Takagi, H., Suzuma, K., Otani, A., Oh, H., Kobayashi, K., and Honda, Y. (1999) 17 Beta-estradiol increases VEGF receptor-2 and promotes DNA synthesis in retinal microvascular endothelial cells. *IOVS., 40,* 2122-9.

Taichman, N.S., Young. S., Cruchley, A.T., Taylor, P., and Paleolog, E. (1997) Human neutrophils secrete vascular endothelial growth factor. *Journal of Leukocyte Biology, 62,* 397-400.

Taniguchi, M., Miura, K., Iwao, H., and Yamanaka, S. (2001) Quantitative assessment of DNA microarrays – comparison with Northern blot analyses. *Genomics, 71*, 34-9.

Torry, D.S., and Torry, R.J. (1997) Angiogenesis and the expression of vascular endothelial growth factor in endometrium and placenta. *American Journal of Reproductive Immunology, 37,* 21-29.

Vazquez, F., Rodriguez-Manzaneque, J.C., Lydon, J.P., Edwards, D.P., O'Malley, B.W., Iruela-Arispe, M.L. (1999) Progesterone regulates proliferation of endothelial cells. *J Biol Chem.*, *274,* 2185-92.

Venkov, C.D., Rankin, A.B., and Vaughan, D.E. (1996) Identification of authentic estrogen receptor in cultures endothelial cells. *Circulation, 94,* 727-33.

Villablanca, A.C., Lewis, K.A., and Rutledge, J.C. (2002) Time- and dose-dependent differential upregulation of three genes by 17β-estradiol in endothelial cells. *J Appl Physiol.*, 92, 1064-73.

Wehling, M. (1997) Specific, nongenomic actions of steroid hormones. *Annu Rev Physiol., 59,* 365-93.

Weston, G.C., Haviv, I., and Rogers, P.A.W. (2002) Microarray analysis of VEGF-responsive genes in myometrial endothelial cells. *Mol Hum Reprod.*, *8*, 855-863.

Wu, W.X., Ma, X.H., Smith, G.C.S., and Nathanielsz, P.W. (2000) Differential distribution of ERα and ERβ mRNA in intrauterine tissues of the pregnant rhesus monkey. *Am J Physiol Cell Physiol.*, *278,* C190-C198.

Zhang, L., Scott, P.A.E., Turley, H., Leek, R., Lewis, C.E., Gatter, K.C., Harris, A.L., Mackenzie, I.A., Rees, M.C.P., and Bicknell, R. (1998) Validation of anti-vascular endothelial growth factor (anti-VEGF) antibodies for immunohistochemical localization of VEGF in tissue sections: expression of VEGF in the human endometrium. *Journal of Pathology*, *185*, 402-408.

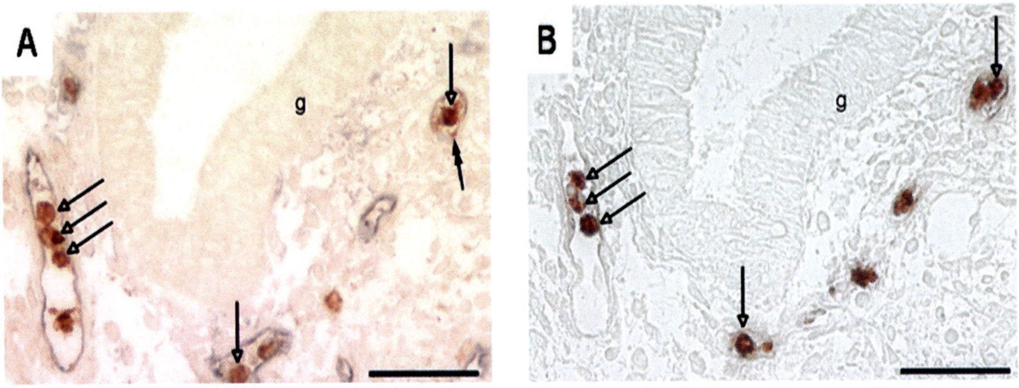

Fig. 16. Same field of view of serial sections (3 µm) of mid-proliferative stage functionalis from human endometrium immunostained with (A) CD34/VEGF showing focal VEGF (red-brown) in cells closely associated with microvessel endometrium (blue) (hollow arrows) and an occasional VEGF expressing cell in nearby stroma and (B) immunostained with anti-human neutrophil elastase, showing that focal VEGF is co-localised in neutrophils (hollow arrows). g: gland, double headed arrow: VEGF bound to endothelial cell. Scale bars = 50 µm. (Reproduced from Gargett et al., 2001 with permission).

In: Trends in Angiogenesis Research
Editor: Roberta V. Zubar, pp. 103-123

ISBN 1-59454-452-2

Chapter IV

SOFTWARE-SUPPORTED QUANTIFICATION OF ANGIOGENESIS IN AN IN VITRO CULTURE SYSTEM. EXAMPLES OF APPLICATIONS IN STUDIES OF BASIC RESEARCH, BIOCOMPATIBILITY AND DRUG DISCOVERY

Kirsten Peters[1*], Harald Schmidt[2], Günter Kamp[2,3], Ronald E. Unger[1], Bettina Hoffmann[4], Frauke Stenzel[5], Günter Ziegler[4,5], Manfred Jung[6], Susanne Stumpf and C. James Kirkpatrick[1]

[1]Institute of Pathology, Johannes Gutenberg-University, Mainz, Germany, [2]AMP-Lab GmbH, Laboratory for Applied Molecular Physiology, Mainz, Germany, [3]Institute of Zoology, Mainz, Germany, [4]Friedrich-Baur-Forschungsinstitut für Biomaterialien, Universität Bayreuth, Germany, [5]BioCer Entwicklungs-GmbH, Bayreuth, Germany, [6]Institute of Pharmaceutical Sciences, Albert Ludwigs-University, Freiburg, Germany

ABSTRACT

Angiogenesis is regulated by complex interactions between endothelial cells and other cell types such as macrophages, fibroblasts, and smooth muscle cells. These intercellular interactions are mediated by cellular compounds such as cytokines, growth factors and extracellular matrix molecules. Although a large number of angiogenic and anti-angiogenic factors have been identified, knowledge concerning the regulation of the dynamic, highly complex and multi-step angiogenic process is incomplete. Due to this complexity studies on angiogenesis in vivo often do not allow insight into cell-specific aspects and a distinction between direct and indirect effects of possible modulators cannot be accurately made. To overcome these difficulties a number of different in vitro

* Correspondence concerning this article should be addressed to Dr. Kirsten Peters. Institute of Pathology, Johannes Gutenberg-University, Langenbeckstr. 1, 55101 Mainz, Germany. Tel.: +49- (0) 6131-174522; Fax: +49- (0) 6131-173448; E-mail address: peters@pathologie.klinik.uni-mainz.de.

cell culture models of angiogenesis have been developed. In these model systems the formation of in vitro capillaries by endothelial cells is induced without the presence of other cell types, blood flow or hydrostatic pressure. These in vitro capillaries are primarily induced by exposing endothelial cells to a 3-dimensional milieu of extracellular matrix proteins and stimulation with pro-angiogenic factors. In this study we have utilized an in vitro model of angiogenesis that exhibits high sensitivity to biological angiogenic stimuli. On the basis of this model system we have defined criteria for a software-supported analysis of microscopic images leading to the quantification of in vitro capillary formation. Here, we describe examples of the application of this model system to examine the effects of biological factors (sensitivity to pro-angiogenic factors such as basic fibroblast growth factor/bFGF, vascular endothelial growth factor/VEGF and low oxygen partial pressure/hypoxia), the effects of pharmacological compounds (protease inhibitors, histone deacetylase inhibitors) and the use of this model system in biocompatibility testing (e.g. metallic implant materials and corrosion products).

Color graphics are presented at the end of the chapter.

Key words: angiogenesis, in vitro, endothelial cells, software-supported image quantification/SSIQ, biocompatibility, bFGF, VEGF, hypoxia, protease inhibitor, histone deacetylase inhibitor, implants, corrosion products, cobalt ions.

Abbreviations: basic fibroblast growth factor/bFGF, capillary-like structures/CLS, endothelial cells/EC, extracellular matrix/ECM, histone deacetylase/HDAC, human dermal microvascular endothelial cells/HDMEC, ImageTool 3.0/IT, software-supported image quantification/SSIQ, Trichostatin A/TSA, vascular endothelial growth factor/VEGF.

1. INTRODUCTION

Endothelial cells (EC) line the inner surface of all blood vessels, forming the interface between blood and tissues and EC are present in nearly every tissue. The endothelial population in an adult human is estimated to weigh approximately 1 kg. Therefore, EC account for a significant share of the total body weight [1]. An important attribute of EC is their ability to form new blood vessels, a process that is called angiogenesis. Angiogenesis is a crucial step during the development of the individual (embryogenesis and growth). Moreover, the degree of the vascular supply is often a determining factor in pathophysiology (e.g. wound healing, tumor angiogenesis, and inflammation) [2].

Angiogenesis is regulated by complex interactions between EC and other cell types such as endothelial progenitor cells, monocytes/macrophages, fibroblasts, tumor cells, smooth muscle cells and pericytes [3,4]. This intercellular cross talk is connected with the release of compounds such as cytokines and growth factors, molecules of the extracellular matrix (ECM), and cell surface adhesion molecules that are known modulators of the angiogenic processes [2,5]. Although new methods allow molecular insight into the angiogenic process the complex regulation of angiogenesis is still poorly understood. Studies on angiogenesis in vivo are hindered by this complexity, the sensitivity to environmental influences, and the inaccessibility of the tissues for biochemical analyses. Furthermore, other cell types influence the angiogenic processes in vivo by the secretion of angiogenesis-stimulating and -inhibiting factors, proteins of the ECM and proteolytic enzymes [6-8]. Thus, studies on angiogenesis in vivo do not allow a distinction to be made between direct and indirect effects of possible modulators of angiogenesis. To overcome these difficulties a number of different models to demonstrate angiogenesis in vitro have been developed [9-14]. A major criterion for these in vitro models of angiogenesis is the formation of capillary-like structures (CLS) by the EC. The formation of CLS initially does not require the presence of other cell types, blood flow or hydrostatic pressure [12]. The in vitro model systems utilize ECM molecules and the establishment of CLS requires additional angiogenic stimuli such as VEGF or bFGF. The different available models of angiogenesis in vitro may reflect varying aspects of angiogenesis in vivo.

Although in vitro models of angiogenesis can to a degree shed light on the complexity of the in vivo situation, the unambiguous quantification of effects remains a major problem. Manual counting of sprouts or the determination of sprout length is generally used for quantification of the angiogenic degree. Since these approaches are laborious they do not allow high throughput. To overcome these problems we have developed a method using software-supported quantification of microscopic images (software-supported image quantification – SSIQ) to determine the degree of angiogenesis [15]. In this study we have utilized a 3-dimensional in vitro model of angiogenesis previously described [16] that mimics a number of the physiological aspects of angiogenesis in vivo. We have defined criteria for the recognition of angiogenic patterns by SSIQ that allow a variable application. The possibility for variability in the determination of quantification criteria is important since different compounds lead to variations in the CLS phenotype and thus to variations in pattern formation. We show examples of detection and quantification of angiogenesis-influencing effects of biological factors, novel pharmacological compounds, and implanted materials and their corrosion products by means of SSIQ.

2. Materials and Methods

2.1 Overview of Experimental Design

Human dermal microvascular EC (HDMEC) were stimulated to establish CLS within a 3-dimensional matrix consisting of type I collagen and fibrin by the addition of pro-angiogenic factors (VEGF/bFGF). 5-7 days after the induction of angiogenesis in vitro the processes of CLS-formation reached an advanced stage. Vital staining of cells resulted in a contrast-rich image of the newly developed CLS. Using this method a bright and contrast-rich depiction of CLS was achieved. The acquired microscopic images were used to assess the degree of angiogenesis by SSIQ. The method was used to quantify the effects of biological factors, novel pharmacological compounds, and implanted materials and their corrosion products respectively on angiogenesis in vitro.

2.2 Materials

All chemicals, enzymes, antibiotics, and biological factors were purchased from Sigma (Germany) unless indicated otherwise. Cell culture plastics were from BD Biosciences Falcon (Germany) and Greiner (Germany).

2.3 Cell Isolation

HDMEC were isolated from juvenile foreskin and the tissues were enzymatically treated as described previously [15]. Before the resulting cell cultures (containing EC and other cell types) were confluent (normally 4 - 6 days following isolation) the HDMEC were separated from the other cells in culture by immunomagnetic isolation with CD31-Dynabeads following the manufacturer's instructions (Dynal Biotech, Germany). To avoid any influences by contaminating cell types an additional second immunomagnetic isolation step was performed after the following passage (passage 1). The resulting cell population was shown to be of endothelial origin since all cells stained positively for the endothelial markers CD31, VE-Cadherin and von Willebrand Factor and were negative for smooth muscle actin and cytokeratins.

2.4 Culture Conditions

The purified HDMEC were cultured in Endothelial Cell Basal Medium MV (PromoCell, Germany) supplemented with 15% heat-inactivated FCS, bFGF (2.5 ng/ml), sodium heparin (10 µg/ml), 100 U/ml penicillin, and 100 µg/ml Streptomycin at 37°C (5% CO_2) on gelatin-coated cell culture surfaces. All assays were conducted with cells in passage 4. Any remaining CD31-Dynabead-positive HDMEC were removed by magnetic isolation from the cell suspension before the final plating-out step. The state of normoxia was set as 10% O_2 (~76 mmHg). Hypoxia was induced by setting the oxygen content at 3% O_2 (~23 mmHg).

2.5 Cytotoxicity Assay

For the evaluation of cytotoxicity the CellTiter 96® AQ_{ueous} non-radioactive assay (Promega, Germany) was performed according to the manufacturer's instructions. This assay gives evidence for the enzymatic conversion of a tetrazolium salt (MTS reagent) by mitochondrial dehydrogenase and thus an indirect evidence for cell viability.

2.6 Determination of Endothelial Proliferative State by Ki67 Staining

The Ki67 antigen is only expressed in cells undergoing division. This antigen can be used to quantify proliferating cells using an enzyme-linked immunoassay based on a peroxidase staining reaction and the subsequent dye quantification by a microplate reader. Therefore, cells were seeded onto fibronectin-coated 96-well microtiter plates (6500 cells/well) and grown to subconfluence. Afterwards cells were subjected to specific cell culture conditions and cultivated for an additional 24 h. The cells were fixed with methanol:ethanol (2:1, 15 min, room temperature) and permeabilized with PBS-buffered 0.1% Triton X-100 (5 min, room temperature).

Ki67 was detected with mouse-anti human Ki67-antibody (Dako, Germany). The secondary antibody was a peroxidase-conjugated rabbit-anti mouse-antibody (Dako). The staining reaction was performed by addition of the peroxidase-substrate (o-phenylene-diamine-dihydrochloride) for 15 min at 37°C. The staining reaction was stopped with 3 M HCl. Absorbance was determined with a microtiter plate spectrophotometer (ThermoLab Systems, Germany) at 492 nm. The Ki67-expression of compound-treated EC was compared to the Ki67-expression of the non-treated EC (relative proliferative state).

2.7 Induction of Angiogenesis in Vitro

HDMEC were embedded in a solution of fibrinogen (1 mg/ml; Chromogenix AB, Sweden) and acid-soluble type I collagen (0.75 mg/ml; ICN, Germany) with a cell number of approximately $0.7x10^6$ cells/ml gel. Gel clotting was achieved by the addition 0.7 U/ml of fibrinogen-cleaving enzyme (Arvin™ - Ancrod, Knoll Pharma, Germany) and collagen fibril formation was achieved by a change of pH (from acid to neutral) by the addition of double-concentrated cell culture medium (IMDM, Invitrogen). The stimulation with recombinant human $VEGF_{165}$ (50 ng/ml; Biomol, Germany) and bFGF (5 ng/ml) led to the establishment of in vitro capillaries within 5 – 7 days.

2.8 Tested Pharmacological Compounds

The synthetic serine protease inhibitor WX-UK1 (inhibitor of the urokinase plasminogen activator (uPA) [17]) was provided by Wilex AG (Germany). Trichostatin A (TSA) is an anti-fungal antibiotic from *Streptomyces hygroscopicus* that functions as an inhibitor of histone deacetylase (HDAC) [18]. The third tested compound, MD85, is a synthetic HDAC inhibitor [19]. HDAC inhibitors lead to cell cycle arrest and are thus inhibitors of proliferative activity.

2.9 Preparation of Metallic Samples

Metallic samples (∅ = 15 mm) were smoothened with SiC-paper (with decreasing grain size, 320-1200, Struers, Germany) in several steps and then finally polished with OP-S-suspension (colloidal silica suspension for final polishing, Struers). The quality of surfaces was controlled by light microscopy. The polished samples were cleaned in an ultrasound bath with the following sequence of solutions: tenside, water, cyclohexane (p.a., Merck, Germany), acetone (technical grade, Merck) and ethanol (p.a., Merck). Polished cpTi-

(titanium grade 2, ZAPP) and Co28Cr6Mo-samples (cast alloy, Eska Implants GmbH) were tested. For testing the effect of metallic samples on angiogenesis in vitro the EC were embedded in the gel of ECM, and this solution was poured onto the test samples. Angiogenic stimulation was performed as described above (see 2.7).

2.10 Staining Procedures

CLS were visualized by vital and nuclear staining. Vital staining was performed with calcein-acetoxymethylester (Calcein-AM, Molecular Probes/Invitrogen, Germany). Calcein-AM was added to the culture medium at a final concentration of 10 μM and incubated at 37°C for 30 min. Staining of nuclei was carried out with Hoechst Dye 33342. Dye was added to the culture medium (final concentration 3 μg/ml culture medium) and co-incubated with calcein-AM for 30 min at 37°C.

2.11 Microscopy and Digitalization

Images for angiogenesis-quantification were acquired with an inverted microscope (Leica DM IRBE) equipped with a digital camera (Kappa DX30). Angiogenesis in vitro in contact to metallic samples was observed by an upright microscope (Leica, DM RX). Calcein-AM-treated samples were excited with the 450-490 nm bandpass filter and emitted light passed through 515 nm longpass filter (I3-filter, Leica). Hoechst 33342-stained nuclei were excited with the 340-380 nm bandpass filter and emitted light passed through a 425 nm longpass filter (A-filter, Leica).

2.12 Image Analysis and Statistical Evaluations

For quantification of angiogenic processes, grey scale images were analyzed with ImageTool 3.0/IT (freeware: http://ddsdx.uthscsa.edu/dig/itdesc.html, University of Texas Health Science Center at San Antonio). Variations in the fluorescence intensity in different samples that were a result of the cell staining technique (enzymatic development of fluorochrome) were standardized with the software Photoshop 7.0 (Adobe Systems Inc., USA) by equalizing the contrast. Stained objects were identified (find objects command) and subsequently classified according to their perimeters (perimeter was the length of the outside boundary of the object). Only objects yielding a perimeter >250 pixels were counted. For each image the perimeters of all objects classified were added, representing an indicator of sprout formation. At least 18 images (usually between 40 and 160 images) from 3 individual experiments were analyzed. Means and standard deviations (SDs) or standard error of the means (SEMs) were calculated from the results of SSIQ. Significant differences between means were calculated from total perimeters with Microsoft Excel. According to the results of the variance ratio analysis (F-test, $p<0.05$) an unpaired t-test for either homoscedastic or heteroscedastic variances was performed ($p< 0.01$).

3. Results

3.1 Angiogenesis in Vitro

EC were able to establish in vitro-capillaries after embedding in a matrix consisting of fibrin and type I collagen. The development of capillary-like structures (CLS) was dependent on the stimulation by pro-angiogenic factors (VEGF/bFGF) (Fig. 1a). The CLS were detectable as an interconnecting network showing a number of branches. CLS-development began immediately after growth factor stimulation and between 5 and 7 days were required for the full expansion. The developing CLS often established a central lumen with varying diameters. The cultivation beyond 5-7 days led to regression of CLS.

The morphogenic processes, occurring during angiogenesis in vitro, were easily observed by phase contrast microscopy. By monitoring the change from isolated, suspended cells in a 3-dimensional milieu to the CLS by time-lapse video microscopy, it was evident that there was an increase of CLS length and branching, dependent on the progression of CLS-formation (see time-lapse video: http://www-klinik.uni-mainz.de/Pathologie/E/Research/3D-Angio%20HighQ.WMV).

3.2 Pattern Identification

For an evaluation of the significant changes in endothelial morphology during CLS-formation a method of software-supported image quantification (SSIQ) was developed. Cells were visualized by treatment with membrane-permeable calcein-AM. After uptake by living cells this compound is converted by intracellular esterase activity into the membrane-impermeable, fluorescent calcein that led to a fluorescent staining of the cytoplasm. In this way, a contrast-rich visualization of CLS in front of a dark background was achieved (Fig. 1a).

In order to enable the unequivocal quantification of angiogenic processes in vitro we utilized the software program ImageTool 3.00 (IT). IT can analyze and process grey scale and color images. Image analysis functions of IT include dimensional (distance, angle, perimeter, area) and grey scale measurements (point, line and area histogram with statistics).

To choose the most applicable analysis parameter for angiogenesis in vitro, we focused on the most characteristic behavior of angiogenesis-stimulated EC in vitro. A major characteristic for the CLS formation was the aggregation of single cells and morphogenesis to elongated objects, where most of the cells appeared optically fused. The utilization of these criteria demonstrated that the longer the interconnecting CLS were the more pronounced angiogenesis in vitro had taken place. From the analysis parameters included in IT the "object perimeter" was most useful for the quantification of these elongated, interconnected objects.

An example for object recognition and classification on the basis of the "perimeter" in IT is shown in Fig. 2. The original image (Fig. 2a) was first analyzed by the "find object" command using the manual thresholding method selecting all pixels with grey levels within a manually adjusted threshold range (red, Fig. 2b). For all images in an experimental series the same threshold value was applied, which was previously defined according to the brightness of the CLS within the respective series. The procedure to determine the threshold resulted in object identification and counting (identified objects are red-framed and counted as indicated, Fig. 2c). All objects identified by the "find objects" procedure were further processed according to the attribute perimeter by the "object classification" plug-in. The classification procedure separated objects with a perimeter above 250 pixels (orange, Fig. 2d) from objects below this value (red, Fig. 2d). Object classification resulted in the elimination of structures which could not be attributed to the angiogenic process (objects < 250 pixels). The analysis of the example image resulted in 24 objects identified by the "find objects" command (Fig. 2e). Only 2 objects accounted for typical CLS (object perimeter > 250 pixels) while the other 22 objects were small, single EC or small rounded clusters of cells. The degree of angiogenesis in vitro was based on the total perimeter calculated from the mean perimeter multiplied by the number of objects.

3.3 Evaluation of the Angiogenesis Model System and Quantification Method by Testing Biological Stimuli of Angiogenesis

In order to evaluate the capacity of the chosen analysis parameter of IT (perimeter) we performed assays where the ECM-embedded EC were stimulated with known pro-angiogenic factors. The collagen/fibrin-embedded EC were stimulated with bFGF (5 ng/ml), VEGF (50 ng/ml), bFGF+VEGF (5 and 50 ng/ml respectively), and bFGF+VEGF+hypoxia (5 and 50 ng/ml respectively, 3% O_2). In the absence of pro-angiogenic factors the formation of CLS was completely absent (Fig. 3a) and only a few single cells were detectable. The supplementation with bFGF led to the establishment of a few elongated objects without branching (Fig. 3b). In comparison to the non-stimulated culture the number of single cells increased under the influence of bFGF-stimulation. The exposure of embedded EC to VEGF led to the development of elongated, branched objects (Fig. 3c). When bFGF and VEGF were supplemented in combination the developing CLS-network was much more pronounced than the effects induced by each factor alone (Fig. 3d). A further enhancement of the CLS-formation was induced by the additional exposure of the bFGF/VEGF-stimulated cultures to hypoxic culture conditions (Fig. 3e).

The application of SSIQ with the chosen analysis parameter perimeter of objects (see 3.2.) to images acquired in these different culture conditions revealed the expected graded increase in angiogenesis in vitro (Fig. 3f): leaving out pro-angiogenic factors led to the complete absence of CLS (0% angiogenesis in vitro compared to the bFGF+VEGF-stimulated culture, set as 100%). The addition of bFGF induced a slight CLS-formation that was analyzed by SSIQ to be about 3%, VEGF alone induced a CLS-formation of about 55% in comparison to the bFGF/VEGF-treated cultures. The additional exposure of bFGF/VEGF-stimulated EC to hypoxia induced a further increase in angiogenesis in vitro to 135%.

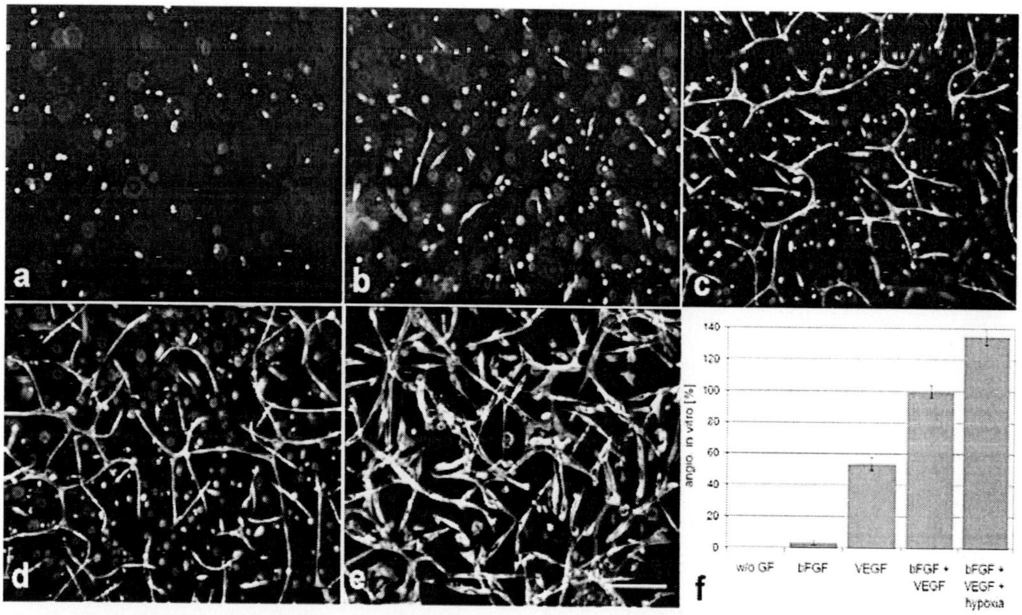

Fig. 3. Vital staining of ECM-embedded (fibrin/type I collagen) EC under different culture conditions. a) w/o growth factors, b) bFGF-supplementation, d) VEGF-supplementation, d) bFGF/VEGF-supplementation, e) bFGF/VEGF-stimulated EC under hypoxia (3% O_2) (grey scale images; scale bar: 600 µm), f) angiogenic degree of the different culture conditions determined by SSIQ (values are given in percent as means ± SEM, bFGF/VEGF-treated cultures were set as 100%).

3.4 Testing of Pharmacological Compounds

The specific intervention of progression of angiogenesis by pharmacological compounds is a desirable aim, since a number of pathological processes are accompanied by blood vessel formation. Therefore, we determined the usefulness of our model system in testing the effect of different drugs on angiogenesis in vitro. Three different pharmacological compounds were chosen, and two of which possessed comparable cellular mechanisms. One compound was the synthetic serine protease inhibitor WX-UK1 and the other two were the HDAC inhibitors TSA (natural inhibitor) and MD85 (synthetic inhibitor) with proliferation-inhibiting mechanisms.

We tested the effect of these pharmacological compounds on angiogenesis in vitro with effective concentrations. For WX-UK1 the effective concentration known to inhibit protease activity was about 10 µM. For TSA and MD85 we performed a proliferation assay, the Ki67 assay, which allows a quantification of cells participating in the cell cycle. Here, TSA-concentrations of 1 µM and MD85-concentrations of 5 µM showed a significant inhibition of EC-proliferation (Fig. 4a). Therefore, we tested the effect of these pharmacological compounds on angiogenesis in vitro with the following concentrations: WX-UK1 – 10 and 20 µM, TSA – 0.1 µM (below the proliferation effect dose) and 1 µM; MD85 – 0.5 µM (below the proliferation effect dose) and 5 µM. Since all assays were performed in the presence of both bFGF and VEGF an inhibition of angiogenesis in vitro by the compound should be manifested by reduced CLS-formation. In comparison to the positive control (Fig. 4b, bFGF/VEGF-stimulated cultures, set as 100 %) WX-UK1-treated cultures showed a reduced CLS amount. Since the lower WX-UK1-concentration (10 μM) showed a weaker effect (Fig. 4c) than the higher WX-UK1 concentration (20 μM, Fig. 4d) a concentration dependency can be assumed. Low concentrations of TSA (0.1 μM) did not show an apparent effect in comparison to the positive control (Fig. 4e). The higher TSA-concentration tested (1 μM) demonstrated the complete absence of formation of CLS (Fig. 4f). Both concentrations of MD85 did not show impairment of CLS formation (shown for 5 μM MD85, Fig. 4g).

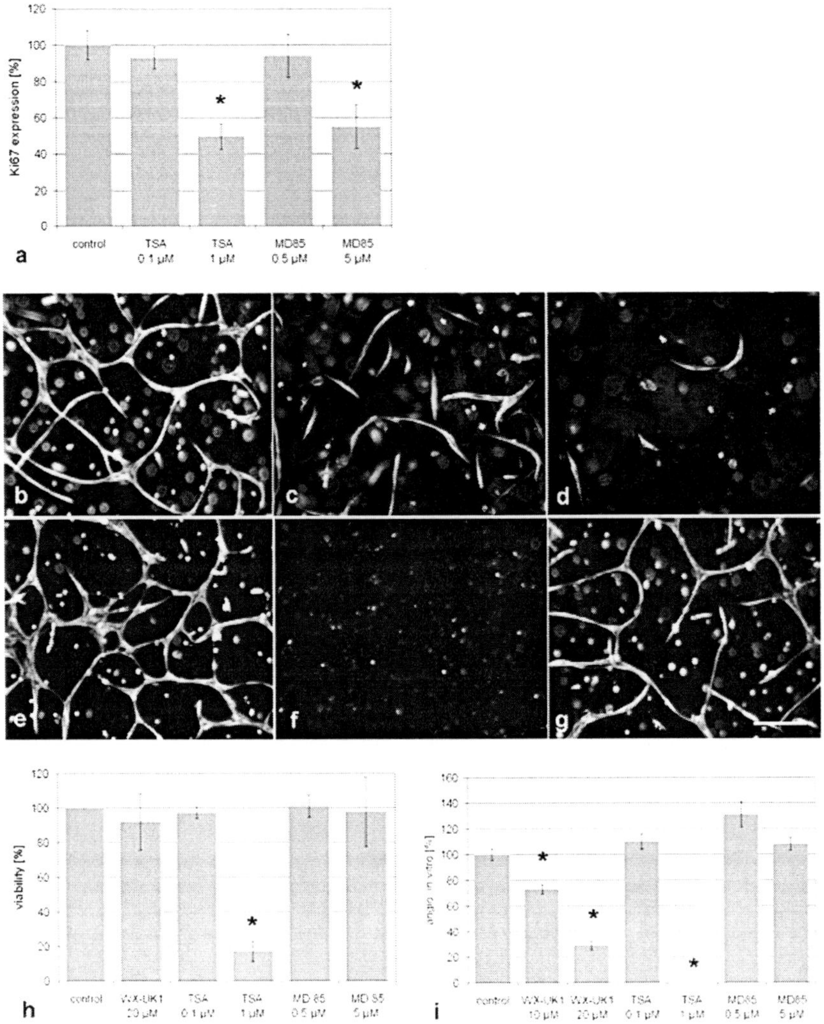

Fig. 4. Effects of pharmacological compounds on EC. a) relative Ki67 expression in TSA- and MD85-treated EC after 24 h (immunocytochemical detection of Ki67, spectrophotometric quantification, significantly different from control: *$p<0.01$), b-g) calcein-AM stained, angiogenesis-stimulated EC (scale bar: 400 μm), b) positive control, c) WX-UK1-treated (10 μM), d) WX-UK1-treated (20 μM), e) TSA-treated (0.1 μM), f) TSA-treated (1 μM), g) MD85-treated (5 μM), h) cytotoxicity testing of the different compounds after 48 h exposure (WX-UK1: 20 μM, TSA: 0.1 and 1 μM, MD85: 0.5 and 5 μM), i) angiogenic degree of the compound-treated angiogenic cultures determined by SSIQ (significantly different from control: *$p<0.01$, values are given in percent of the control as means ± SD).

In order to exclude the possibility that unspecific cytotoxic effects of the tested compounds were responsible for the angiogenesis inhibition we performed cytotoxicity assays (Fig. 4h). These assays revealed that all tested compounds did not show cytotoxicity within 48 h except for high concentrations of TSA (1 μM). Here, cell viability was significantly reduced after 48 h TSA-exposure. Thus, the impairment of CLS-formation by TSA was due to the reduction of cell viability and not to specific effect on angiogenesis in vitro.

The analysis of the acquired images by SSIQ (Fig. 4i) revealed a concentration-dependent, significant inhibition of angiogenesis in vitro by WX-UK1 (10 μM: 73%; 20 μM: 29% in comparison to the untreated control set as 100%). Low, non-cytotoxic concentrations of TSA did not significantly influence angiogenesis in vitro (0.1 μM: 110%), the higher, cytotoxic concentration of TSA led to a complete breakdown of angiogenic processes (0%). Both concentrations of MD85 did not induce significant changes on angiogenesis in vitro in comparison to the untreated control. In contrast, 0.5 μM MD85 induced a non-significant increase in the angiogenic degree (129%).

3.5 Testing of Implant Materials and their Corrosion Products

Not only is it essential that a biomaterial does not elicit cytotoxic effects, but it is also important that an implant material does not impair angiogenesis. If reduced angiogenesis should occur in the peri-implant tissue during the wound healing process an impairment of implant stability could be a possible consequence. Therefore, we expanded the utilization of our model system in performing angiogenesis assays in direct contact with different metallic implant materials. For this purpose cpTi and Co28Cr6Mo-alloy samples were chosen. Furthermore, we tested the effect of possible corrosion products arising from CoCr-alloys, divalent cobalt ions (Co^{2+}) and trivalent chromium ions (Cr^{3+}).

CLS-formation on cpTi-surfaces showed a characteristic phenotype (Fig. 5a). This phenotype was comparable to the positive controls (see Fig. 1a); i.e. aggregation of the cells into elongated, stretched formations and bifurcations of these. Performing the angiogenesis assay in direct contact to the Co28Cr6Mo surfaces revealed that nearly no CLS but rather monolayer-like areas were formed (Fig. 5b). To examine if corrosion products of the Co28Cr6Mo-alloy were responsible for the changes in the EC phenotype on Co28Cr6Mo surfaces, we tested the effects of Co^{2+} and Cr^{3+}. Co^{2+} induced a pronounced impairment of angiogenesis in vitro, whereas Cr^{3+} did not influence the processes (data not shown). However, in contrast to the effects on the Co28Cr6Mo-surface the number of CLS decreased by Co^{2+}-exposure; monolayer-like areas were not visible (concentrations tested were between 0.01-0.3 mM Co^{2+}). Thus, the effects of Co^{2+} differed from the effects on angiogenesis in vitro induced by the Co28Cr6Mo-alloy.

The application of SSIQ to these experiments turned out to be problematic: When applying the generally utilized analysis parameter "total perimeter" there was an increase detectable for the Co28Cr6Mo-alloy in comparison to the cpTi-sample (Fig. 5c, ca. 22000 pixels compared to ca. 12500 on cpTi). This increase would imply an increase in the angiogenic degree which was not in accordance with the apparent phenotype, since on Co28Cr6Mo-surfaces no CLS were visible. The problem in quantification was induced by the unusual effect that although CLS-formation was obviously inhibited, EC on Co28Cr6Mo-surfaces built up monolayer-like areas identified by IT as objects with perimeters above 250 pixels. Interestingly, the analysis parameter "mean object number" confirmed this problem since it was enhanced on Co28Cr6Mo-surfaces in comparison to the cpTi-surface (Fig. 5c). This increase of object number with simultaneously increased perimeter was contradictory to the results observed so far.

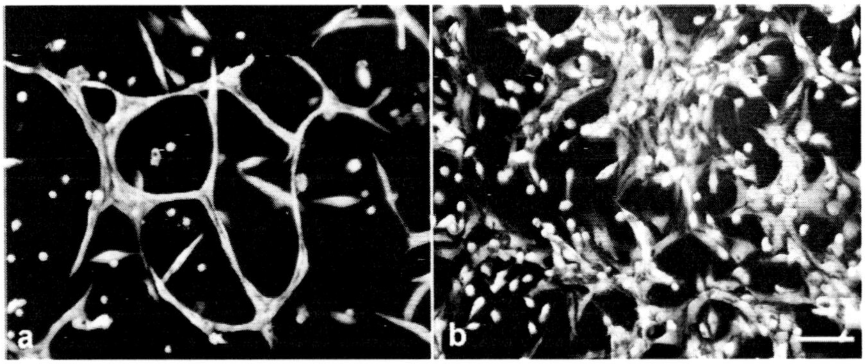

c

		mean object number	total perimeter	compactness
cpTi	mean	**6**	**12476**	**0.36**
	SD	2	3368	0.04
Co28Cr6Mo	mean	**15**	**21964**	**0.51**
	SD	6	8191	0.04
T-test		**3.13E-08**	**3.53E-02**	**7E-13**

Fig. 5. Angiogenesis in vitro in contact with metallic samples. a) angiogenesis-stimulated EC in contact with a cpTi sample, b) angiogenesis-stimulated EC in contact with a Co28Cr6Mo sample (calcein-AM staining, scale bar: 200 µm), c) object analysis of different analysis parameters in angiogenesis in vitro (mean object number, total perimeter, compactness) by IT (means and standard deviation/SD; significance was tested by t-test (homoscedastic or heteroscedastic according to the results of the F-test), significance was determined to be $p<0.01$).

To circumvent these problems and to obtain a quantification method regardless of this unusual phenotype we searched for an additional quantification parameter of IT with the ability to distinguish between CLS and monolayer-like areas. The most suitable analysis parameter in IT for this specific aspect was the parameter "compactness". This parameter is defined in IT as *square root (4 x area/circle Pi)/major axis length*. The "compactness" provided a measure of the object's circleness. At compactness values of 1 the object is roughly circular. When the compactness value decreases from 1 the object becomes less circular. When applied to the angiogenic structures this would indicate that as more distinct CLS develop, the smaller the "compactness" of the identified objects. This was reflected in the compactness values on the metallic samples: whereas on cpTi-samples the compactness values were 0.36, on Co28Cr6Mo-samples the values were 0.51 (Fig. 5c). Therefore, the "compactness" was low when CLS with a great amount of extensions developed, whereas the "compactness" was higher when monolayer-like structures were detectable. Thus, this change in the selection of a quantification parameter allowed the analysis of this exceptional endothelial phenotype.

4. Discussion

4.1 General Considerations

The complexity and inaccessibility of angiogenesis to in vivo observation and analysis requires the use of in vitro models. Different models to examine angiogenesis in vitro have been developed [9-14]. However, unequivocal quantification of angiogenic processes is difficult. Therefore, these systems are not applicable for screening procedures and can only be evaluated optically or by analogue morphometric measurement. To circumvent these limitations we have developed an in vitro model of angiogenesis that allows a digital quantification and is suitable for screening procedures. This model works with an angiogenesis-relevant cell type (human microvascular EC) in a 3-dimensional matrix consisting of fibrin and type I collagen, resembling the ECM of a tumor or an early granulation tissue. This in vitro assay mimics many aspects of the complex processes of angiogenesis in vivo (dependency on pro-angiogenic factors, EC migration, lumen formation, interendothelial communication, changes in intercellular junctions, and morphogenesis of CLS). It was determined that an optimal time point for analysis in the 3D-angiogenesis system was between 5 – 7 days after induction of angiogenesis in vitro. At this time point, generally regardless of donor, a similar reproducible pattern of CLS formation occurred. This reproducibility in pattern is essential in that changes to CLS morphology can be attributed to the test compounds.

4.2 Angiogenic Pattern Determination for SSIQ

We have extended the usefulness of this model system by applying SSIQ, which allows an exact quantification of even minor changes. This quantification is based on the analysis of the phenotypic changes during the morphogenesis of CLS: As previously mentioned, EC within CLS formed during angiogenesis in vitro exhibited a specific pattern that is characterized by a change from a large number of single, suspended EC in the 3-dimensional scaffold of ECM at the beginning, to only few, elongated, interconnected structures (CLS) with optically fused cells. This change in morphology can be reflected by different parameters of IT-software.

Our aim was to find an analysis parameter(s) in IT that would be uniquely suitable for all quantification applications in angiogenesis in vitro. The "perimeter" command in IT was found to be most applicable. By using this analysis parameter a shift could be detected from large quantities of objects with perimeters below 250 pixels (single cells suspended in the 3D-ECM), to only a few objects with perimeters above 250 pixels (distinct CLS). Therefore, a stimulation of angiogenesis in vitro resulted in an increase of "total perimeter" and in case of the inhibition of angiogenesis a reduction of "total perimeter" was observable.

However, under certain conditions the "total perimeter" value failed in the quantification of CLS. This was observed in case of metallic materials (see 3.5) where the establishment of an exceptional endothelial phenotype did not allow the quantification by the analysis parameter "total perimeter". Under these conditions, the more complex analysis parameter "compactness" of objects was used for quantification. This example shows that a simple analysis and quantification are not generally possible. In some cases unexpected and unusual phenotypic variations can prevent automatic analyses. Therefore, to best utilize a quantification method it is imperative to obtain experience in evaluating different conditions that affect CLS formation to determine which IT parameters should be used.

4.3 Evaluation of the Model System and the Quantification Method by Exposure to Biological Pro-Angiogenic Factors

In order to evaluate the significance of the utilized model system we tested the effects of different pro-angiogenic stimuli such as the exposure to bFGF, VEGF and hypoxia. If these different stimuli or combinations thereof demonstrate similar effects as observed in vivo, the quantification by SSIQ should reveal a graded increase in angiogenesis in vitro.

EC which are suspended within the three-dimensional ECM but without the supplementation of bFGF and VEGF die within 5-7 days (i.e. nearly no calcein positive cells detectable). In contrast, the exposure of the ECM-embedded EC to VEGF revealed a clear induction of CLS development in vitro. The ability of VEGF (also referred to as VEGF-A) to induce angiogenesis is well-documented [20]. VEGF-A signaling is thought to be the critical rate-limiting step in physiological angiogenesis. The isoform $VEGF_{165}$, utilized in this study, is the predominant isoform of four different known VEGFs [21] and is believed to have optimal characteristics of bioavailability and angiogenic potency due to its heparin-binding domain [22].

The second tested compound bFGF is a multifunctional signaling factor with a broad spectrum of tissue distribution, target cells and bioactivities. We have shown that bFGF induced only a slight increase in CLS formation in response to bFGF-exposure. bFGF is known to modulate several cellular functions simultaneously [23]. One of those functions is the impact of bFGF on angiogenesis. Since the action of bFGF is known to be nonspecific in that it acts on many other cell types, a direct effect of bFGF on EC in angiogenesis remains controversial [24]. However, in vitro data showed bFGF-induced endothelial proliferation [25] and chemotactic movement [26]. Interestingly, the exposure to both bFGF and VEGF simultaneously led to a significant increase in the degree in angiogenesis in vitro. This increase is beyond an additive impact of both factors and indicates a synergistic effect of the combination of bFGF and VEGF. This synergistic effect is in agreement with the effects previously shown in vitro [27] and in vivo [28].

Furthermore, the state of low oxygen pressure (hypoxia) induced a significant increase in the degree of angiogenesis in vitro. The stimulation of angiogenesis by hypoxic conditions is a physiological response in that the increase of blood vessel density circumvents an insufficient oxygen supply [29]. This effect is assumed, in addition to other factors, to be mediated by an increase of responsiveness of EC to the different angiogenic factors. For example Li et al. [30] showed that the responsiveness of EC to the pro-angiogenic factor bFGF was increased in hypoxia by promoting preferential synthesis of heparan sulfate and increasing the number of bFGF-binding sites on heparan sulfate chains. In addition, hypoxia induced an increased level of the VEGF receptor-1/Flt-1 expression in human EC [31].

Thus, all three pro-angiogenic factors and combinations of these factors induced an appropriate, graded response in our model system of angiogenesis in vitro, which was in accordance with the state of knowledge. Without the exposure to these fundamental factors angiogenesis in vitro did not occur.

4.4 Utilization of SSIQ in Testing Pharmacological Compounds for their Angiogenesis-influencing Potential

Since angiogenesis is a sequence of events that is fundamental to many pathologic processes (e.g. cancer, diabetic retinopathy, chronic inflammation) therapeutic intervention in angiogenesis by pharmacological compounds is considered as a promising strategy. Therefore, we tested our model system regarding its usefulness in testing the effect of different pharmacological compounds on angiogenesis in vitro. We have chosen three different compounds of which two possessed comparable cellular mechanisms.

One of these compounds was the synthetic serine protease inhibitor WX-UK1. WX-UK1 is a known inhibitor of uPA [17] and shows efficacy in inhibiting invasion capacity of carcinoma cells in vitro [32]. WX-UK1 is currently in clinical development phase I/IIa for the treatment of various solid tumors by blocking primary tumor growth and metastasis formation. Since a regulated, spatially focalized degradation of the ECM by the uPA system (and other factors) is also required for tissue remodeling processes such as angiogenesis [33], the inhibition of a major proteolytic system could be an important step in inhibiting angiogenesis. Testing the effects of WX-UK1 on angiogenesis in vitro revealed a dose-dependent decrease. Non-cytotoxic WX-UK1 concentrations induced an inhibition of angiogenesis in vitro of more than 70%. Thus, WX-UK1 was able to block angiogenesis in vitro, presumably by blocking the uPA-system, leading to an impairment of proteolytic activity of the EC embedded in ECM consisting of type I collagen and fibrin. Taken together, WX-UK1 exerts effects by inhibiting invasive capacity of carcinoma cells and inhibiting angiogenic morphogenesis of EC to CLS in vitro. This comprehensive effect on different cancer-relevant aspects in different cell types without cytotoxic effects in vitro appears promising for the utilization of WX-UK1 in treatment of cancer in vivo.

The other tested compounds were inhibitors of histone deacetylase (HDAC): TSA (natural inhibitor) and MD85 (synthetic inhibitor). These compounds induce an accumulation of acetylated histone proteins and thus induce an arrest in cell cycle progression. This inhibitory effect on the proliferative activity of (cancer) cells resulted in the classification of HDAC inhibitors as a novel group of anticancer agents [34]. To test if HDAC inhibitors also exert effects on angiogenic processes of EC in vitro, we performed the angiogenesis assays in the presence of both inhibitors in concentrations known to inhibit EC proliferation and also below the effective concentration.

Whereas MD85 did not show a significant effect on angiogenic differentiation in vitro, high concentrations of TSA induced a complete failure in CLS-formation. However, these effects on angiogenesis and EC proliferation in vitro were accompanied by an impairment of cell viability (detected after 48 h). Thus, we determined that TSA did not exert direct, specific effects on angiogenesis in vitro (which needs 5-7 days to mature) in the concentrations tested. Only a few studies have examined the effects of TSA on EC in vitro. In these studies TSA concentrations of 0.1 – 1 µM were mostly used for short term exposure in testing TSA-induced effects on e.g. VEGF- and NO-signalling [35-37]. However, the experiments on the effects of TSA in different models of angiogenesis in vitro needed longer exposure times (up to 11 days). Two studies showed TSA-induced inhibition of angiogenesis in vitro estimated by optical evaluation [36,37]. Interestingly, these studies did not show evidence for EC viability after long term exposure to TSA. Since in our experiments 0.1 µM TSA did not show any effects (either on proliferation and angiogenesis or on impairment of cell viability) and 1 µM induced strong effects in both functional assays with simultaneously strong cytotoxicity, it appears that TSA possesses a narrow window of effective concentration at least in EC. Furthermore, these data demonstrate the importance of cell viability testing on the relevant cell type in drug development. Thus, the effects of HDAC inhibitors on angiogenesis need further investigation since complex regulatory mechanisms are presumed.

4.5 SSIQ for Testing Biocompatibility of Implant Materials and their Corrosion Products

The basic requirement for the long term success of implanted materials is biocompatibility. Biocompatibility is defined as the ability of a material to perform with an appropriate host response in a specific application. Wound healing, which is necessary after implantation, involves the processes of angiogenesis. Therefore, appropriate host responses in angiogenesis should not be impaired by an implanted material. If reduced angiogenesis in the peri-implant tissue should occur during the wound healing processes an impairment of implant stability could be a possible consequence.

We tested the effects of two metallic materials, polished cpTi- and Co28Cr6Mo-samples. Whereas angiogenesis on cpTi-surfaces evolved comparable to the positive control, the Co28Cr6Mo-surface induced a unique EC phenotype in that no CLS and a number of monolayer-like areas developed. We also tested possible corrosion products of the CoCr-alloy. Co^{2+}-ions induced an impairment of CLS-formation and Cr^{3+} did not induce any effects in angiogenesis in vitro. However, the monolayer-like EC phenotype developed on the Co28Cr6Mo-surface did not evolve.

This raises the question of which features of a metallic material can be recognized by cells and might be responsible for the deviations on the Co28Cr6Mo-alloy. A possible candidate could be Co^{2+}-ions, since these have been detected in the peri-implant tissues of CoCr-alloys in high concentrations ($\leq$0.9 mM) [38]. Co^{2+}-ions are known to induce a broad spectrum of alterations in (endothelial) cell function. This includes impairment of angiogenesis in vitro [16] and impairment of EC adhesion [39]. Furthermore, Co^{2+}-exposure leads to an NF-κB-dependent activation in EC [40]. In addition, Co^{2+} has been shown to be involved in the development of reactive oxygen species [41]. Long term exposure of Co^{2+} leads to the initiation of apoptosis in EC [39].

However, other aspects such as surface charge, thickness of the oxide layer, chemical composition of the outermost surface layer, corrosion behavior, protein adsorption and synergistic effects of different released metal ions may be involved in the varying cell response of these materials. These factors all influence each other in a complex way. Co28Cr6Mo and cpTi have different oxide layers, which differ both in thickness and composition [42-45]. Titanium exhibits a passive layer, which is electron non-conducting, whereas the Co28Cr6Mo passive layer is electron conducting [46]. Thus, different electrochemical reactions at the interface are possible. It is known that redox-reactions with biomolecules occur at metal-conducting passive layers, which change protein conformation and can lead to immunological reactions [46]. Whereas the oxide layer of titanium consists of TiO_2, TiO and Ti_2O_3 [42], the Co28Cr6Mo-alloy, consisting mainly of Cr_2O_3 with $CoCr_2O_4$ and CoO species [47], is known to release Co-ions and Cr- and Mo-oxides remain in the outermost layer [45]. Thus, the different compositions result in distinct surface charges (zeta potential), which influences the protein adsorption and at least the cell adhesion [44].

4.6 Conclusions

Our data show that the 3-dimensional in vitro model of angiogenesis described is highly sensitive to biological stimuli, is reproducible and the measurement of angiogenesis in vitro by SSIQ is a versatile, reliable tool in the quantification of angiogenesis-influencing effects. However, all in vitro models are merely an attempt to simplify the complex in vivo situation, and the models will inevitably show deviations from the in vivo situation. Nevertheless, the in vitro angiogenesis system described here has demonstrated responses to factors in vitro similar to known responses in vivo and therefore should be useful in basic research, pharmacological studies and biomaterial evaluation. In addition, models such as described should contribute to a reduction in animal experimentation.

Acknowledgements

This work was supported by the German Research Foundation (Deutsche Forschungsgemeinschaft), Priority Program "Biosystem" (322 1100). We want to thank Susanne Barth and Anne Sartoris for their excellent technical assistance and the Knoll AG, Ludwigshafen (Germany) for the generous gift of Arvin™. Furthermore, we wish to thank the Wilex AG (Munich, Germany) for allowing us to present the results of the WX-UK1 in vitro-angiogenesis study.

REFERENCES

[1] Cines, DB; Pollak, ES; Buck, CA; Loscalzo, J; Zimmerman, GA; McEver, RP; Pober, JS; Wick, TM; Konkle, BA; Schwartz, BS; Barnathan, ES; McCrae, KR; Hug, BA; Schmidt, AM; Stern, DM. Endothelial cells in physiology and in the pathophysiology of vascular disorders. *Blood,* 1998, 91, 3527-3561.

[2] Carmeliet, P. Angiogenesis in health and disease. *Nat Med,* 2003, 9, 653-660.

[3] Gerhardt, H; Betsholtz, C. Endothelial-pericyte interactions in angiogenesis. *Cell Tissue Res*, 2003, 314, 15-23.

[4] Jung, YD; Ahmad, SA; Liu, W; Reinmuth, N; Parikh, A; Stoeltzing, O; Fan, F; Ellis, LM. The role of the microenvironment and intercellular cross-talk in tumor angiogenesis. *Semin Cancer Biol,* 2002, 12, 105-112.

[5] Battegay, EJ. Angiogenesis: mechanistic insights, neovascular diseases, and therapeutic prospects. *J Mol Med*, 1995, 73, 333-346.

[6] Pepper, MS; Montesano, R; Mandriota, SJ; Orci, L; Vassalli, JD. Angiogenesis: a paradigm for balanced extracellular proteolysis during cell migration and morphogenesis. *Enzyme Protein*, 1996, 49, 138-162.

[7] Folkman, J. Fundamental concepts of the angiogenic process. *Curr Mol Med*, 2003, 3, 643-651.

[8] O'Reilly, MS; Wiederschain, D; Stetler-Stevenson, WG; Folkman, J; Moses, MA. Regulation of angiostatin production by matrix metalloproteinase-2 in a model of concomitant resistance. *J Biol Chem*, 1999, 274, 29568-29571.

[9] Korff, T; Augustin, HG. Integration of endothelial cells in multicellular spheroids prevents apoptosis and induces differentiation. *J Cell Biol*, 1998, 143, 1341-1352.

[10] Nehls, V; Drenckhahn, D. A novel, microcarrier-based in vitro assay for rapid and reliable quantification of three-dimensional cell migration and angiogenesis. *Microvasc Res,* 1995, 50, 311-322.

[11] Montesano, R; Orci, L; Vassalli, P. In vitro rapid organization of endothelial cells into capillary-like networks is promoted by collagen matrices. *J Cell Biol*, 1983, 97, 1648-1652.

[12] Folkman, J; Haudenschild, C. Angiogenesis in vitro. *Nature,* 1980, 288, 551-556.

[13] Kadish, JL; Butterfield, CE; Folkman, J. The effect of fibrin on cultured vascular endothelial cells. *Tissue Cell*, 1979, 11, 99-108.

[14] Auerbach, R; Lewis, R; Shinners, B; Kubai, L; Akhtar, N. Angiogenesis assays: a critical overview. *Clin Chem*, 2003, 49, 32-40.

[15] Peters, K; Schmidt, H; Unger, RE; Otto, M; Kamp, G; Kirkpatrick, CJ. Software-supported image quantification of angiogenesis in an in vitro culture system: application to studies of biocompatibility. *Biomaterials*, 2002, 23, 3413-3419.

[16] Peters, K; Schmidt, H; Unger, RE; Kamp, G; Prols, F; Berger, BJ; Kirkpatrick, CJ. Paradoxical effects of hypoxia-mimicking divalent cobalt ions in human endothelial cells in vitro. *Mol Cell Biochem*, 2005, 270, 157-166.

[17] Sturzebecher, J; Vieweg, H; Steinmetzer, T; Schweinitz, A; Stubbs, MT; Renatus, M; Wikstrom, P. 3-Amidinophenylalanine-based inhibitors of urokinase. *Bioorg Med Chem Lett,* 1999, 9, 3147-3152.

[18] Yoshida, M; Kijima, M; Akita, M; Beppu, T. Potent and specific inhibition of mammalian histone deacetylase both in vivo and in vitro by trichostatin A. *J Biol Chem*, 1990, 265, 17174-17179.

[19] Jung, M; Brosch, G; Kolle, D; Scherf, H; Gerhauser, C; Loidl, P. Amide analogues of trichostatin A as inhibitors of histone deacetylase and inducers of terminal cell differentiation. *J Med Chem*, 1999, 42, 4669-4679.

[20] Leung, DW; Cachianes, G; Kuang, WJ; Goeddel, DV; Ferrara, N. Vascular endothelial growth factor is a secreted angiogenic mitogen. *Science,* 1989, 246, 1306-1309.

[21] Ferrara, N; Gerber, HP; LeCouter, J. The biology of VEGF and its receptors. *Nat Med,* 2003, 9, 669-676.

[22] Keyt, BA; Berleau, LT; Nguyen, HV; Chen, H; Heinsohn, H; Vandlen, R; Ferrara, N. The carboxyl-terminal domain (111-165) of vascular endothelial growth factor is critical for its mitogenic potency. *J Biol Chem*, 1996, 271, 7788-7795.

[23] Szebenyi, G; Fallon, JF. Fibroblast growth factors as multifunctional signaling factors. *Int Rev Cytol,* 1999, 185, 45-106.

[24] Yancopoulos, GD; Davis, S; Gale, NW; Rudge, JS; Wiegand, SJ; Holash, J. Vascular-specific growth factors and blood vessel formation. *Nature*, 2000, 407, 242-248.

[25] Gajdusek, CM; Luo, Z; Mayberg, MR. Basic fibroblast growth factor and transforming growth factor beta-1: synergistic mediators of angiogenesis in vitro. *J Cell Physiol*, 1993, 157, 133-144.

[26] Kumar, R; Yoneda, J; Bucana, CD; Fidler, IJ. Regulation of distinct steps of angiogenesis by different angiogenic molecules. *Int J Oncol*, 1998, 12, 749-757.

[27] Pepper, MS; Ferrara, N; Orci, L; Montesano, R. Potent synergism between vascular endothelial growth factor and basic fibroblast growth factor in the induction of angiogenesis in vitro. *Biochem Biophys Res Commun*, 1992, 189, 824-831.

[28] Asahara, T; Bauters, C; Zheng, LP; Takeshita, S; Bunting, S; Ferrara, N; Symes, JF; Isner, JM. Synergistic effect of vascular endothelial growth factor and basic fibroblast growth factor on angiogenesis in vivo. *Circulation*, 1995, 92, II365-371.

[29] Pugh, CW; Ratcliffe, PJ. Regulation of angiogenesis by hypoxia: role of the HIF system. *Nat Med*, 2003, 9, 677-684.

[30] Li, J; Shworak, NW; Simons, M. Increased responsiveness of hypoxic endothelial cells to FGF2 is mediated by HIF-1alpha-dependent regulation of enzymes involved in synthesis of heparan sulfate FGF2-binding sites. *J Cell Sci*, 2002, 115, 1951-1959.

[31] Gerber, HP; Condorelli, F; Park, J; Ferrara, N. Differential transcriptional regulation of the two vascular endothelial growth factor receptor genes. Flt-1, but not Flk-1/KDR, is up-regulated by hypoxia. *J Biol Chem*, 1997, 272, 23659-23667.

[32] Ertongur, S; Lang, S; Mack, B; Wosikowski, K; Muehlenweg, B; Gires, O. Inhibition of the invasion capacity of carcinoma cells by WX-UK1, a novel synthetic inhibitor of the urokinase-type plasminogen activator system. *Int J Cancer*, 2004, 110, 815-824.

[33] Mazar, AP; Henkin, J; Goldfarb, RH. The urokinase plasminogen activator system in cancer: implications for tumor angiogenesis and metastasis. *Angiogenesis*, 1999, 3, 15-32.

[34] Jung, M. Inhibitors of histone deacetylase as new anticancer agents. *Curr Med Chem*, 2001, 8, 1505-1511.

[35] Zeng, L; Zhang, Y; Chien, S; Liu, X; Shyy, JY. The role of p53 deacetylation in p21Waf1 regulation by laminar flow. *J Biol Chem*, 2003, 278, 24594-24599.

[36] Deroanne, CF; Lapiere, CM; Nusgens, BV. In vitro tubulogenesis of endothelial cells by relaxation of the coupling extracellular matrix-cytoskeleton. *Cardiovasc Res*, 2001, 49, 647-658.

[37] Rossig, L; Li, H; Fisslthaler, B; Urbich, C; Fleming, I; Forstermann, U; Zeiher, AM; Dimmeler, S. Inhibitors of histone deacetylation downregulate the expression of endothelial nitric oxide synthase and compromise endothelial cell function in vasorelaxation and angiogenesis. *Circ Res*, 2002, 91, 837-844.

[38] Blumenthal, NC; Cosma, V; Jaffe, W; Stuchin, S. A new technique for quantitation of metal particulates and metal reaction products in tissues near implants. *J Appl Biomater*, 1994, 5, 191-193.

[39] Peters, K; Unger, RE; Barth, S; Gerdes, T; Kirkpatrick, CJ. Induction of apoptosis in human microvascular endothelial cells by divalent cobalt ions. Evidence for integrin-mediated signaling via the cytoskeleton. *J Mater Sci Mater Med*, 2001, 12, 955-958.

[40] Wagner, M; Klein, CL; van Kooten, TG; Kirkpatrick, CJ. Mechanisms of cell activation by heavy metal ions. *J Biomed Mater Res,* 1998, 42, 443-452.

[41] Yamamoto, K; Inoue, S; Yamazaki, A; Yoshinaga, T; Kawanishi, S. Site-specific DNA damage induced by cobalt(II) ion and hydrogen peroxide: role of singlet oxygen. *Chem Res Toxicol*, 1989, 2, 234-239.

[42] Okazaki, Y; Tateishi, T; Ito, Y. Corrosion resistance of implant alloys in pseudo physiological solution and role of alloying elements in passive films. *Mater Trans*, 1997, 38, 78-84.

[43] Okazaki, Y; Gotoh, E. Comparison of metal release from various metallic biomaterials in vitro. *Biomaterials,* 2005, 26, 11-21.

[44] Hanawa, T; Hiromoto, S; Asami, K. Characterization of the surface oxide film of a CoCrMo alloy after being located in quasi-biological environments using XPS. *Appl Surf Sci*, 2001, 183, 68-75.

[45] Hanawa, T. Metal ion release from metal implants. *Mat Sci Eng C,* 2004, 24, 745-752.

[46] Thull, R (1998). *Tissue-implant interaction. In Metals as biomaterials*, J. A. Helsen, and H. J. Breme, eds. (New York), pp. 291-313.

[47] Strandman, E; Landt, H. Oxidation resistance of dental chromium-cobalt alloys. *Quintessence Dent Technol*, 1982, 6, 67-74.

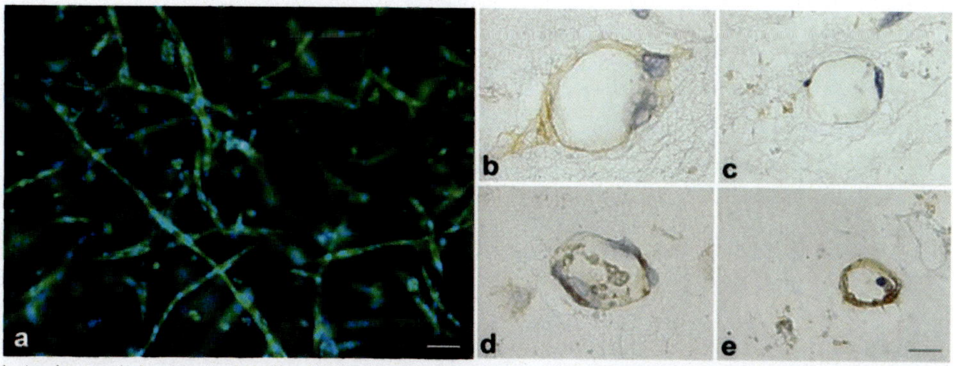

Fig. 1. Angiogenesis in vitro (induced by VEGF/bFGF). a) digital overlay of a vital and a nuclear staining (green: vital staining, blue: nuclear staining, scale bar: 200 µm). b-e) lumen formation in angiogenesis in vitro (immunocytochemical staining for the endothelial marker CD31 (brown) and nuclei (blue); light gray fibrils: ECM; scale bar: 50 µm). Results shown are from one representative donor. Similar patterns were observed with other HDMEC donors.

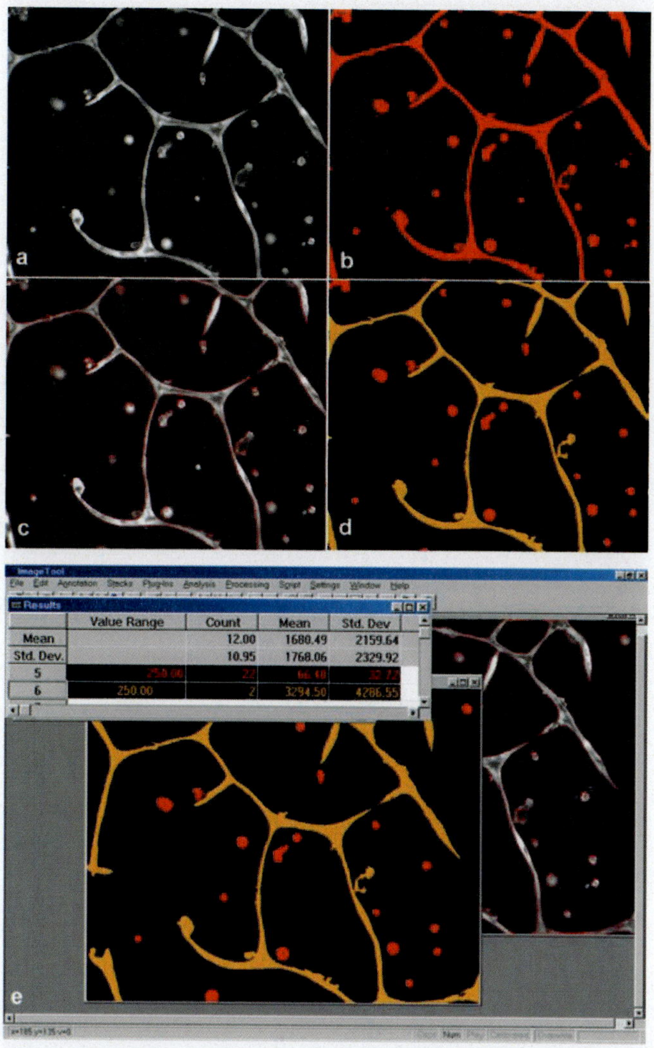

Fig. 2. Pattern identification in angiogenesis in vitro by IT. a) original image of a positive control (bFGF/VEGF-stimulated cells), b) marked objects (red) after using the "find object" command, c) object identification and counting, d) object classification (objects with perimeter below 250 pixels: red; objects with perimeter above 250 pixels: orange), e) calculation after classification (screen shot).

In: Trends in Angiogenesis Research
Editor: Roberta V. Zubar, pp. 125-138

ISBN 1-59454-452-2

Chapter V

Restin, a Potent Angiogenesis Inhibitor Derived from Type XV Collagen

Ren Xu* and Ren-Bao Gan

[1]Institute of Biochemistry and Cell Biology, Shanghai Institute of Biological Sciences, Chinese Academy of Sciences, ShangHai, China

Abstract

Extracellular matrix (ECM) has been found to be involved in the regulation of angiogenesis, thus making ECM a candidate source of angiogenesis inhibitors. Recently several angiogenesis inhibitors have been identified from ECM components, including endostain, restin, tumstatin, canstatin, and vastatin. Restin, which is highly homologous to endostatin, is derived from the C terminus of collagen XV. Here we show that purified recombinant restin specifically inhibits the proliferation of BAE cells stimulated by basic fibroblast growth factor (bFGF) in a dose-dependent manner. Treatment with recombinant restin can also induce apoptosis in the BAE cells. A human hepatoma cell line, overexpressing secreted restin, was subcutaneously injected into nude mice; the growth of the restin-expressing tumors was much slower than that of control tumors. These data indicate that restin is able to inhibit angiogenesis both *in vitro* and *in vivo*, and that it also has a potential anti-tumor activity.

Key words: angiogenesis inhibitor; restin; collagen XV; extracellular matrix; anti-tumor

---

* Correspondence concerning this article should be addressed to Dr. Ren Xu. Present address: Life Science Division, Lawrence Berkeley National Laboratory, 1 Cyclotron Road, 977 R225A, Berkeley, CA 94706, USA. E-mail address: rxu@lbl.gov. Tel: 01-510-4864368; Fax: 01-510-4865586.

INTRODUCTION

Extracellular matrix (ECM) is a complex mixture of proteins that surround cells providing both chemical and mechanical support to maintain tissue function in mammals (Badylak, 2002). ECM contains collagen, laminin, elastin, fibronectin, and proteoglycans. The components of ECM are variable from one tissue to another; thus ECM allows the formation of distinct microenvironments that act to regulate cell proliferation and differentiation in different tissue, in addition to providing a scaffold for cell attachment and migration.

The relationship between ECM and angiogenesis has been investigated for decades with culturing endothelial cell. Banerjee and his colleagues showed that endothelial cells form capillary-like structure when the cells are plated on collagen (Banerjee et al., 1985). The research of Hsieh P has demonstrated that ECM isolated from chick embryo fibroblast or human and rabbit corneal stromal cells induces polarization and elongation of the corneal endothelial cells in culture (Hsieh and Baum, 1985). These studies suggest that the tissue-morphogenesis of endothelial cells depends on the ECM signals. Integrins expressed on endothelial cells act as receptors for ECM molecules, such as collagen and laminin. Additionally, integrins also severed as a linker between extracellular matrix and cell cytoskeleton (Lawler et al., 1988). Signal cascades induced by ligand-integrin binding regulate the migration and proliferation of endothelial cells, as well as controlling the morphology of the cells and cytoskeleton.

ECM also regulates angiogenesis by sequestering angiogenic growth factors. Vascular endothelial growth factor (VEGF), also know as vascular permeability factor (VPF), which has five isoforms and has been implicated in tumor-associated angiogenesis. All the VEGF isoforms, except $VEGF_{121}$, can bind to heparin in the ECM, and these isoforms may dissociate slowly from the ECM providing prolonged angiogenic stimulation or be released from the ECM as a result of the activity of proteases (Houck et al., 1992) (Poltorak et al., 1997). Basic fibroblast growth factor (bFGF), another angiogenesis regulator, also has heparin-binding activity. Although the binding between bFGF and the heparin is not directly involved in regulating the function of endothelial cells, heparin may serve as a carrier molecular for bFGF, and facilitate the distribution of bFGF while protecting it from degradation (Moscatelli, 1988).

One important step of angiogenesis involves degradation of the ECM surrounding pre-existing vessels, facilitating the migration of endothelial cell toward an angiogenic stimulus and the proliferation of endothelial cell. During this process, growth factors, such as VEGF and bFGF, are released from the ECM; meanwhile angiogenesis inhibitors are also generated. The identification of angiogenesis inhibitor endostatin revealed that ECM plays an important role in the negative control of angiogenesis. Endostatin, originally purified from hemangioendothelioma conditioned media, specifically inhibits endothelial proliferation and migration *in vitro*, and potently inhibits angiogenesis and tumor growth in nude mice (O'Reilly et al., 1997). N-terminal amino acid sequencing demonstrated that endostain corresponds to a 185 amino acid C-terminus fragment of the collagen XVIII alpha 1 chain; furthermore, cathepsin L was shown to be responsible for the generation of endostatin with the predicted N-terminus (Felbor et al., 2000).

Ramchandran's and our group have identified restin, a highly homologous domain from collagen XV, by searching the protein databases using the endostatin protein sequence. Restin is composed of 184 amino acids, from the C terminal non-collagenous (NC) domain of collagen XV (Ramchandran et al., 1999; Xu et al., 2002). The comparison between collagen XVIII and collagen XV indicates that the two proteins have similar structure and function. Both type XVIII collagen and type XV collagen are localized in the basement membrane, which is a specialized form of ECM underneath of endothelial and epithelial cells (Kalluri, 2003). Type XV collagen is composed of 1363 amino acids, and contains a highly interrupted collagenous region of 577 residues, and non-collagenous amino- and carboxyl-terminal domains of 530 and 256 residues respectively (Myers et al., 1996). Type XV collagen is present in many human tissues and is associated with vascular, neural and mesenchymal basement membrane zones (Hagg et al., 1997). Collagen XV null mice had capillary degradation present in the tissues where type XV collagen normally resides in the endothelia, this effect being particularly prominent in the heart and skeletal muscle (Eklund et al., 2001). Amenta *et al* also found that the lost of type XV collagen is associated with the development of invasive breast tumours (Amenta et al., 2003). Taken together, these studies suggest that the expression of type XV collagen contributes to angiogenesis through inducing the formation or maintaining the function of capillaries.

In this study, we investigated the biological activity of mouse restin *in vitro* and *in vivo*. Treatment of BAE cells with recombinant restin specifically inhibits proliferation stimulated by basic fibroblast growth factor (bFGF). FITC-Annexin V binding assays showed that recombinant restin also induces apoptosis in the BAE cells. To determine the protein activity *in vivo*, a human hepatoma cell line was transfected with a secretory expression plasmid containing the restin gene. The growth of the tumor formed by these cells was measured and the growth of the tumors expressing restin was much slower than that of control tumors. These data suggest that restin is an angiogenesis inhibitor both *in vitro* and *in vivo*, and that the protein also has a potential anti-tumor activity.

Material and Methods

Plasmids and cell lines pQE32 (Qiagen); pcDNA3 (Invitrogen). E.*coli* DH5α and E. *coli* M15 (Qiagen). Cell line: Bovine aortic endothelial (BAE) cells (primary cells isolated from bovine aorta); hepatoma cell line Bel7404 (provided by Professor Mujun Zhao).

cDNA amplification and Plasmid construction Total RNA was extracted using TRIZOL reagent (GIBCO BRL) from Mouse fresh muscle. Then, the restin cDNA was generated from the RNA sample using Superscript^{TM} RNase H$^-$ transcriptase (GIBCO BRL) according to the manufacturer's instructions. PCR was performed with Ex-Taq DNA polymerase (TaKaRa) according to the manufacturer's instructions. The synthetic oligonucleotides were obtained from Shanghai Sangon Co. Ltd. (Shanghai China). The primers used were as follows: sense primer: 5'ATTTTAAGTGCCAACTATGAGAGGCCT.3'; anti sense primer 5'TTATTACTTCCTAGTGTCTGTCATGAA AC 3', two stop codens were included in the antisense primer. The amplified cDNA fragment was ligated into the vector pQE32 (Qiagen), resulting in the construction of an *Escherichia coli* expression plasmid pQEXV. To make the secretory mammalian cell expression plasmid for restin, the restin gene was fused to human plasminogen signal peptide sequence by PCR, and then cloned into eukaryotic expression vector pcDNA3. Both of the recombinant plasmids were proved to be correct by sequencing.

Purification and refolding of recombinant Restin from E.coli After recombinant plasmid pQEXV was transformed into E. *coli* M15 (Qiagen), restin expression was induced by 1 mM IPTG. After centrifugation, the cell pellet was resuspended in 20 mM Tris-HCl, pH8.0, 50 mM KCl, 0.5 mM EDTA, 5mM DTT and lysozyme was added to the final concentration of 0.5 mg/ml. The cells were incubated at 4° C for 30 min, then were disrupted by sonic homogenizer for 10 sec for ten times with 30 sec interval each time. After centrifugation at 4° C, 15000 g for 30 min, the pellet was collected and resuspended in 8 M urea, 0.1 M NaH_2PO_4, 10 mM Tris-HCl, pH8.0. Centrifuged again, the supernatant was loaded on a Ni^{2+}-nitrilotriacetic acid-agarose column (Qiagen). The recombinant protein was eluted from the column according to the manufacturer's instructions. To achieve refolding, the purified protein was adjusted to pH8.0 and DTT was added to the final concentration of 10 mM. Following incubation at room temperature for 2 hours, the solution was added to refolding buffer (0.1 M Tris-HCl, pH 8.0, 0.5 M arginine, 5 mM EDTA, 1 mM GSSG, 5 mM GSH) with the ratio of 1:200 (v/v). After 24 hours incubation at room temperature, the soluble protein was dialyzed against PB buffer (10mM Na_2HPO_4, 10mM NaH_2PO_4, PH 7.2) for 24-48 hours.

Bovine aortic endothelial cell proliferation and migration assays Bovine aortic endothelial cells were maintained in DMEM supplemented with 10% heat-inactivated FCS. Monolayer of BAE cells growing in 60-mm dish were dispersed in 0.05% trypsin solution. Cells were resuspended in DMEM containing 2% FCS. Approximately 3000 cells in 200 μl were plated into each well of 96-well tissue culture plates and incubated at 37° C (in 5% CO_2). Cells adhered to the plate for about 12 hours. The medium was replaced with 200 μl of fresh DMEM containing 2% FCS, 5 ng/ml bFGF; at the same time, different concentrations of recombinant restin or endostatin were added to each well. After 72 hours' incubation, 10 μl MTT (100 mg/ml) was added to each well and incubated for another 4 hours at 37° C, 5% CO_2.. The absorbency of A_{570nm}, which correlates to the number of cells, was measured with microplate reader (Model 450, Bio-Rad).

To check whether the recombinant restin suppresses BAE cell migration induced by bFGF, migration assays were performed using transwell membrane (8 μm pore size) in 24 well plates (Corning/Costar). BAE cells were diluted in DMEM containing 2% FBS, and 1.0×10^4 cells were seeded on upper chamber wells. After the cells adhered to the upper chamber well, bFGF was added (10 ng/ml) to the medium in lower chamber, and recombinant restin and endostatin were added (2 μg/ml) in the upper chamber. The chamber was incubated at 37℃ with 5% CO_2 for 12 h. After discarding the non-migrated cells and washing the upper chambers with PBS, the membrane was fixed in methanol, and the migrated cells were dyed with 0.2% trypan blue. Cells of three fields in each well were counted on an Olympus microscope. The results were expressed as mean±SEM, and statistical significance was accessed by student's unpaired *t* test, with $p<0.05$ consider significant.

Annexin V-FITC binding assay Annexin V-FITC (CLONTECH, Palo Alto, CA) binding assays were performed according to the manufacturer's instructions. 2.5×10^5 cells were plated in a 60 mm dish in DMEM containing 10% FCS. After 24 h incubation at 37℃, 5% CO_2, the medium was changed with DMEM supplement with 2% FCS, 2 μg/ml recombinant restin or endostatin. After 24 hours of treatment, the medium containing detached cells was collected, and attached cells were trypsinized, combined with detached cells and centrifuged at 3,000 × *g*. Then the cells were washed with PBS and resuspended in binding buffer (10 mM HEPES/NaOH, pH 7.4, 140 mM NaCl, 2.5 mM $CaCl_2$). Annexin V-FITC was added to a final concentration of 100 ng/ml, and the cells were incubated in the dark for 10 min. 10 μl of propidium iodide (PI) was added to each sample before flow cytometric analysis. For each sample, minimums of 10000 cells were counted. Data analysis was performed with standard Cell Quest software.

Stable transfection of Bel7404 cell line The human hepatoma cell line Bel7404 was growth in DMEM containing 5% FBS. The cells were transfected with pcDNAXV and pCDNA3 by Lipofectin Reagent (Gibcol BRL) according to the manufacturer's instructions. Briefly, after Bel7404 cells were cultured on 6-well plates to 60% confluence, 3 μg of pCDNAXV and pCDNA3 was mixed with lipofectamine and added to the serum-free medium. The medium was then changed with fresh growth medium containing 600 μg/ml of G418 in 24 hours. After two weeks of selection, the stable transfectants were isolated and amplified. The transcription of restin in stable transfected cells was tested by RT-PCR and western-blot, with pCDNA3 transfected cells as a negative control. The expression and secretion of restin were detected by western-blot. The conditioned medium of the stable tansfectants was concentrated with Centricon (Amicon), and then the proteins were separated on a 15% SDS-PAGE gel. After the proteins were transferred to nitrocellulose membrane, rabbit anti-endostain serum was used to do the western blotting as the first antibody.

Proliferation assay of stable transfectants The stable transfectants were plated in 96-well plates at 3000 cells per well. MTT assay was performed as described above from the first day to the sixth day after the cells were plated; three wells of each transfectant were analyzed everyday.

Nude mice experiment Stable transfected 7404 cells were growth in 100 mm dish to 90% confluence. After trypsinization, the cells were resuspended in PBS, and 2 million cells were subcutaneously injected into 4-week-old male nude mice (n=5). About 7 days later, tumors formed under the skin. The diameter of the tumor was measured every two days, and the volume of the tumor was calculated by standard formula, $\text{length} \times \text{width}^2 \times 0.52$, as described before (Banerjee et al., 1985).

RESULTS

Cloning the Restin Gene into Prokaryotic and Eukaryotic Expression Vectors. The mouse restin cDNA was amplified by RT-PCR from mouse muscle total RNA. The cDNA encodes 184 amino acids corresponding to the amino acids 1132 to 1315 of collagen XV. The amplified cDNA fragment was cloned into the *E.coli* expression vector pQE32, with six histidines and two stop codes before and after the gene respectively. The expression of recombinant protein in E.*Coli* was regulated by T5 promoter. To obtain the secreting expression of restin in mammalian cells, the restin gene was fused to human plasminogen signal peptide sequence by PCR; and then, the gene was cloned into eukaryotic expression vector pcDNA3 to get pcDNAXV. DNA sequencing indicated that the desired plasmids had been obtained.

Purification and characterization of mouse Restin. Recombinant his-tagged mouse restin was expressed in E.coli and purified using a Ni^{2+}-nitrilotriacetic acid-agarose column and then was refolded *in vitro*. Under reducing conditions, recombinant restin migrated in SDS-PAGE with the molecular mass 22 kDa, consistent with the predicted molecular mass (Figure 1).

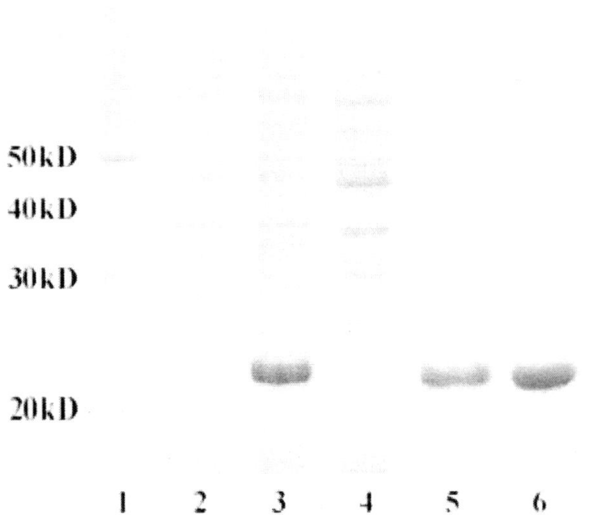

Figure 1. 15% SDS-PAGE analysis the expression and purification of the recombinant restin (Coomassie blue stains); 1, molecular weight marker; 2, uninduced cells; 3, induced cells; 4, soluble protein; 5, insoluble protein; 6, purified protein.

Recombinant restin inhibits BAE cell proliferation and migration BAE cells were derived from fetal bovine aorta, and were able to survive and proliferate on plastic in 10% FBS without any specific growth factor. After the BAE cells were plated on 96-well plates for 24 hours, the cells were incubated with different concentrations of recombinant restin and endostatin for 3 days. MTT assay results showed that the proliferation of BAE cells was inhibited by restin in a dose-dependent manner, however, the inhibitory activity of restin was lower than that of endostatin (Figure 2A). We did not observe any inhibitory activities on fibroblast cell line Balb/3T3 (data not shown), so the inhibitory activity of recombinant restin was specific to endothelial cells. Furthermore, FACS analysis demonstrated that treatment of BAE cells with restin caused a cell cycle arrest mainly in G_0/G_1 phase and a decreased cell number in S phase (data not shown). Morphological changes of BAE cells were also observed in restin-treated endothelial cells; the cells were elongated and formed spindle-like structures.

To investigate whether restin can inhibit the migration of BAE cells, migration assays were performed in transwell (8 μm pore size) (Corning/Costar). After the cells attached to the upper chamber filter, bFGF and recombinant protein were added to the medium and incubated for 12 hours. bFGF induced the migration of endothelial cells, while this induction was significantly inhibited by recombinant restin and endostatin (Fig. 2B). In consistent with the proliferation assay results, the inhibitory activity of restin for migration is lower than that of endostain.

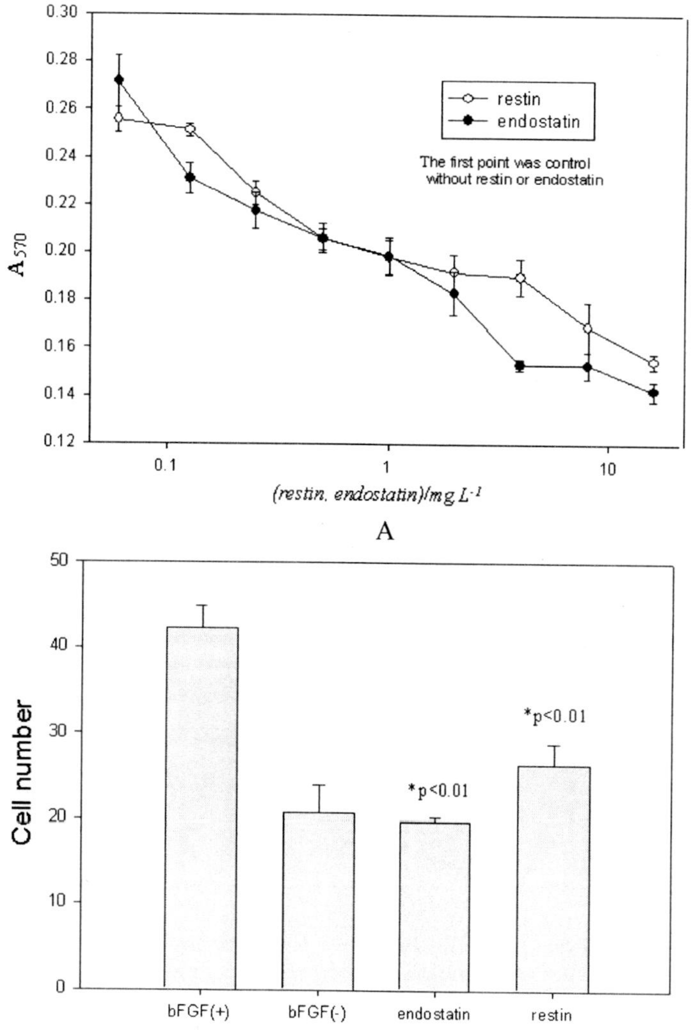

B

Figure 2 . Recombinant mouse restin and endostatin inhibit the proliferation and migration of BAE cells stimulated by bFGF. A) MTT assays detect the inhibitory activity of recombinant restin in BAE cells. BAE cells were plated in 96 well plates, after 72 hours treatment with restin and endostatin, 10 μl MTT (100 mg/ml) was added to each well, and the absorbance of A_{570nm} was measured with a microplate reader (Model 450, Bio-Rad). Values represent the means of triplicates (n=3). B) Migration assays. After 1.0×10^4 BAE cells were plated and attached on the upper chamber membrane, bFGF was added (10 ng/ml) in lower-chamber medium, and recombinant restin and endostatin were added (2 μg/ml) in upper-chamber medium. After 12 hours incubation, the migrated cells were dyed with trypan blue and counted. The results were expressed as mean±SEM, and statistical significance was assessed by student's unpaired *t* test, with $p<0.01$ consider significant.

Annexin V-FITC binding assays After the initiation of apoptosis, phosphatidyl-serine (PS) is translocated from cytoplamic face of the plasma membrane to the cell surface; therefore, PS is used as an early apoptosis marker for many cell types. Annexin V has a strong affinity for PS and serves as a probe for detecting apoptosis (Koopman et al., 1994). In this assay, BAE cells were first treated with recombinant restin and endostatin for 24 h, then the Annexin V-FITC labeled cells were counted by FACS analysis. The results demonstrated that the recombinant proteins induced a significant shift in fluorescence intensity, indicating that the BAE cells underwent apoptosis (Figure 3). The apoptosis induced by restin was lower than the amount of apoptosis induced by endostain at the same protein concentration.

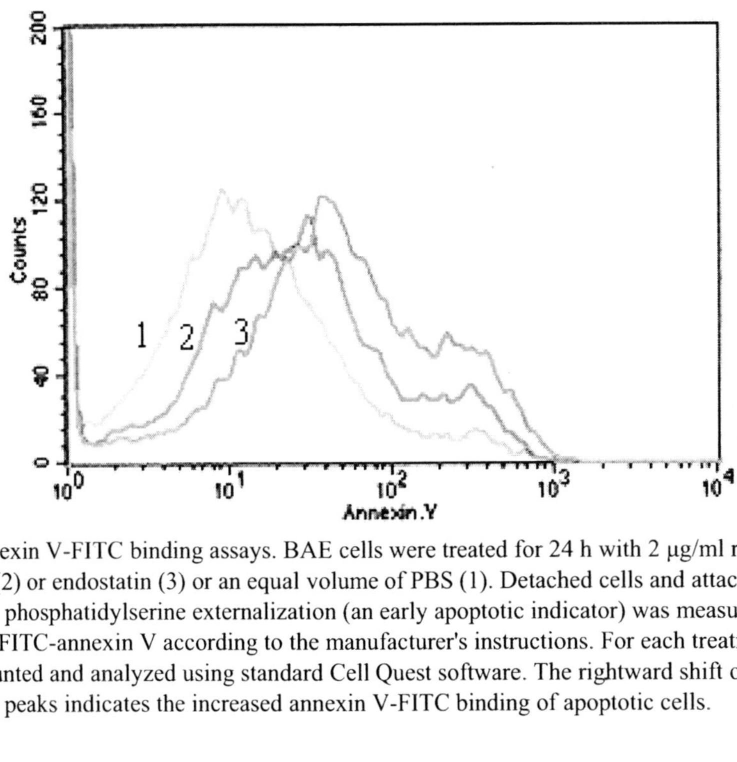

Figure 3. Annexin V-FITC binding assays. BAE cells were treated for 24 h with 2 μg/ml recombinant mouse restin (2) or endostatin (3) or an equal volume of PBS (1). Detached cells and attached cells were collected, and phosphatidylserine externalization (an early apoptotic indicator) was measured by labeling with FITC-annexin V according to the manufacturer's instructions. For each treatment, 10,000 cells were counted and analyzed using standard Cell Quest software. The rightward shift on the x axis of the 2 and 3 peaks indicates the increased annexin V-FITC binding of apoptotic cells.

Stable transfected hepatoma cell line Bel7404 establishment Human hepatoma cell line Bel 7404 can form tumors after subcutaneous injection into the mice, and was used here for the *in vivo* study. The Bel7404 cells were transfected with the secretion expression plasmid pCDNAXV, and pCDNA3 was transfected as a negative control. After two weeks selection with G418, the stable transfectants were isolated and amplified for the sequent experiments.

RT-PCR and western blot were used to check the transcription and secretion of recombinant restin in the stable transfected cells. Total RNA was extracted from pCDNAXV stable transfected cells (Bel7404R cells) and control cells (Bel7404C cells, transfected with pCDNA3), and RT-PCR result showed that murine restin gene was expressed only in the Bel7404R cells (Figure 4A). The conditioned media of Bel7404R and Bel7404C cells was concentrated, and proteins in the media were checked by Western-blotting to confirm restin expression and secretion. Results showed that restin was expressed and secreted in Bel7404R cells (Figure 4B). These stably transfected cell lines were used in the further experiments to detect the biological activity of restin in nude mice.

Proliferation assay of the stable transfected cell lines The Bel7404R and Bel7404C cells, stably transfected with pCDNAXV or pCDNA3, were plated into 96-well plate. Then the number of the cell was measured from the first day to sixth day by MTT assays. The proliferation curves of stable transfectants were calculated by Sigma-plot. We did not detect any differences in the proliferation rates between the cell line Bel7404R and Bel7404C in culture, and no morphology changes in the cell lines were detected following transfection (Figure 4C). These data suggest that the expression and secretion of restin in Bel7404 cells do not directly inhibit the proliferation of the hepatoma cell.

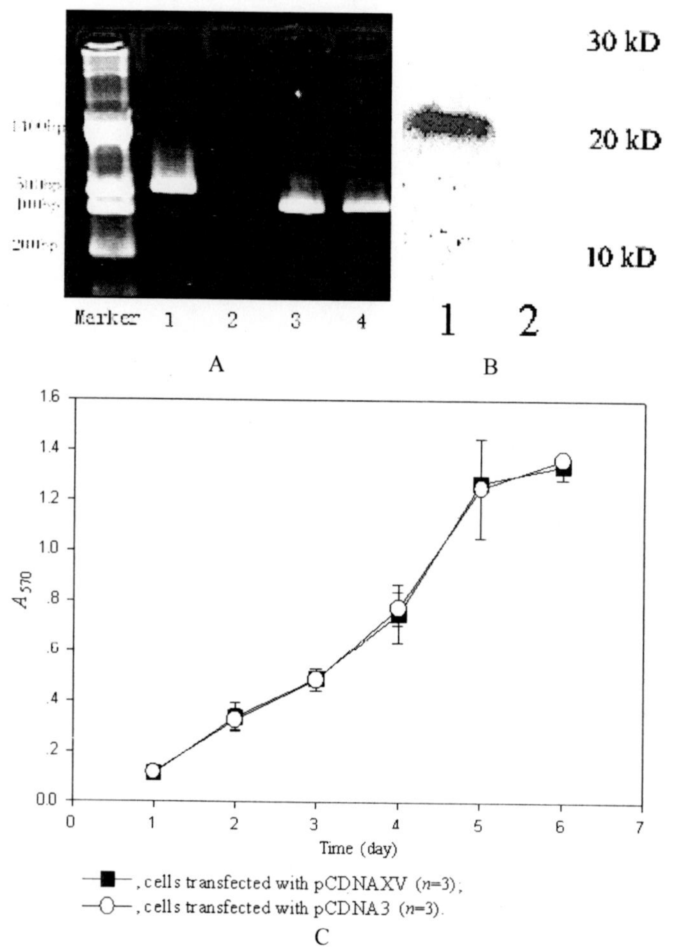

Figure 4. A) RT-PCR check the transcription of restin in stably transfected Bel7404 cells; lane 1 and lane 2 are the PCR products amplified from cDNA sample of 7404R and 7404C cell with restin primers; lane 3 and lane 4 are the PCR products amplified with GAPDH primers. B), Restin expression and secretion was detected by western blot using anti-endostatin antibody after the condition medium of the stable transfected cells was concentrated; 1, condition medium of Bel7404R cells; 2, conditioned medium of Bel7404C cells. C) Growth curve of Bel7404R and Bel7404C cells; the cells were plated into 96-well plates, and the number of the cell was measured from the first day to sixth day by MTT assay. Values represent the means of three wells (n=3).

Tumor model in nude mice Bel7404R and Bel7404C cells were plated on 100 mm tissue culture plates. After the cells were trypsinized and resuspended in PBS, 2.0X10^6 cells were injected into nude mice subcutaneously. Tumors formed under the mice skin after 7 days, and volume of the tumors was measured and calculated using standard formula: length$\times$width$^2\times$0. 52 (Banerjee et al., 1985). Comparing the tumor growth rate from the two groups, we observed that the tumors formed by Bel7404R cells grew much slower than the control group (Figure 5A). The significant difference of tumor volumes between the two groups was first detected 12 days after injection. Based on these results, restin does not inhibit the tumor formation under mice skin, and does not suppress tumor growth until tumor volume is beyond 30 mm^3. These observations might be explained by the fact that tumor formation and the initial growth of the tumor are not dependent on the angiogenesis.

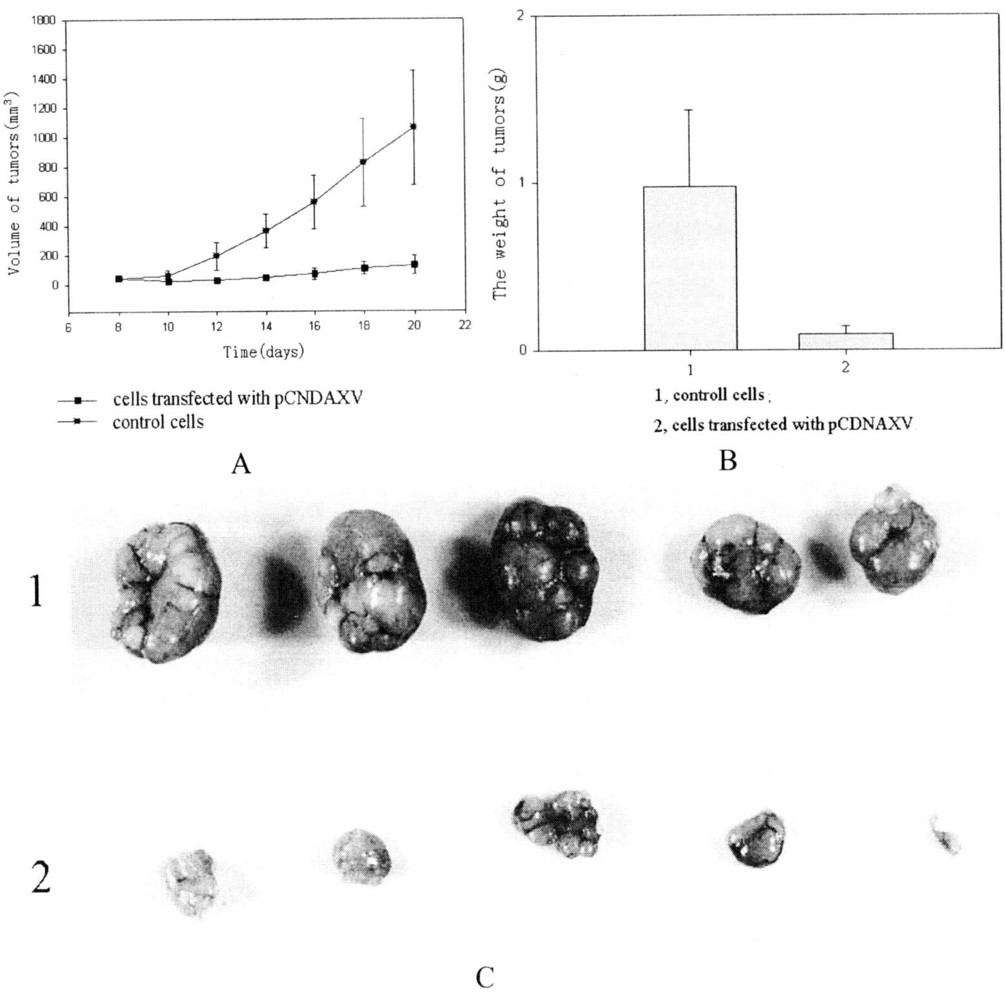

Figure 5. A) The growth curve of tumor in nude mice. The diameter of the tumor was measured every two days after Bel7404R and Bel7404C cells were subcutaneously injected into nude mice and formed tumors under mice skin, and the tumor volume was calculated by standard formula: length$\times$width$^2\times$0. 52. B) The weight of tumor was measured after the mice were sacrificed. C) 1, the tumors formed by Bel7404C cells; 2, the tumors formed by Bel7404R cells.

DISCUSSION

At least five angiogenesis inhibitors originating from collagens have been identified in the last decade. They are endostatin, which derived from type XVIII collagen; tumstatin, derived from alpha3 chain of type IV collagen; canstatin, a fragment of the alpha2 chain of type IV collagen; vastatin, the C-terminus of type VIII collagen; restin, a protein homologous to endostatin derived from type XV collagen (Kamphaus et al., 2000; O'Reilly et al., 1997; Ramchandran et al., 1999; Xu et al., 2002; Xu et al., 2001). Endostatin, tumstatin, and vastatin have been shown to inhibit endothelial cell proliferation and migration *in vitro*. However, Ramchandran *et al.* showed that recombinant human restin only inhibited endothelial cell line ECV304 migration *in vitro*, but no inhibitory activity for the proliferation of endothelial cells (Ramchandran et al., 1999).

In the present study, we tested the biological activity of recombinant mouse restin on BAE cells. We first investigated whether mouse restin inhibits the proliferation and migration of endothelial cells. In contrast to previous report, our results showed that recombinant mouse restin specifically inhibited the proliferation of BAE cells (Figure 2), although the activity was lower than that of endostatin; furthermore, we also noticed the cell cycle was arrested mainly at G_0/G_1 by treatment with restin. We also found that the recombinant protein inhibited the migration of endothelial cells, as previously shown by Ramchandran. Two possibilities may explain the discrepancy between our results and previous report. Alignment analysis demonstrates that 15% of amino acids are different between mouse and human restin; therefore, the structure and function of mouse and human restin may be slightly different. The other possibility is that the biological activity of restin may be different in different endothelial cell lines; primary BAE cells were used here, and C-PAE cells were used in Ramchandran study.

Since endostatin and tumstatin were found to induce endothelial cell apoptosis *in vitro*, we further tested whether mouse restin also induced apoptosis in BAE cells. Our results showed that BAE cells underwent apoptosis after 24 hours treatment with the recombinant protein. Comparing the *in-vitro* biological activity of recombinant restin and endostatin, we found that both specifically inhibit the proliferation and migration of endothelial cells, and induce cell apoptosis; however, the anti-angiogenesis activity of restin is less than that of endostatin.

How restin inhibits the proliferation and induces apoptosis is still undefined. However, studies with endostatin and tumstatin provide us with interesting clues to guide future research. Sudhakar and Wickstrom have studied the integrin binding ability of endostatin and tumstatin. They found that tumstatin binds to $\alpha v\beta 3$ integrin in a RGD peptide independent manner, whereas endostatin competes with RGD peptide to bind $\alpha 5\beta 1$ integrin (Sudhakar et al., 2003; Wickstrom et al., 2002). Furthermore, Endostatin treatment induces disassembly of focal adhesions and actin stress fibers, and disturbs the deposition of the fibronectin matrix through a mechanism involving Src and tyrosyl phosphatase activity (Wickstrom et al., 2002). As restin is highly homologous to endostatin, we speculate that it might inhibit endothelial cell proliferation and migration through binding to integrins. So it is important to identify which type of integrin is the receptor of restin in the future.

It is well documented that solid tumor growth and metastasis is dependent on angiogenesis to provide oxygen and nutrition; and therefore, some antiangiogenic agents have been used to suppress caner growth and metastasis (Albo et al., 2004). Both endostatin and tumstatin have been shown to inhibit the growth and metastasis of different types of solid tumor in nude mice (Kamphaus et al., 2000; O'Reilly et al., 1997). In addition to detecting the anti-angiogenesis activity of restin *in vitro*, we also investigated whether restin can repress tumor growth by inhibiting angiogenesis in nude mice.

The usual method to detect the anti-tumor activity of angiogenesis inhibitors *in vivo* is subcutaneous injecting the recombinant protein after tumor is established in mice. However, using this method requires large amounts of recombinant protein, because the dose for mice experiments is about 1-10 mg/kg/day (O'Reilly et al., 1997). To avoid the time consuming process of collecting recombinant protein, we have constructed a eukaryotic expression plasmid containing the restin gene. To ensure that restin can be expressed and secreted out of eukaryotic cells, the gene was fused with a signal peptide. This technique has been used to research angiogenesis stimulators, such as VEGF and FGF4 *in vivo* (Kurebayashi et al., 1993; Zhang et al., 1995). After the plasmid was stably transfected into Bel7404 cells, we injected the cells into nude mice subcutaneously. Although both control cells and the cells secreting restin form tumors after one week (suggesting that the expression of restin has no effect upon the tumorigenic ability of Bel7404 cells); the growth of the tumors secreting restin is much slower than the control tumors (as shown in figure 5). These results suggest that restin is able to suppress tumor growth by inhibiting angiogenesis *in vivo*. It also suggests that the technique used in this study might be applicable to test the anti-angiogenesis activity of other proteins *in vivo*. Compared with traditional methods (subcutaneously injection of recombinant protein), this technique has the following advantages: first the time consuming process of expression and purification of the recombinant protein is avoided; second the inhibitor is secreted by tumor cells, thus it can specific inhibit the angiogenesis induced by tumors; and third the inhibitor is secreted 24 hours every day and maintains the inhibition activity all the time, rather than the recombinant protein is degraded after injection.

ACKNOWLEDGEMENTS

We thank Dr. Paraic Kenny, Melissa Adriance for valuable discussion for the manuscript.

REFERENCES

Albo, D., T.N. Wang, and G.P. Tuszynski. 2004. Antiangiogenic therapy. *Curr Pharm Des. 10*:27-37.

Amenta, P.S., S. Hadad, M.T. Lee, N. Barnard, D. Li, and J.C. Myers. 2003. Loss of types XV and XIX collagen precedes basement membrane invasion in ductal carcinoma of the female breast. *J Pathol. 199*:298-308.

Badylak, S.F. 2002. The extracellular matrix as a scaffold for tissue reconstruction. *Semin Cell Dev Biol. 13*:377-83.

Banerjee, D.K., R.L. Ornberg, M.B. Youdim, E. Heldman, and H.B. Pollard. 1985. Endothelial cells from bovine adrenal medulla develop capillary-like growth patterns in culture. *Proc Natl Acad Sci U S A. 82*:4702-6.

Eklund, L., J. Piuhola, J. Komulainen, R. Sormunen, C. Ongvarrasopone, R. Fassler, A. Muona, M. Ilves, H. Ruskoaho, T.E. Takala, and T. Pihlajaniemi. 2001. Lack of type XV collagen causes a skeletal myopathy and cardiovascular defects in mice. *Proc Natl Acad Sci U S A. 98*:1194-9.

Felbor, U., L. Dreier, R.A. Bryant, H.L. Ploegh, B.R. Olsen, and W. Mothes. 2000. Secreted cathepsin L generates endostatin from collagen XVIII. *Embo J. 19*:1187-94.

Hagg, P.M., P.O. Hagg, S. Peltonen, H. Autio-Harmainen, and T. Pihlajaniemi. 1997. Location of type XV collagen in human tissues and its accumulation in the interstitial matrix of the fibrotic kidney. *Am J Pathol. 150*:2075-86.

Houck, K.A., D.W. Leung, A.M. Rowland, J. Winer, and N. Ferrara. 1992. Dual regulation of vascular endothelial growth factor bioavailability by genetic and proteolytic mechanisms. *J Biol Chem. 267*:26031-7.

Hsieh, P., and J. Baum. 1985. Effects of fibroblastic and endothelial extracellular matrices on corneal endothelial cells. *Invest Ophthalmol Vis Sci. 26*:457-63.

Kalluri, R. 2003. Basement membranes: structure, assembly and role in tumour angiogenesis. *Nat Rev Cancer. 3*:422-33.

Kamphaus, G.D., P.C. Colorado, D.J. Panka, H. Hopfer, R. Ramchandran, A. Torre, Y. Maeshima, J.W. Mier, V.P. Sukhatme, and R. Kalluri. 2000. Canstatin, a novel matrix-derived inhibitor of angiogenesis and tumor growth. *J Biol Chem. 275*:1209-15.

Koopman, G., C.P. Reutelingsperger, G.A. Kuijten, R.M. Keehnen, S.T. Pals, and M.H. van Oers. 1994. Annexin V for flow cytometric detection of phosphatidylserine expression on B cells undergoing apoptosis. *Blood. 84*:1415-20.

Kurebayashi, J., S.W. McLeskey, M.D. Johnson, M.E. Lippman, R.B. Dickson, and F.G. Kern. 1993. Quantitative demonstration of spontaneous metastasis by MCF-7 human breast cancer cells cotransfected with fibroblast growth factor 4 and LacZ. *Cancer Res. 53*:2178-87.

Lawler, J., R. Weinstein, and R.O. Hynes. 1988. Cell attachment to thrombospondin: the role of ARG-GLY-ASP, calcium, and integrin receptors. *J Cell Biol. 107*:2351-61.

Moscatelli, D. 1988. Metabolism of receptor-bound and matrix-bound basic fibroblast growth factor by bovine capillary endothelial cells. *J Cell Biol. 107*:753-9.

Myers, J.C., A.S. Dion, V. Abraham, and P.S. Amenta. 1996. Type XV collagen exhibits a widespread distribution in human tissues but a distinct localization in basement membrane zones. *Cell Tissue Res. 286*:493-505.

O'Reilly, M.S., T. Boehm, Y. Shing, N. Fukai, G. Vasios, W.S. Lane, E. Flynn, J.R. Birkhead, B.R. Olsen, and J. Folkman. 1997. Endostatin: an endogenous inhibitor of angiogenesis and tumor growth. *Cell. 88*:277-85.

Poltorak, Z., T. Cohen, R. Sivan, Y. Kandelis, G. Spira, I. Vlodavsky, E. Keshet, and G. Neufeld. 1997. VEGF145, a secreted vascular endothelial growth factor isoform that binds to extracellular matrix. *J Biol Chem. 272*:7151-8.

Ramchandran, R., M. Dhanabal, R. Volk, M.J. Waterman, M. Segal, H. Lu, B. Knebelmann, and V.P. Sukhatme. 1999. Antiangiogenic activity of restin, NC10 domain of human collagen XV: comparison to endostatin. *Biochem Biophys Res Commun. 255*:735-9.

Sudhakar, A., H. Sugimoto, C. Yang, J. Lively, M. Zeisberg, and R. Kalluri. 2003. Human tumstatin and human endostatin exhibit distinct antiangiogenic activities mediated by alpha v beta 3 and alpha 5 beta 1 integrins. *Proc Natl Acad Sci U S A. 100*:4766-71.

Wickstrom, S.A., K. Alitalo, and J. Keski-Oja. 2002. Endostatin associates with integrin alpha5beta1 and caveolin-1, and activates Src via a tyrosyl phosphatase-dependent pathway in human endothelial cells. *Cancer Res. 62*:5580-9.

Xu, R., L. Xin, Y. Fan, H.R. Meng, Z.P. Li, and R.B. Gan. 2002. *Mouse restin inhibits bovine aortic endothelial cell proliferation and causes cell apoptosis.* Sheng Wu Hua Xue Yu Sheng Wu Wu Li Xue Bao (Shanghai). 34:138-42.

Xu, R., Z.Y. Yao, L. Xin, Q. Zhang, T.P. Li, and R.B. Gan. 2001. NC1 domain of human type VIII collagen (alpha 1) inhibits bovine aortic endothelial cell proliferation and causes cell apoptosis. *Biochem Biophys Res Commun. 289*:264-8.

Zhang, H.T., P. Craft, P.A. Scott, M. Ziche, H.A. Weich, A.L. Harris, and R. Bicknell. 1995. Enhancement of tumor growth and vascular density by transfection of vascular endothelial cell growth factor into MCF-7 human breast carcinoma cells. *J Natl Cancer Inst. 87*:213-9.

In: Trends in Angiogenesis Research
Editor: Roberta V. Zubar, pp. 139-152

ISBN 1-59454-452-2

Chapter VI

Endothelial Cell Adhesion Molecules, Inflammation and Atherosclerosis in Chronic Renal Failure

Aikaterini Papagianni* and Dimitrios Memmos
University Department of Nephrology, Hippokration General Hospital, Thessaloniki, Greece

Abstract

Atherosclerotic cardiovascular disease is greatly increased in patients with chronic renal failure (CRF) and contribute to the high mortality rate observed in these patients. The prevalence of atherosclerotic disease is especially marked in patients undergoing renal replacement therapy but the probable effect of hemodialysis (HD) treatment is not yet established. Recently, emerging evidence suggests that cellular adhesion molecules (CAM), expressed on the surface of vascular endothelial cells in response to proinflammatory cytokines, play a major role in the atherogenic process. In this chapter, we report the research results of adhesion molecule ICAM-1 (intercellular adhesion molecule-1), VCAM-1 (vascular cell adhesion molecule-1) and E-selectin levels and atherosclerotic vascular changes, as assessed by high resolution ultrasonography of the common carotid arteries, in patients with stage 5 CRF prior to the start of renal replacement therapy. Eighty-five CRF patents and 65 age- and sex-matched apparently healthy normotensive controls participated in the study. Compared with controls, CRF patients had significantly increased serum CRP, ICAM-1 and VCAM-1 ($p<0.0001$, $p<0.0001$ and $p<0.0001$ respectively), but not E-selectin, levels, as well as carotid intima-media thickness (IMT) and plaque score values ($p<0.001$ and $p<0.0001$ respectively). In univariate analyses, IMT was significantly correlated with age, systolic blood pressure (BP), previous history of cardiovascular disease, logCRP and serum ICAM-1 ($p=0.0001$, $p=0.01$, $p=0.01$, $p=0.02$ and $p=0.004$ respectively). Multivariate

* Correspondence concerning this article should be addressed to: Aikaterini Papagianni, MD, University Department of Nephrology, Hippokration General Hospital, 50 Papanastasiou Str, 54642 Thessaloniki Greece, e-mail: aikpapag@otenet.gr

analysis showed that ICAM-1 was a strong independent correlate of IMT values ($p=0.001$). Plaque score was correlated with age, systolic BP and logCRP ($p=0.0001$, $p=0.02$ and $p=0.03$ respectively). Multivariate analysis showed that the latter was an independent contributor to plaque score values ($p=0.006$). Adhesion molecule levels failed to be a significant correlate of plaque score. Comparison of adhesion molecule levels and carotid atherosclerotic changes between the 85 CRF patients and 91 age- and sex-matched HD patients showed that the latter had significantly increased serum CRP, ICAM-1 and VCAM-1 levels ($p<0.001$, $p<0.001$ and $p<0.0001$ respectively), as well as IMT and plaque score values ($p<0.05$ and $p<0.001$ respectively). The above results suggest that CRF patients have advanced atherosclerosis and increased CAM levels before starting renal replacement therapy. Serum ICAM-1 appeared a significant independent predictor of carotid IMT and could be a useful molecular marker of early atherosclerotic vascular changes in these patients. HD treatment is associated with further activation of the inflammatory response and acceleration of the atherogenesis. Further research aimed at identifying novel markers of atherosclerosis would provide additional targets for preventive and therapeutic interventions in this high-risk population.

Key words: adhesion molecules, atherosclerosis, chronic renal failure, inflammation, intima-media thickness,

INTRODUCTION

Atherosclerotic cardiovascular disease (CVD) is greatly increased in patients with chronic renal failure (CRF) and contribute to the high mortality rate observed in these patients [1-3]. The prevalence of CVD is especially marked in patients undergoing renal replacement therapy, but the probable effect of hemodialysis (HD) treatment has yet to be established. The premature and accelerated development of atherosclerosis is multifactorial and may be explained partly by the higher prevalence of classic (diabetes, hypertension, dyslipidemia) and uremia-related (anemia, hemodynamic overload, inflammation, oxidative stress) cardiovascular risk factors in CRF patients. However, the combination of all the above factors do not fully explain the excess burden of atherosclerosis indicating that other factors, yet to be defined, are also likely triggered in this patient population [3].

Recently, emerging evidence suggests that endothelial cell adhesion molecules (CAM) play a major role in the initiation and progression of atherosclerosis through their effects on leukocyte activation, cell migration and smooth muscle cell proliferation [4]. E-selectin is a member of selectin family that is expressed transitory only on the surface of cytokine-activated endothelial cells where it mediates leukocyte rolling, a step that immediately precedes adhesion. Intercellular adhesion molecule-1 (ICAM-1) and vascular cell adhesion molecule-1 (VCAM-1) are two members of the Ig-like supergene family of adhesion molecules that are normally expressed by endothelial cells. Cytokine activation produces a dramatic upregulation of their expression on the cell surface where they support the firm adhesion and subsequent transmigration of leukocytes [5]. We have previously demonstrated that serum CAM levels are increased in patients on chronic HD treatment and are associated with carotid atherosclerosis [6]. In this chapter, we report the research results of adhesion molecule ICAM-1, VCAM-1 and E-selectin levels and carotid atherosclerotic vascular changes in patients with CRF prior to the start of renal replacement therapy. Moreover, the differences in CAM levels and atherosclerotic changes between CRF patients on conservative treatment and patients on chronic HD are also reported.

SUBJECTS AND METHODS

Subjects

Between May 2001 and November 2003, 85 adult patients with stage 5 CRF (38 male, mean age 64 years, range 30 to 82 years) from the outpatient clinic of the University Department of Nephrology at Hippokration General Hospital consecutively entered the study. The mean ± SD clearance of urea and creatinine at the time of examination was 7.8 ± 2.4 mil/min (range 4 to 14 ml/min) The causes of CRF were diabetic nephropathy in 27 cases, glomerulonephritis in 17 cases, tubulointerstitial nephritis in 6, polycystic kidney disease in 9, renovascular hypertension in 7 and was undetermined in 19 cases. None of the patients was receiving antibiotics, corticosteroids or cytotoxic drugs at the time of the study. Seventy-six patients (89.4%) were receiving one or more antihypertensive drugs (calcium channel blockers, angiotensin-converting enzyme inhibitors, angiotensin II receptor antagonists, oral nitrates or beta-blockers) at the time of the study. Fifty-nine patients (69.4%) were on recombinant human erythropoietin therapy and the mean dosage was 100 ± 32 IU/KgBW/week. Thirty-three patients (38.8%) had clinical signs or previous history of cardiovascular diseases and they were grouped as CVD. Of the 33 patients, 23 had a history of myocardial infarction, coronary artery bypass or clinical signs of angina pectoris, 3 had suffered from stroke and 12 had peripheral vascular disease. The control group consisted of 65 age- and sex-matched apparently healthy subjects (30 male, mean age 63 years, range 29 to 81 years) who were recruited from hospital staff members and their relatives. These control subjects did not have any history of hypertension, diabetes mellitus and renal or vascular disease, and were receiving no drugs at the time of the study. The study protocol conformed to the ethical guidelines of our institution and an informed consent was obtained from each participant.

Blood Pressure Measurements

Blood pressure (BP) was measured after 15 min of recumbency and five measurements 2 min apart were averaged.

Laboratory Methods

Blood samples from patients and control subjects were taken from a peripheral vein under fasting conditions. Serum samples were separated from clotted blood by immediate centrifugation (1500g for 10 min), aliquoted and stored at -70°C until assay. Serum levels of the circulating adhesion molecules ICAM-1, VCAM-1 and E-selectin were measured by an enzyme-linked immunosorbent assay (ELISA) using commercially available standard kits (Quantikine human sICAM-1, sVCAM-1 and sE-selectin, Research & Diagnostic Systems Europe Ltd, Abington UK). The sensitivity of the ELISA system was 2 ng/ml, 2 ng/ml and 1 ng/ml for the above molecules respectively. Serum albumin, total cholesterol, triglycerides and HDL-cholesterol was determined by routine techniques using an automated analyzer. LDL-cholesterol was calculated using the Friedewald formula. Serum CRP levels were measured by end-point nephelometry. The detection limit was 3.13 mg/l and in the statistical evaluation all values <3.13 mg/l were treated as 3 mg/l.

Carotid Ultrasonography

Ultrasonographic studies were performed with a Aloka Sonos SSD-1700 (Aloka, Tokyo Japan) instrument using a 7.5 MHz high-resolution probe. Intima-media thickness (IMT) was defined as a low-level echo grey band that does not project into the arterial lumen and was measured at the diastolic phase as the distance between the leading edge of the first and second echogenic line. IMT was measured bilaterally on the longitudinal views of the far wall of the distal segment of common carotid artery, the carotid bifurcation, and the initial tract of the internal carotid artery on both sides. Measurements were performed 0.5, 1 and 2 cm below and above the bifurcation (six measurements on each side) in a plaque free arterial segment. The average measurement of the obtained values was taken as IMT and it was considered abnormal when it exceeded 0.82 mm [7]. Carotid plaques were defined (and counted) either as faint grey echoes (soft plaques) or bright white echoes (calcified plaques) protruding into the arterial lumen. Plaque thickness was measured in a suitable longitudinal or transverse view. Plaque score was computed by summing maximum thickness in millimeters of plaques in each segment on both sides.

Adhesion Molecule Levels and Carotid Atherosclerosis in HD Patients

We have previously reported adhesion molecule ICAM-1, VCAM-1 and E-selectin levels and atherosclerotic vascular changes, as assessed by high resolution ultrasonography of the common carotid arteries, in 112 patients on chronic HD treatment. This patient material has been recently published [6]. Ninety-one patients were randomly selected from our data-base so that the two groups were closely matched for age and gender.

Statistical Analysis

Data are expressed as means ± SD and with range. The significance of differences in means between the two groups was assessed by Student's *t* test or Mann-Whitney test as appropriate. Differences in proportions were tested with the use of chi-square statistic. Correlations were tested by regression analysis. Not-normally distributed variables were log-transformed before entering regression analysis. Multiple regression analysis with a forward elimination procedure was used to assess the combined influence of variables on IMT and plaque score values. The following variables were used: age, sex, smoking, diabetes mellitus, history of CVD, systolic and diastolic blood pressure, serum albumin, cholesterol, triglycerides, HDL, LDL, fibrinogen, logCRP, ICAM-1, VCAM-1 and E-selectin levels.

RESULTS

The somatometric, hemodynamic and biochemical characteristics of controls and CRF patients are shown in Table 1. Triglycerides were significantly increased and HDL was significantly decreased in CRF patients compared with control subjects. In addition, systolic BP was elevated in CRF patients whereas mean diastolic BP did not differ significantly between the two groups. BMI and smoking status were also similar in the two groups (Table 1).

Table 1. Somatometric, hemodynamic and biochemical characteristics of 65 control subjects and 85 chronic renal failure patients.

	CONTROLS	CRF PATIENTS	P
Age (years)	63 ± 11	64 ± 12	NS
Sex (M/F)	30/35	38/47	NS
BMI (kg/m^2)	24.9 ± 2.7	25.5 ± 3.9	NS
Smoking (% of patients)	22 (33.8%)	28 (32.9%)	NS
Systolic BP (mmHg)	139.0 ± 11.7	147.6 ± 17.8	0.01
Diastolic BP (mmHg)	78.9 ± 7.2	80.6 ± 11.2	NS
Hemoglobulin (g/dl)	14.3 ± 0.6	10.2 ± 1.6	0.001
Albumin (g/dl)	4.7 ± 0.6	3.9 ± 0.6	0.001
Cholesterol (mg/dl)	200 ± 24	218 ± 49	NS
Triglycerides (mg/dl)	117 ± 39	187 ± 94	0.001
HDL (mg/dl)	49.2 ± 9.9	39.5 ± 8.6	0.001
LDL (mg/dl)	127 ± 20	141 ± 46	NS

Compared with control subjects, CRF patients had significantly increased IMT and plaque score (0.71 ± 0.08 vs 0.87 ± 0.16 mm, $p<0.001$ and 0.51 ± 0.80 vs 2.91 ± 3.75 mm, $p<0.0001$ respectively). IMT was increased (> 0.82 mm) in 51 (60.0%) of CRF patients. Atherosclerotic plaques were detected in 53 (62.4%) of CRF patients and in 20 (30.8%) of controls. The difference in plaque occurrence between the two groups was significant ($p<0.0001$). The number of plaques ranged from 1 to 3 in control subjects and in 1 to 8 in CRF patients.

Ultrasonographic Findings and Risk Factors for Atherosclerosis

IMT and plaque score were significantly correlated with age both in control subjects (r=0.53, p=0.0001 and r=0.48, p=0.0001 respectively) and CRF patients (r=0.47, p=0.0001 and r=0.42, p=0.0001 respectively). In the latter group, the number of plaques in individual patients was also significantly correlated with age (r=0.46, p=0.0001). In addition, IMT was significantly correlated with systolic BP in both groups (r=0.42, p=0.005 and r=0.26, p=0.01 respectively). In CRF patients, plaque score was also correlated with systolic BP (r=0.24, p=0.02). Ultrasonographic parameters did not show any significant correlation with other classic cardiovascular risk factors in both groups, such as gender, smoking status, total cholesterol, triglycerides, HDL and LDL-cholesterol levels, or diabetes mellitus in CRF patients. In univariate analysis, a previous history of CVD was significantly correlated with IMT (p=0.01). Morover, compared with patients with negative history of vascular diseases, patients with CVD had significantly increased IMT, but not plaque score values (0.92 ± 0.17 vs 0.84 ± 0.14 mm, p<0.01 and 3.65 ± 4.57 vs 2.41 ± 3.04 mm, p=NS respectively).

Ultrasonographic Findings and Inflammation

Compared with control subjects, CRF patients showed a significant increase in serum fibrinogen and CRP values (2.72 ± 0.7 vs 4.17 ± 1.2 g/l, p<0.0001 and 3.92 ± 0.8 vs 7.75 ± 7.2 mg/l, p<0.0001). Fourty-three out of the 85 CRF patients (50.6%) had increased fibrinogen levels (normal 2 to 4 g/l) and 33 patients (38.8%) had abnormal CRP (normal <3.13 to 5mg/l). Fibrinogen values were significantly correlated with logCRP (r=0.39, p=0.0003). In univariate analyses, IMT and plaque score were significantly correlated with logCRP values (r=0.26, p=0.02 and r=0.24, p=0.03 respectively) (Fig. 1). In addition, compared with patients with normal CRP, patients with elevated CRP (>5mg/l) had significantly increased IMT (0.84 ± 0.13 vs 0.92 ± 0.18, p<0.05) and plaque score (2.09 ± 2.41 vs 4.27 ± 4.94 mm, p<0.01). Multivariate analysis showed that logCRP values were a strong independent correlate of plaque score values (r=0.32, p=0.006) (Table 2).

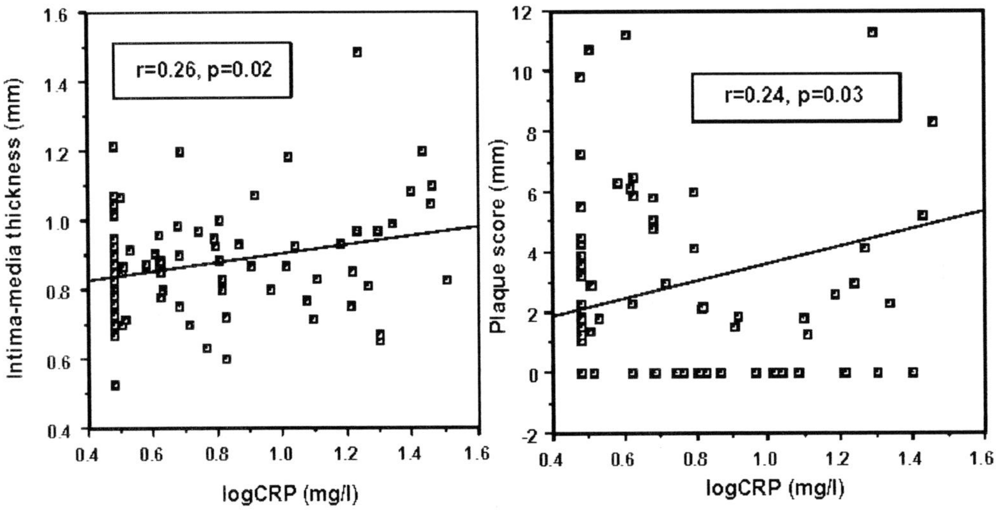

Figure 1. Correlation between logCRP and intima-media thickness (left panel) and plaque score (right panel) values in 85 patients with chronic renal failure.

Table 2. Multivariate analysis of carotid plaque score.

Independent variables	r	P
Age	0.44	0.0001
Systolic BP	0.22	0.04
logCRP	0.32	0.006
Out of model		
Sex	-0.12	0.20
Diabetes mellitus	-0.16	0.16
History of CVD	-0.21	0.29
Albumin	-0.04	0.69
Triglycerides	0.06	0.55
HDL-cholesterol	0.18	0.69
Fibrinogen	0.16	0.15

Data are partial correlation coefficients and *P*. Carotid plaque score multiple r=0.57, p=0.0003

Ultrasonographic Findings and Endothelial Adhesion Molecules

Compared with control subjects, CRF patients showed a significant increase in serum ICAM-1 (248 ± 77 vs 412 ± 101 ng/ml, p<0.0001) and VCAM-1 (1004 ± 184 vs 1751 ± 619 ng/ml, p<0.0001), but not in E-selectin concentrations (82 ± 40 vs 87 ± 45 ng/ml, p=NS). No differences were observed in adhesion molecule levels between diabetic and non-diabetic patients. In addition, serum CAM levels were not correlated with age, gender or estimated GFR. However, serum ICAM-1 and VCAM-1 levels were significantly correlated with log CRP (r=0.31, p=0.003 and r=0.35, p=0.001 respectively). The correlations were even higher when only the 58 patients with an exact CRP value (≥3.13 mg/l) were entered in the regression analysis (r=0.37, p=0.004 and r=0.36, p=0.005 respectively) (Fig. 2).

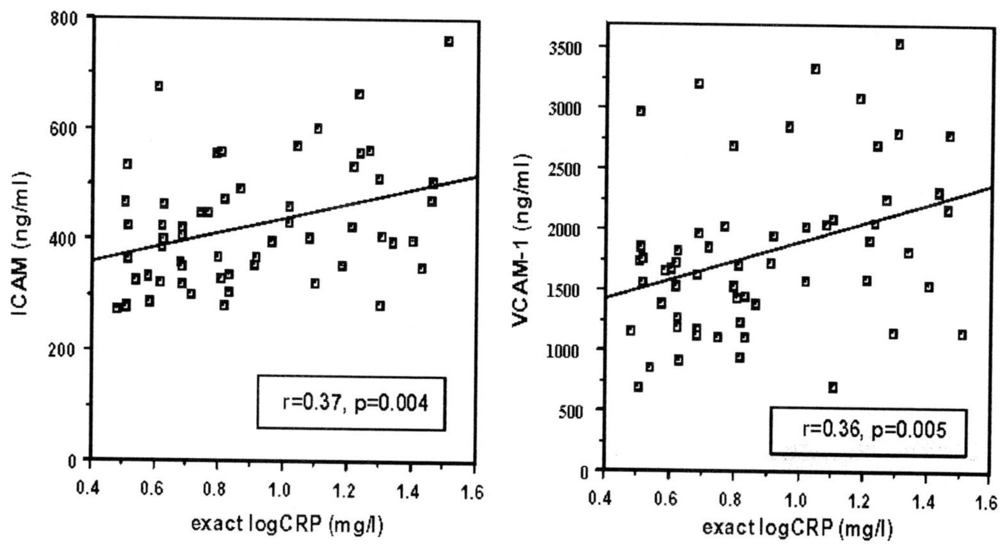

Figure 2. Correlation between exact logCRP and serum ICAM-1 (left panel) and VCAM-1 (right panel) levels in 85 patients with chronic renal failure.

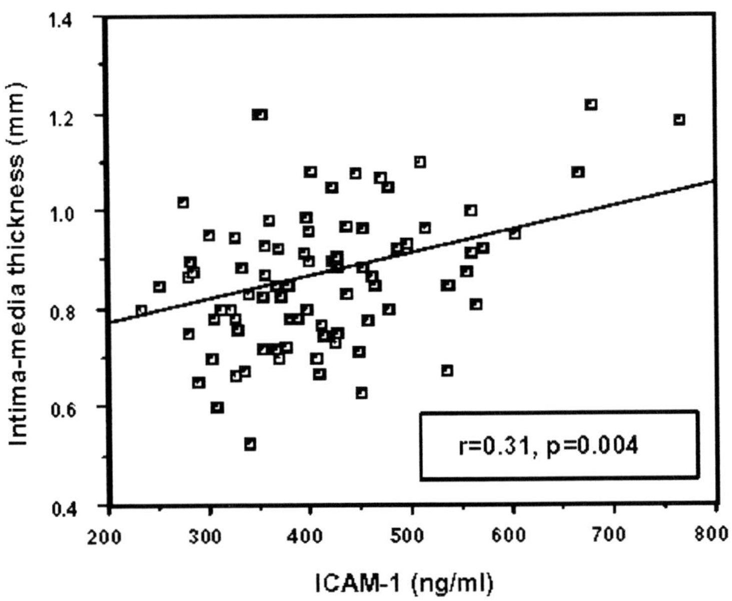

Figure 3. Correlation between intima-media thickness values and serum ICAM-1 levels in 85 patients with chronic renal failure.

In univariate analysis, IMT values were significantly correlated with ICAM-1 (r=0.31, p=0.004) (Fig. 3), but not VCAM-1 or E-selectin levels. Moreover, compared with patients with normal IMT, patients with increased IMT values (>0.82 mm) had significantly elevated ICAM-1 (376 ± 71 vs 436 ± 111 ng/ml, p<0.01) but not VCAM-1 (1710 ± 592 vs 1814 ± 660 ng/ml, p=NS), or E-selectin (81 ± 41 vs 83 ± 41 ng/ml, p=NS). Multivariate analysis showed that serum ICAM-1 concentrations were a strong independent correlate of IMT (r=0.30, p=0.001) (Table 3). Because of the highly significant relationship between ICAM-1 and logCRP values, the latter parameter was an independent correlate of IMT (r=0.28, p=0.01), only if serum ICAM-1 was excluded from the model. History of CVD failed to be a significant correlate of IMT in multivariate analysis (Table 3).

Table 3. Multivariate analysis of carotid IMT.

Independent variables	r	P
Age	0.47	0.0001
Systolic BP	0.24	0.02
ICAM-1	0.30	0.001
Out of model		
Sex	-0.13	0.20
Diabetes mellitus	-0.14	0.12
History of CVD	-0.15	0.15
Albumin	-0.05	0.57
Triglycerides	0.10	0.23
HDL-cholesterol	0.05	0.58
Fibrinogen	0.08	0.37
logCRP	0.18	0.07

Data are partial correlation coefficients and *P*. Carotid plaque score multiple r=0.68, p=0.0001

Adhesion molecule levels failed to be a significant contributor to plaque score values either on univariate or multivariate analyses. However, compared with patients with no atherosclerotic plaques, patients with at least one plaque had significantly increased serum ICAM-1 (382 ± 83 vs 430 ± 108 ng/ml, $p<0.05$), but not VCAM-1 (1667 ± 537 vs 1803 ± 663 ng/ml, p=NS) or E-selectin levels (82 ± 41 vs 82 ± 40 ng/ml, p=NS).

Ultrasonographic Findings and Endothelial Adhesion Molecules in CRF and HD Patients

Serum CAM levels and atherosclerotic vascular changes were investigated in 91 patients on chronic HD treatment (42 male). Mean age was 63 ± 12 years (range 29 to 82 years) and mean HD duration was 76 ± 75 months (range 5 to 372 months). Thirty-seven patients (40.6%) had a previous history or clinical signs of cardiovascular disease. Compared with CRF patients, HD patients had significantly increased IMT and plaque score values (0.87 ± 0.16 vs 0.92 ± 0.17 mm, $p<0.05$ and 2.91 ± 3.75 vs 5.25 ± 4.51 mm, $p<0.001$ respectively). Atherosclerotic plaques were detected in 53 CRF (62.4%) and in 80 HD patients (87.9%). The difference in plaque occurrence between the two groups was significant ($p<0.001$). Moreover, compared with CRF patients, HD patients had significantly increased serum CRP values 7.75 ± 7.2 vs 12.4 ± 11.8 mg/l, $p<0.001$), as well as ICAM-1 (412 ± 101 vs 506 ± 198 ng/ml, $p<0.001$) and VCAM-1 (1752 ± 619 vs 2419 ± 631 ng/ml, $p<0.0001$), but not E-selectin levels (87 ± 45 vs 91 ± 58 ng/ml, p=NS).

Discussion

The degree of atherosclerosis can be evaluated from various aspects such as incidence of death from atherosclerotic disease, narrowing of arterial lumen, histological grading, and stiffening and thickening of arterial wall. However, the introduction of high-resolution ultrasonography has provided a reliable, reproducible, and non-invasive method for detecting and monitoring the progression of subclinical atherosclerosis [8]. The investigation of the carotid atherosclerotic changes with this technique is valuable as there is evidence that they could provide an indirect estimate of the atherosclerotic burden in other vessels, including coronary arteries [9, 10]. In agreement with a previous report, the present research demonstrated that IMT values were significantly increased in CRF patients compared with age and sex-matched controls [11]. In addition, the former group had significantly increased plaque score and incidence of plaque occurrence. Overall the above findings provide further evidence that advanced atherosclerotic vascular changes are present in patients with CRF prior to the start of renal replacement therapy and support the hypothesis of an accelerated "atherogenesis" in this patient population.

Over the last years, the idea that inflammation plays a key role in atherosclerosis has received considerable attention. Consequently, several markers of inflammation have been examined as potential tools for predicting the presence of vascular disease or the risk of vascular events [12]. Of the variety of circulating markers, CRP, the major acute phase response protein, has been the best studied, with the most consistent relationship to future risk for cardiovascular events in general population [13, 14]. Moreover, accumulating data from studies in end-stage renal disease patients demonstrated a particularly strong association between elevated CRP levels and all-cause and cardiovascular mortality [15, 16]. In accordance with previous reports, the present research showed a significant correlation between IMT and CRP values [17, 18]. In addition, CRP was a significant contributor to plaque score both on univariate and multivariate analyses. The above results support the concept that chronic inflammation plays a critical role in atherosclerosis and further strengthen the value of CRP as a surrogate marker for atherosclerotic vascular damage.

Recently, mounting evidence suggests an important role for endothelial cell adhesion molecules in the pathogenesis of atherosclerosis. Adhesion molecules ICAM-1, VCAM-1 and E-selectin have been detected by immunohistochemistry in human atherosclerotic lesions and their expression was found to be correlated with intimal infiltration by T-lymphocytes and monocytes/macrophages [19]. However, their relative contribution to the initiation and progression of atherosclerotic lesions as well as their potential value to serve as biological markers for predicting the presence and the severity of vascular damage in patients with CRF has not been investigated. In the present chapter, we have reported that serum ICAM-1 and VCAM-1 concentrations are increased in patients with CRF compared with normotensive controls. Elevated serum concentrations of adhesion molecules have previously been documented in CRF patients, both on conservative treatment and on renal replacement therapy [20-22]. The causes of increased serum CAM in these patients are probably multifactorial, involving both inadequate clearance and enhanced synthesis. Previous srudies have demonstrated a strong linear correlation between serum creatinine and levels of adhesion molecules suggesting that inadequate clearance might be an important contributor to elevated serum CAM levels [21]. However, in the present study no significant correlations were observed between renal function and serum adhesion molecule levels. These results are in good agreement with a previous report in end-stage renal disease patients [22] and might be explained by the fact that only patients with advanced CRF were evaluated. Moreover, significant correlations were found between CRP and serum ICAM-1 and VCAM-1 levels suggesting that the chronic inflammation of uremia may be a major cause of elevated serum levels of these proteins in CRF patients. Indeed, several studies have demonstrated that renal failure promotes activation of the inflammatory response. Among the factors which have been proposed to promote this inflammation, are included increased oxidative stress and accumulation of advanced glycation end products and products of carbonyl stress, all as a consequence of the failure of renal clearance [23-26].

The most important finding reported in the present chapter was the significant association between carotid IMT and serum ICAM-1 levels. Multivariate analysis showed that ICAM-1 was a strong independent correlate of IMT, whereas CRP became a significant correlate of IMT only when ICAM-1 levels were excluded from the analysis. Furthermore, this association appeared to be minimally influenced by a number of traditional or uremia-related risk factors for atherosclerosis, including previous cardiovascular complications. The above data concur with our results in HD patients and indicate that ICAM-1 is a valuable marker integrating information otherwise present in a number of other less strongly related markers of infammation, including CRP and fibrinogen values. Moreover, they support the concept that measurements of this molecule could help to construct a better model for predicting atherosclerotic disease than models based only on classic risk factors and other markers of inflammation. Finally, based on the relative independence of the association between ICAM-1 and IMT of a number of risk factors, it is tempting to speculate that this correlation underlies a pathogenetic link. Interestingly, two previous studies in end-stage renal disease and dialysis patients [6, 22] have demonstrated that serum ICAM-1 is a strong independent predictor of mortality. Overall, the above results may indicate that this protein could be a marker of a process that contributes to the high mortality of this patient population. However, clearly larger additional studies are necessary to confirm the above intriguing hypothesis and to allow a better appreciation of the value of this molecule for risk stratification in patients with chronic renal failure.

Adhesion molecule concentrations failed to be a significant correlate of plaque score both on univariate and multivariate analyses. The relative contribution of these molecules to the initiation and progression of atherosclerotic vascular damage has yet to be defined. However, the natural history of atherosclerotic vascular changes is well documented and known to progress through the stage of intimal thickening to fully developed plaques and obstructive lesions. Consequently, the above results may indicate that these molecules rather have a more important role on the early pathophysiological events than on the more advanced stages of atherosclerosis. Furthermore, these data may imply that ICAM-1 levels could be more useful as molecular markers of early atherosclerosis.

Atherosclerosis is particularly advanced in CRF patients treated with hemodialysis, but whether atherosclerosis is accelerated in long-term maintenance HD is not well established. Some authors have reported a positive correlation between carotid artery IMT and duration of HD tretament [27, 28], whereas others failed to confirm such a significant correlation [29, 30]. The present research demonstrated that compared with CRF patients on conservative treatment, age- and sex-matched chronic HD patients have significangtly increased IMT, plaque score and incidence of plaque occurence. These results which have not previously reported appeared discrepant with a recent study which has shown no difference in IMT values between CRF and dialysis patients [11]. However, in the above study only the greatest thickness of intima-media complex was used for analysis, whereas plaque score measurements were not performed. Interestingly, in our research maximum intima-media thickness was also similar in CRF and HD groups (data not shown). Consequently, our findings can support the concept that HD treatment further promotes the vascular changes in these patients although the underlying mechanisms are at present unclear. In addition, compared with CRF patients, HD patients had significantly increased serum CRP as well as ICAM-1 and VCAM-1 levels. In support of the above findings, previous studies have suggested that the dialysis procedure, with extracorporeal circulation of blood may cause inflammation. Potential causes of inflammation in dialysis patients are dialysis against non-biocompatible membranes, ther use of non-sterile dialysate and the back-leak of dialysate across the dialysis membrane [31, 32]. However, it has been demonstrated that although optimized HD therapy using ultrapure dialysate and biocompatible membranes reduces CRP, it does not normalize it [33], suggesting that uremia may be an important cause of inflammation in CRF patients. Moreover, these findings confirm our previous study which have shown that HD treatment *per se* induces a striking increase in serum ICAM-1 and VCAM-1 levels independently of the type of dialysis membrane used [34].

Conclusions

The research results reported in the present chapter have shown that increased serum CAM levels and advanced atherosclerosis are present in CRF patients prior to the start of renal replacement therapy. In patients with chronic renal failure, both on conservative treatment and on hemodialysis, ICAM-1 levels are linked to an inflammatory state and are potentially a useful surrogate marker of early carotid atherosclerosis Hemodialysis appreared associated with further activation of the inflammatory response and acceleration of the atherosclerotic process. However, whether HD treatment promotes atherosclerosis, at least partially, via a stimulatory effect on adhesion molecules warrants further investigation. Further research aimed at identifying novel markers of atherosclerosis would provide additional targets for preventive and therapeutic interventions in this particularly high-risk patient population.

References

[1] Ma KW, Greene EL, Raij L. Cardiovascular risk factors in chronic renal failure and hemodialysis populations. *Am J Kidney Dis* 1992; 19*:* 505-513

[2] Lameire N, Bernaert P, Lambert M-C, Vijt D. Cardiovascular risk factors and their management in patients on continuous ambulatory peritoneal dialysis. *Kidney Int* 1994 ; 46 (Suppl 48): S31-S38

[3] Cheung AK, Sarnak MJ, Yan G et al. Atherosclerotic cardiovascular disease risks in chronic hemodialysis patients. *Kidney Int* 2000; 58: 353-362

[4] Persson J, Blann AD, McCollum CN. Circulating endothelial cell/leukocyte adhesion molecules in atherosclerosis. *Thromb Haemost* 1994; 72: 151-154

[5] Carlos TM, Harlan JM. Leukocyte-endothelial adhesion molecules. *Blood* 1994; 84: 2068-2101

[6] Papagianni A, Kalovoulos M, Kirmizis D et al. Carotid atherosclerosis is associated with inflammation and endothelial cell adhesion molecules in chronic haemodialysis patients. *Nephrol Dial Transplant* 2003; 18: 113-119

[7] Aminbakhsh A, Mancini GB. Carotid intima media thickness measurements. What defines an abnormality? A systematic review. *Clin Invest Med* 1999; 22: 149-157

[8] Persson J, , Fromgren J, Israelsson B, Berglund G. Ultrasound determined intima-media thickness and atherosclerosis. Direct and indirect validation. *Arterioscler Thromb* 1994; 14: 261-264

[9] Allan PL, Mowbray PI, Lee AJ, Fowkes FG. Relationship between carotid intima-media thickness and symptomatic and asymptomatic peripheral vascular disease: The Edinburgh Artery Study. *Stroke* 1997; 28: 348-353

[10] Craven TE, Ryu JE, Espeland MA et al. Evaluation of the associations between carotid artery atherosclerosis and coronary artery stenosis: A case control study. *Circulation* 1990; 82: 1230-1242

[11] Shoji T, Emoto M, Tabata T et al. Advanced atherosclerosis in predialysis patients with chronic renal failure. *Kidney Int* 2002; 61: 2187-2192

[12] Ridker PM. Evaluating novel cardiovascular risk factors: Can we do better predict heart attacks? *Ann Int Med* 1999; 130: 933-937

[13] Lagrand WK, Visser CA, Hermens WT et al. C-reactive protein as a cardiovascular risk factor: More than an epiphenomenon? *Circulation* 1999; 1000: 96-102

[14] Morrow DA, Ridker PM. C-reactive protein, inflammation, and coronary risk. *Med Clin North Am* 2000; 84: 149-161

[15] Zimmermann J, Herrlinger S, Pruy A, Metzger T, Wanner C. Inflammation enhances cardiovascular risk and mortality in hemodialysis patients. *Kidney Int* 1999; 55: 648-658

[16] Yeun JY, Levine RA, Mantalidok V et al. C-reactive protein predicts all-cause and cardiovascular mortality in hemodialysis patients. *Am J Kidney Dis* 2000; 35: 469-476

[17] Stenvinkel P, Heimbürger O, Paultre F et al. Strong association between malnutrition, inflammation and atherosclerosis in chronic renal failure. *Kidney Int* 1999; 55: 1899-1911

[18] Zoccali C, Benedetto FA, Mallamaci F et al. Inflammation is associated with carotid atherosclerosis in dialysis patients. *J Hypertens* 2000; 18: 1207-1213

[19] O'Brien KD, McDonald TO, Chait A, Allen MD, Alpers CE. Neovascular expression of E-selectin, intercellular adhesion molecule-1 and vascular cell adhesion molecule-1 in human atherosclerosis and their relation to intimal leukocyte content. *Circulation* 1996; 93: 672-682

[20] Rabb H, Calderon E, Bittle PA, Ramirez G. Alterations in soluble intercellular adhesion molecule-1 and vascular cell adhesion molecule-1 in hemodialysis patients. *Am J Kidney Dis* 1996; 27: 239-243

[21] Bonomini M, Heale M, Santarelli P, Stuard S, Settefrati N, Abertazzi A. Serum levels of soluble adhesion molecules in chronic renal failure and dialysis patients. *Nephron* 1998; 79: 399-407

[22] Stenvinkel P, Lindholm B, Heimbürger M, Heimbürger O. Elevated serum levels of soluble adhesion molecules predict death in pre-dialysis patients: association with malnutrition, inflammation and cardiovascular disease. *Nephrol Dial Transplant* 2000; 15: 1624-1630

[23] Pereira BJ, Shapiro L, King AJ, Falagas ME, Strom JA, Dinarello CA. Plasma levels of IL-1β, TNF-a and their specific inhibitors in undialyzed chronic renal failure, CAPD and hemodialysis patients. *Kidney Int* 1994; 45: 890-896

[24] Martin-Mateo MC, Sanchez-Portugal M, Iglesias S, de Paula A, Bustamante J. Oxidative stress in chronic renal failure. *Ren Fail* 1999; 21: 155-167

[25] Miyata T, Wada Y, Cai Z et al. Implication of an increased oxidative stress in the formation of advanced glycation end products in patients with end-stage renal failure. *Kidney Int* 1997; 51: 1170-1181

[26] Miyata T, van Ypersele de Strihou C, Kurokawa K, Baynes JW. Alterations in nonenzymatic biochemistry in uremia: Origin and significance of "carbonyl stress" in long-term uremic complications. *Kidney Int* 1999; 55: 389-399

[27] Burdick L, Periti M, Salvaggio A et al. Relation between carotid artery atherosclerosis and time on dialysis. A non-invasive study in vivo. *Clin Nephrol* 1994; 42: 121-126

[28] Guz G, Nurhan Ozdemir F, Sezer S et al. Effect of apolipoprotein E polymorphism on serum lipid, lipoproteins and atherosclerosis in hemodialysis patients. *Am J Kidney Dis* 2000; 36: 826-836

[29] Hojs R. Carotid intima-media thickness and plaques in hemodialysis patients. *Artif Organs* 2000; 24: 691-695

[30] Kawagishi T, Nishizawa Y, Konishi T et al. High-resolution B-mode ultrasonography in evaluation of atherosclerosis in uremia. *Kidney Int* 1995; 48: 820-826

[31] Tielemans C, Husson C, Schurmans T et al. Effects of ultrapure and non-sterile dialysate on the inflammatory response during in vitro hemodialysis. *Kidney Int* 1996; 49: 236-243

[32] Schouten WEM, Grooteman MPC, van Houte A-J, Schoorl M, van Limbeek J, Nubé MJ. Effects of dialyser and dialysate on the acute phase response in clinical biocarbonate dialysis. *Nephrol Dial Transplant* 2000; 15: 379-384

[33] Schindler R, Boenisch O, Fischer C, Frei U. Effect of the haemodialysis membrane on the inflammatory reaction in vivo. *Clin Nephrol* 2000; 53: 452-459

[34] Papagianni A, Alexopoulos E, Giamalis P et al. Circulating levels of ICAM-1, VCAM-1 and MCP-1 are increased in haemodialysis patients. Association with inflammation, dyslipidaemia and vascular events. *Nephrol Dial Transplant* 2002; 17: 435-441

In: Trends in Angiogenesis Research
Editor: Roberta V. Zubar, pp. 153-182

ISBN 1-59454-452-2

Chapter VII

THE EFFECTS OF THE ENDOTHELINS - AN ANGIOGENIC FAMILY OF MOLECULES - IN SOLID CANCERS

Matthew J. Grimshaw*

Cancer Research UK Breast Cancer Biology Group, Thomas Guy House, Guy's Hospital, London, UK

ABSTRACT

Endothelins are a family of small, structurally related, vasoactive peptides that have a variety of physiological roles in many tissues. The 'endothelin axis' consists of three 21 amino acid peptides (ET-1, ET-2 and ET-3), two G-protein-coupled receptors (ET-RA and ET-RB), and two activating peptidases (endothelin-converting enzymes, ECE-1 and ECE-2). Endothelins have numerous potential roles in tumours, including inducing mitogenesis and invasion of tumour cells, and protecting cells from apoptosis. The endothelins are also implicated in tumour angiogenesis, both directly through stimulation of endothelial cell growth, motility and the formation of tubule structures, and indirectly through the induction of vascular endothelial growth factor (VEGF) via the transcription factor hypoxia-inducible factor (HIF)-1. As well as facilitating neovascularisation, the endothelins may also modulate blood flow through the established tumour vasculature due to their vasoactive nature. The expression of the endothelin axis is complex and tumour-specific; many types of tumour have deregulated expression of one or more of the endothelins or their receptors compared to the normal (non-neoplastic) tissue, but expression may be increased or decreased depending upon tumour type. Several different cell types within solid tumours may contribute to endothelin expression including not only the tumour cells but also fibroblasts, the immune infiltrate and endothelial cells of the vasculature. There is increased expression of the endothelins and their receptors in both ovarian and breast tumours, and this may induce VEGF expression by tumour cells

* Correspondence concerning this article should be addressed to Dr. Matthew J. Grimshaw, Cancer Research UK Breast Cancer Biology Group, 3rd Floor, Thomas Guy House, Guy's Hospital, London, UK. SE1 9RT. Tel: 00 44 20 718 84230; Fax: 00 44 20 718 80919; Email: matthew.grimshaw@cancer.org.uk.

and endothelial cells. Endothelin expression correlates not only with the level of VEGF expression but also the degree of vascularity in the tumour. The association between endothelins, poor prognosis and angiogenesis may mean that the endothelin axis is a valid therapeutic target for the treatment of several types of solid tumours. This review summarises our current knowledge of the role of endothelins in angiogenesis in solid tumours and discusses the potential further directions of such research as well as the possibility of anti-endothelin-based therapy of cancer.

Color graphics are presented at the end of the chapter.

Key words: Endothelin, angiogenesis, tumour, HIF, VEGF.

1. INTRODUCTION

There is a growing interest in the many potential roles of the 'endothelin axis' in cancer [1]. Endothelins are small (21 amino acid) vasoactive peptides that have a great number of physiological roles in many tissues, notably in development and vascular homeostasis (table 1) [2]. Endothelins bind, with varying affinity, to two similar G protein-coupled receptors, ET-RA and ET-RB [3]; binding of the ligands may modulate several overlapping signalling pathways including the PKC and MAPK pathways and the mobilisation of intracellular calcium [1].

Numerous tumours - including carcinomas of the breast, lung, prostate and ovary - produce one or more of the endothelins and their receptors [1]. Endothelins play a role in regulating growth of several tumour cell types including ovarian cancer cell lines and tumours [4], inhibit apoptosis of tumour cells [5], and also affect differentiation, inflammation and invasion [1]. Many malignant cells express increased levels of endothelins compared to their non-neoplastic counterparts, and the tumour microenvironment, particularly hypoxia and inflammatory cytokines, may further induce endothelin expression by the tumour and stroma cells. Cells that may express endothelins include not only the tumour cells themselves but also fibroblasts, endothelial cells and tumour-associated macrophages (TAMs).

Endothelins may also play a key role in the neovascularisation of several types of tumour. There are several mechanisms by which endothelins may stimulate tumour angiogenesis including a direct mitogenic effect on endothelial cells and also indirect effects via vascular endothelial growth factor (VEGF) and the transcription factor hypoxia inducible factor (HIF)-1. Further pro-angiogenic cytokines, such as basic fibroblast growth factor (bFGF, FGF2), may also be stimulated by endothelins.

Small-molecule inhibitors of the endothelin receptors already exist and have been used in phase III trials for the treatment of several diseases, including prostate cancer, and may therefore present an avenue of anti-angiogenic therapy for the treatment of cancer that can quickly be exploited.

This review summarises our knowledge of the association between endothelins and angiogenesis in solid tumours - focussing on the extensively studied ovarian carcinoma, and our own work on breast cancer - and the possible future directions of such research.

2. The Endothelin Axis

The endothelin axis consists of three 21 amino acid peptides (ET-1, ET-2 and ET-3), two G-protein-coupled receptors (ET-RA and ET-RB), and two endothelin-converting enzymes (ECE-1 and ECE-2) [2]. ET-1 was initially found in the conditioned medium of cultured endothelial cells and its activity as a potent vasoconstrictive peptide was described [6]; when ET-1 was injected intravenously into rats, a sustained and long-lasting pressor response was observed, suggesting a role for the endothelins in the maintenance of blood pressure and the generation of hypertension. ET-2 and ET-3 were rapidly described following ET-1's discovery [7] and, while the vasoconstrictive activity of the endothelin axis has been most extensively studied, further potential roles in a variety of tissues have been described (table 1) [2]. Endothelins are expressed embryonically and play a crucial role in differentiation and development; the use of knockout mice to assess the roles of individual components of the endothelin axis in, for instance, tumour development has been hindered by the fact that endothelin and/or receptor knockout mice die in utero or soon after birth. In blood vessels, the endothelin system has a basal vasoconstricting role and participates in the development of diseases such as hypertension and atherosclerosis. In the heart, endothelins mediate cardiac hypertrophy and remodelling in congestive heart failure. In the lungs, the endothelin system regulates the tone of airways and blood vessels, and is involved in the development of pulmonary hypertension. In the kidney, endothelin peptides control water and sodium excretion and acid-base balance, and participate in acute and chronic renal failure. In the brain, the endothelin axis modulates cardiorespiratory centres and the release of hormones.

Expression and Processing of Endothelins

The three endothelin peptide isoforms - which are highly conserved in human, rat and mouse [9] - derive from three separately regulated genes yet have a similar structure [7]: 21 amino acid peptides with a hydrophobic C-terminus and two cysteine bridges at the N-terminus (figure 1a). The peptide sequences of ET-2 and ET-3 differ from ET-1 by two and six residues respectively [6,8,9].

Human ET-1 derives from a 212 amino acid precursor, preproendothelin-1 (figure 1b), which is intracellularly cleaved by the membrane-bound metalloproteinases ECE-1 and -2 [10]. Further enzymes, yet to be identified, are also thought to be involved [12]. Removal of the signal sequence generates the 195 amino acid proendothelin-1, which is further processed to release the intermediate 38 amino acid 'Big ET-1'. Endothelin-converting enzymes hydrolyse Big ET-1 to yield the active 21 amino acid ET-1.

The gene for each endothelin has a distinct pattern of tissue expression (table 2): ET-1 is expressed by endothelial cells of many organs, ET-2 in epithelial cells of the kidney and intestine, and ET-3 is found in the brain [2]. There is a relatively low basal level of synthesis of endothelins but these genes are readily inducible by inflammatory stimuli such as exposure to cytokines or hypoxia [5,13]. It is of note, however, that endothelins and their receptors are also expressed by 'mobile' inflammatory cells such as monocytes and macrophages [13,14].

Table 1. Physiological roles of the endothelin axis

Endothelin/Receptor	Tissue	Role
ET-1 and -3 ET-RA and -RB	Embryonic tissue.	Development of *e.g.* craniofacial structures.
ET-1 ET-RA and -RB	Vasculature	Vascular homeostasis.
ET-1 ET-RA and -RB	Heart	Inotropic and chronotropic effects.
ET-1 ET-RA and -RB	Lung	Airway tone.
ET-1 ET-RA and -RB	Kidney	Renal blood flow, reabsorption of water and sodium, acid-base balance.
ET-1 and -3 ET-RA and -RB	Brain	Cardiorespiratory control, hormone release.
ET-1 and -2 ET-RA and -RB	Immune system	Differentiation and activation, and trafficking of immune cells.

The endothelins have a large variety of physiological roles and an exhaustive list is inappropriate here, but shown are an example of some of the major roles of endothelins in several different organs.

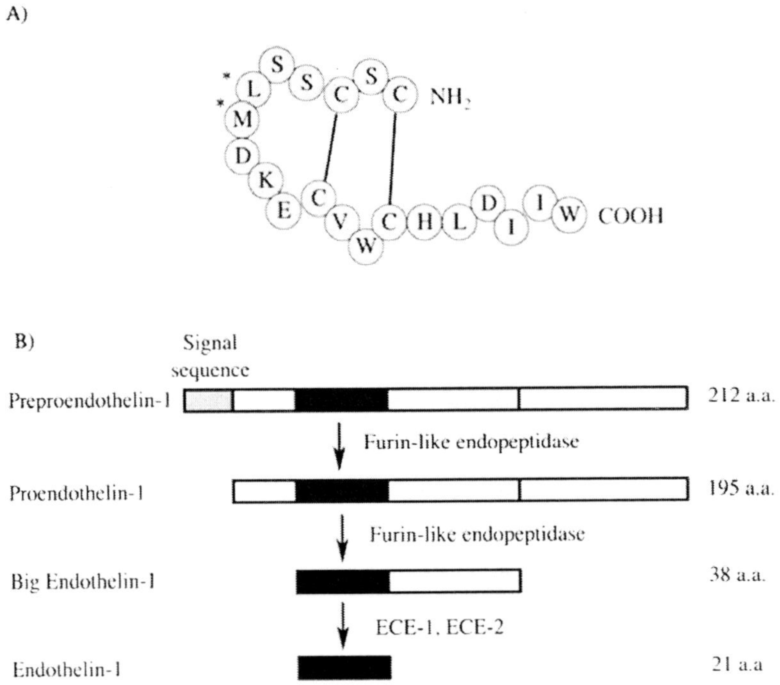

Figure 1. Processing and structure of endothelin-1. A) ET-1 is a 21 amino acid peptide with a hydrophobic C-terminus and two disulphide bonds at the N-terminus. ET-2 and ET-3 are structurally similar to ET-1, differing by two and six amino acids respectively. The amino acids which differ in the ET-2 sequence are indicated by '*' B) The 212 amino acid (a.a.) human preproendothelin-1 is processed by proteases to form 'big-ET' intermediates, which are further cleaved to yield the mature endothelin.

Endothelin Receptors and Signalling

Two receptors for endothelins have been characterized and designated ET-RA (also known as EDNRA or ET_AR) and ET-RB (EDNRB, ET_BR). It has been postulated that further sub-types of the endothelin receptors exist, but the pharmacological evidence for this is so far lacking [15,16]. Both receptors are expressed in a wide variety of tissue types, in some cases with distinct expression and in others showing a degree of overlapping expression (table 2). ET-RA is expressed by, amongst others, vascular smooth muscle cells (VSMCs), osteoblasts and adipocytes; ET-RB is expressed by all these cells and also by endothelial cells [2]. Each contains transmembrane domains comprising seven stretches of 20-27 hydrophobic amino acid residues, and has an N-terminal signal sequence and a long N-terminal extracellular domain.

Table 2. Expression of the endothelin axis in normal tissues

	ET-1	ET-2	ET-3	ET-RA	ET-RB
Endothelial cells	+	-	-	-	+
VSMCs	-	-	-	+	+
Epithelial cells	+	-	-	+	+
Lung epithelial cells	+	-	+	+	+
Kidney epithelial cells	+	+	+	+	+
Cardiomyocytes	+	-	-	+	+
Hepatocytes	+	-	-	+	+
Neurons	+	-	+	+	+
Adipocytes	-	-	-	+	+
Monocytes	+	+	-	+	-
Macrophages	+	+	-	+	+
Dendritic cells	+	+	+	+	+

Expression of members of the endothelin axis is widespread, but there is a distinct and restricted pattern of expression dependent upon tissue-type and also location (e.g. epithelial cells).

Endothelins bind to the two receptors with varying affinity: ET-RA binds ET-1 ≥ ET-2 > ET-3, but ET-RB shows no selective affinity for any endothelin subtype. Binding of the ligands to these G protein-coupled receptors may modulate several overlapping signalling pathways resulting in the activation of phospholipase C and MAPK pathways, an increase in intracellular calcium and the induction of immediate early genes [1,17].

Endothelin Receptor Antagonists

The role of endothelins in vasoconstriction and the development of hypertension etc. has led to the development of several antagonists of the endothelin receptors (table 3). These antagonists are now also being put to use in the dissemination of the roles of the endothelins in various cancers and, in some cases, are in clinical trials for the treatment of solid tumours.

Of the antagonists available, it is the modified peptide-based antagonists BQ123 (ET-RA antagonist) [18,19] and BQ788 (ET-RB antagonist) [20] that have been used extensively both in vitro and in vivo, while small molecule antagonists such as Atrasentan (ET-RA antagonist from Abbott Laboratories) [21] have been used in pre-clinical and clinical settings, particularly for the treatment of prostate cancer [22] (see Therapeutic Opportunities below).

BQ123 is a chemically synthesised analogue of the naturally occurring endothelin receptor antagonists BE-18257A and BE-18257B, which were isolated from Streptomyces misakiensis. These compounds inhibit ^{125}I-labelled-ET-1 binding to ET-RA in porcine aortic VSMCs with IC50 values of 1.4 and 0.47 μM, respectively. ^{125}IET-1 binding to ET-RB is not inhibited by either of these compounds even at 100 μM. The analogue, BQ123, also induces extremely potent inhibition of ^{125}IET-1 binding to ET-RA (IC50 of 7.3 nM), but barely inhibits ^{125}IET-1 binding to ET-RB (IC50 of 18 μM) [18].

BQ788 [N-cis-2,6-dimethylpiperidinocarbonyl-L-gamma-methylleucyl-D -1-methoxycarbonyltryptophanyl-D-norleucine] is a potent and selective ET-RB antagonist. In vitro, this compound potently and competitively inhibits ^{125}IET-1 binding to ET-RB (IC50, 1.2 nM) but only poorly inhibits the binding to ET-RA (IC50, 1.3 μM). In isolated rabbit pulmonary arteries, BQ788 shows no agonist activity up to 10 μM and competitively antagonizes the vasoconstriction induced by an ET-RB-selective agonist, BQ3020 [20].

Table 3. Antagonists of the endothelin receptors

Name	Company	Receptor antagonised	Notes
BQ123	Various	ET-RA	Not in clinical development. Used extensively as a research tool.
BQ788	Various	ET-RB	Not in clinical development. Used extensively as a research tool.
Atrasentan (ABT-627)	Abbott	ET-RA	In phase III clinical trials for prostate cancer.
A-192621	Abbott	ET-RB	
A-182086	Abbott	ET-RA and ET-RB	
Bosentan	Actelion	ET-RA and ET-RB	Approved for treatment of pulmonary hypertension.
YM598	Yamanouchi Pharmaceutical	ET-RA	In phase II trials for prostate cancer
AZD4054	AstraZeneca	ET-RA	In phase II trials for prostate cancer.

A selection of the endothelin receptor antagonists currently in use either in basic research (the modified peptide antagonists BQ123 and BQ788) or in pre-clinical/clinical trials (small molecule antagonists such as Atrasentan).

Several small molecule inhibitors of the endothelin receptor antagonists have also been identified and are now in development clinically (table 3). One antagonist under development is Atrasentan (also known as ABT-627) which is a selective ET-RA antagonist under development by Abbott Laboratories (IL, USA) for the treatment of cancer, particularly prostate cancer, for which it is in phase III trials [22]. Phase II trials for renal, ovarian, lung, colorectal, breast and brain cancers are also underway.

3. Endothelin Expression in Cancer

Numerous tumours, including carcinomas of the lung [23], breast [5], prostate [24] and ovary [4] produce one or more of the endothelins and their receptors [1] (table 4). Endothelins play an autocrine and paracrine role in regulating growth of several tumour types including ovarian cancer cell lines and tumours [4]. Endothelins may also inhibit apoptosis [5], as well promoting invasion [25] and angiogenesis [26]. However, the actions of endothelins in cancer are incompletely described and appear to be tumour-specific [27]. In several types of tumour, expression of the endothelin axis - particularly the receptors - is decreased in neoplastic tissue. For instance, in carcinomas of the breast both ET-RA and -RB are increased, yet in prostate cancer ET-RB is decreased or absent [28] and the ET-RB gene is often methylated [29], while in lung cancer ET-RA is down-regulated [23]. The function of the ET-RB receptor in tumours is particularly enigmatic; in some cases, such as breast cancer, ligand-binding to ET-RB initiates or is involved in several pro-tumour actions, such as promoting invasion [30], yet in prostate cancer, the loss of ET-RB expression is postulated to increase ET-1 peptide in the tumour due to the loss of ET-RB's endothelin-clearance function [29].

Table 4. Expression and effects of endothelins in solid tumours

Tumour	Endothelin axis expression	Role of endothelins	Refs
Ovarian cancer	ET-1 is upregulated in tumour cells. ET-RA is expressed by tumour cells and VSMCs. ET-RB is expressed by endothelial cells.	Autocrine growth factor via ET-RA. Receptors correlate with vascularity. VEGF stimulation via HIF-1. MMP induction. Promotes invasion.	[4, 32, 34-36]
Breast cancer	ET-1, -2, ET-RA and -RB increased in breast cancer. Tumour cells and immune infiltrate express ET and ET-R. ET expression induced by hypoxia.	Protection from hypoxia-associated apoptosis. TAM trafficking and activation. MMP induction. Promotes migration and invasion. VEGF stimulation via HIF-1.	[5, 14, 30]
Prostate cancer	High ET-1 and ET-RA expression. Decreased ET-RB expression.	Promotes growth. Inhibits apoptosis.	[29, 89]
Melanoma	ET-RA decreased. ET-RB increased.	Promotes proliferation. Promotes invasion	[44, 45, 90, 91]
Colon cancer	Increased ET-RA and ET-RB.	Inhibits apoptosis.	[92]
Kaposi's sarcoma	ET-RA and ET-RB expressed.	Promotes growth. Promotes migration and invasion.	[46, 47]

Endothelin axis expression is tumour-type dependent, and there are many potential roles for endothelins in several types of tumours.

Below is a description of the data published so far regarding the expression and roles of the endothelin axis in several types of solid tumours with particular reference to angiogenesis (table 5).

Endothelins in Ovarian Carcinoma

Ovarian cancer is one of the few cancers in which the role of endothelins has been extensively studied. Endothelins have several roles in ovarian tumours, including promoting growth and invasion, and stimulate both tumour and stroma cells. Ovarian carcinomas predominantly express ET-RA and secrete ET-1 [4]. Endothelins act as an autocrine growth factor for ovarian carcinoma cells via ET-RA [31,32] and also have a paracrine growth effect on the fibroblastic cells of ovarian cancer [33]. As well as affecting ovarian tumour growth, endothelins - acting through ET-RA - promote invasion of the tumour cells by up-regulating secretion and activation of matrix metalloproteinases (MMPs) [34].

Table 5. Microenvironmental factors which potentially influence endothelin expression in solid tumours.

Stimuli	Endothelin	Cell type	Ref
Endothelin	ET-1, ET-RA, ET-RB	Breast tumour cells	[30]
VEGF	ET-1	Endothelial cells	[53]
Hypoxia	ET-2, ET-RA, ET-RB	Breast tumour cells	[5]
Immune infiltrate	ET-1	Macrophages/breast tumour cells	(Hagemann et al - submitted)
Lipopolysaccharide	ET-1	Macrophages	[13]
TNF-α	ET-2	Renal adenocarcinoma	[93]
IL-1β, TNF-α, TGF-β	ET-1	Prostate cancer cell line	[55]
TGF-β	ET-1	VSMC Endothelial cells	[94] [95]

Factors, potentially present within the tumour microenvironment (or the analogous inflammatory microenvironment) that may induce expression of members of the endothelin axis and the cell type in which this induction has been shown.

ET-RA is found in both tumour cells and intratumoural vessels, whereas ET-RB is expressed mainly in endothelial cells and a further action of endothelins in ovarian cancer is the induction of angiogenesis via HIF-1α and VEGF [35,36]. In primary and metastatic ovarian tumours, ET-1 expression correlates with neovascularisation and VEGF expression, while high levels of ET-1 are detected in the ascitic fluids and correlate with VEGF ascitic concentration [35]. Conditioned media from ovarian carcinoma cell lines, as well as ascitic fluids, cause an increase in endothelial cell migration and ET-RA antagonists inhibit this angiogenic response.

ET-1 stimulates VEGF production in vitro through ET-RA, by an extent comparable to hypoxia. ET-1 stabilises HIF-1α protein leading to accumulation and activation of the HIF-1 transcription complex under both normoxic and hypoxic conditions, suggesting a role for

HIF-1 in the induction of VEGF expression [36]. These effects are inhibited by the selective ET-RA antagonist, BQ123.

In HEY and OVCA433 ovarian carcinoma cells, the induction of VEGF by ET-1 involves Src-mediated epidermal growth factor receptor (EGFR) transactivation. [37]. Cyclooxygenase (COX)-1 and COX-2 are implicated in the development and progression of several malignancies, and ET-1 increases the expression of COX-1 and COX-2 by ovarian carcinoma cells. These effects depend on ET-RA activation and involve multiple MAPK signalling pathways, including p42/44 MAPK, p38 MAPK, and transactivation of EGFR. COX inhibitors block ET-1-induced VEGF release. Further, inhibition of human ovarian tumour growth in nude mice after treatment with the ET-RA antagonist Atrasentan is associated with reduced COX-2, VEGF and microvessel density expression [38].

Endothelins in Breast Cancer

The role of endothelins in breast carcinogenesis has recently received attention both in our laboratories and others. As in other tumours, endothelins have several distinct roles in breast tumours and promote tumour growth and invasion via several different mechanisms and pathways [39]. There is increased expression of several members of the endothelin axis in breast cancer. In the normal breast, ET-1 and ET-RA mRNA expression can be detected; however, in invasive ductal carcinoma (IDC) of the breast there is increased expression of ET-1, ET-2, ET-RA and ET-RB [5,40]. IDCs also have a higher degree of endothelin expression than either benign fibroadenoma or ductal carcinoma in situ (DCIS); lymph node metastases of breast cancer have higher a higher degree of endothelin staining still. Elevated expression of ET-1 is more common in IDCs with larger size, high histological grade and the presence of lymphovascular invasion [41], and there is increased endothelin in the serum of breast cancer patients with lymph node metastases compared to those with no lymph node involvement (Hagemann et al. - submitted).

Cells expressing endothelins and their receptors in IDC include the tumour cells [5], the $CD68^{+}$ macrophage infiltrate [14], and the endothelial cells [26]. The increase in breast tumour cell invasion stimulated by endothelins is due, at least in part, to increased activity of MMPs: endothelins induce MMP-1, -2, -9 and -14 activity in macrophage culture and MMP-14 activity in MCF-7 culture. TIMP-1 release by macrophages and MCF-7 cells is also reduced by endothelins. Induction of MMP activity in macrophages is modulated via both receptors and can be inhibited by either BQ123 or BQ788; the non-selective MMP inhibitor FN439 also blocks endothelin-mediated invasion [25].

In keeping with the polyfunctional nature of endothelins, there are numerous potential consequences of endothelin expression in breast tumours that may lead to a more aggressive tumour cell phenotype.

One of the potential functions of endothelins in breast cancer is the modulation of angiogenesis. In biopsies of invasive breast cancer, the expression of ET-1, ET-RA and ET-RB is associated with increased VEGF expression and vascularity [42]. In vitro, VEGF production by breast cancer cell lines is induced by ET-1 and ET-2, but not ET-3 (our unpublished data). Endothelin-induced VEGF production is via ET-RA and is HIF-1α-dependent. We have also found that macrophage VEGF production is stimulated by endothelins, but in this case all the endothelin isotypes increase VEGF production and both endothelin receptors are involved (our unpublished data). Not only is breast cancer cell line VEGF production induced by endothelins, but further angiogenic factors including bFGF are also stimulated.

Endothelins in Prostate Cancer

The role of endothelins has been studied in the normal and transformed prostate. Endothelins are produced in the normal prostate gland by epithelial cells and are found in high concentrations in seminal fluid. Clinical trials of endothelin receptor antagonists in prostate cancer are now underway and show encouraging results [22]. ET-RA and ET-RB are found in normal prostate tissue, but in the malignant prostate there is a loss of ET-RB (a key component of ET-clearance) and increased levels of ET-1 [29]. Proposed roles for endothelins in prostate cancer include growth promotion, apoptosis inhibition, bone formation, and stimulation of nociceptive receptors. ET-1 can act alone as a mitogen, but its effects are greatest as a co-mitogen with a variety of growth factors, including bFGF, insulin-like growth factors, and platelet derived growth factor [28]. ET-1 also alters the balance of osteoblast and osteoclasts to favour new bone formation, which is a characteristic of the metastatic disease [43]. Several studies indicate that the refractory pain of metastatic cancer is related to the direct nociceptive effects of ET-1. Phase III clinical trials indicate that ET-RA antagonists used in prostate cancer are well tolerated but with mild side-effects related to ET-1's vasoconstrictive effects [22].

There is as yet little data regarding the role of endothelins in prostate cancer angiogenesis. However, there is a high level of ET-1 production and ET-RA expression, and it is likely that endothelins make a significant contribution to prostate cancer angiogenesis.

Endothelins in Melanoma

The activity of endothelins in melanoma has also been studied; however, the data regarding the expression and action of endothelins in melanoma has been contradictory, particularly when comparing melanoma cell lines in vitro and tumours in vivo. However, the data has shown that the endothelin axis may be a promising therapeutic target for the treatment of melanomas, and that endothelins may play a role in melanoma angiogenesis.

Activation of ET-RB in cultured melanocyte precursors promotes cell proliferation while inhibiting differentiation, two hallmarks of malignant transformation; ET-RB has a similar role in malignant transformation of melanoma. The selective ET-RB antagonist BQ788 can inhibit the growth of human melanoma cell lines and this inhibition is associated with increases in pigmentation and in the dendritic shape that is characteristic of mature melanocytes [44]. In vivo, BQ788 significantly slows growth (including a complete growth arrest in half of the mice treated) of human melanoma tumours in nude mice [44]. In contrast, although all the cell lines expressed both ET-RA and ET-RB mRNA, ET-RA antagonists did not have these effects.

In several melanoma cell lines, inhibition of ET-RB also leads to an increase in cell death and endothelins play a role in preventing melanoma cell apoptosis, particularly in metastatic melanoma cells [45]. Microarray analysis showed that BQ788 treatment leads to a reduction in the expression of survival factors, including BCL-2A1, and DNA repair enzymes and that the reduction is more pronounced in cells derived from metastatic than primary melanoma. Decreased cell viability correlates with reduced ET-RB expression, and reducing ET-RB protein levels (using small interfering RNAs) increases cell death.

Endothelins are also involved in angiogenesis in mouse models of melanoma; reduction of ET-RB expression by BQ788 is accompanied by a strong induction of VEGF expression and repression of the angiogenic suppressor gravin [45]; these changes in gene expression correlated with increased angiogenesis in tumours injected with the ET-RB antagonist in vivo.

Endothelins in Kaposi's Sarcoma

Kaposi's sarcoma is a highly angiogenic tumour that expresses endothelins. Both of the endothelin receptors are expressed in the tumour cells and the intratumoural vessels found in Kaposi's sarcoma tissue [46]. The tumourigenic KS IMM cell line (derived from a Kaposi's sarcoma) is susceptible to ET-1 mitogenic activity. ET-1 induces a dose-dependent increase in ^{3H}thymidine incorporation and addition of either BQ123 or BQ788 blocks the ET-1-induced mitogenic response and reduces the basal growth rate of unstimulated cells, suggesting that both receptors mediate the proliferative signal [46].

In the KS IMM cell line, ET-1 increases secretion and activation of MMP-2, -3, -7, -9 and -13, as well as of membrane-type 1-MMP (MT1-MMP) [47]. Addition of both ET-RA and ET-RB antagonists together completely blocks ET-1-induced MMP activity. ET-1 induces a dose-dependent enhancement in KS IMM cell migration and MMP-dependent invasiveness that can be inhibited by antagonists of either endothelin receptor. Treatment with both antagonists also suppresses ET-1-induced phosphorylation of the focal adhesion proteins, FAK and paxillin, which are essential for cell motility. The small molecule ET-R(A/B) antagonist, A-182086, completely inhibits cell proliferation and tumour growth in KS IMM xenografts.

Endothelins and the Stroma

The tumour stroma plays an important role in tumour angiogenesis. Growth factors and cytokines produced by macrophages and other cells are crucial for stroma formation and neovascularisation, and lytic enzymes provided by stromal cells may be essential for invasion. Many of the effects of the tumour stroma come about through the action of secreted soluble substances including the endothelins. Endothelins are both released by stromal cells and act upon them to induce, for instance, cytokine release. The interactions between the stroma and the endothelin axis may play an important role in tumour angiogenesis. However, as with endothelin production by tumour cells, the consequences of stroma/endothelin interactions are likely to be tumour-type dependent.

Macrophages are terminally differentiated cells that produce a number of potent angiogenic cytokines and growth factors including VEGF, TNF-α, IL-8, and bFGF. Tumour-associated macrophages (TAMs) are able to promote tumour growth directly by secreting breast tumour mitogens, such as epidermal growth factor, and indirectly by stimulating tumour angiogenesis and metastasis [48]. They also modulate events in the extracellular matrix through the secretion of extracellular matrix-degrading enzymes and -modulating enzymes.

Endothelins have a role in recruiting TAMs, which may influence tumour angiogenesis. Macrophages produce endothelins [13] and the TAMs contribute to the endothelins in the breast tumour microenvironment [14]. In contrast, no immunoreactive endothelin can be detected in cell extracts from human neutrophils and lymphocytes [13]. Co-culture of tumour cells with macrophages leads to increased endothelin production (Hagemann et al. - submitted). Macrophages express both endothelin receptors and chemotax towards endothelins via ET-RB and a pertussis-toxin sensitive MAPK-mediated signalling pathway [14]. Exposure of macrophages to endothelins in vitro leads to increased cell surface CD68 and HLA-ABC indicating an 'activated' phenotype, whilst in patient biopsies 'foamy' activated macrophages co-localise with regions containing tumour cells that express endothelins [5,14].

Endothelins also stimulate macrophages to produce both VEGF and IL-8 and this is via both receptors (our unpublished data). MMP activity in macrophage culture is induced by endothelins and this has been shown to facilitate breast tumour cell invasion in vitro [30]; however, MMP activity is also a prerequisite for angiogenesis and it is likely that endothelin-induced MMP production by macrophages promotes tumour angiogenesis in breast tumours and other malignancies.

ET-1 and ET-3 induce proliferation and chemotaxis of pulmonary artery fibroblasts while all endothelin isotypes stimulate the growth of fibroblast cell lines derived from ovarian carcinomas [33]. These fibroblasts express both ET-RA and ET-RB, and antagonism of either receptor inhibits ET-1 stimulated growth suggesting the involvement of both receptor types in ET-1 growth regulation. However, ovarian carcinoma-derived fibroblast cell lines do not secrete detectable protein, and endothelin-mediated mitogenesis requires a source of endothelin; ovarian carcinoma cells may be such a source and co-culture experiments of fibroblasts with carcinoma cells demonstrated that growth of both populations of cells is increased compared with either grown in isolation [33]. In this system, growth of the fibroblast cell line was partially inhibited by both BQ123 and BQ788, whilst growth of the carcinoma cell line was inhibited by BQ123 only. These data indicate that endothelins may stimulate growth of the fibroblast population within ovarian cancer tumours and this paracrine effect may contribute to the overall growth of the tumour.

Induction of Endothelin Expression by the Tumour Microenvironment

Solid tumours do not consist of a homogeneous structure or environment: one region of tumour, compared to another, may differ in the levels of hypoxia, cytokine concentration, immune infiltrate, vascularisation, necrosis etc. [49-51]. The breast tumour microenvironment, particularly hypoxia, modulates expression of numerous 'pro-tumour' genes [52], including those of the endothelins and their receptors [5].

The expression of endothelins is increased in unstimulated breast tumour cells compared to benign cells (Hagemann et al. - submitted); which aspect of transformation leads to increased endothelin expression is as yet unknown. However, the levels of endothelin synthesis by tumour cells may be stimulated by numerous factors that may be present within an inflammatory or tumour microenvironment (table 5).

As well as hypoxia, soluble factors such as cytokines modulate the expression of the endothelin axis in breast tumours. Of particular importance is the finding that endothelins themselves stimulate endothelin receptor production by breast tumour cells [25] and endothelial cells.

As discussed above, endothelins stimulate VEGF expression and secretion, but the reverse is also true: VEGF stimulates ET-1 production by bovine aortic endothelial cells [53]. VEGF also increases ECE-1 expression in aortic endothelial cells [54].

Within the vasculature, ET-RA is upregulated in smooth muscle cells by insulin and nitric oxide, while in endothelial cells ET-RB is upregulated by TNF-α and bFGF. In the PC3 human prostate cancer cell line, ET-1 is up-regulated by IL-1β, TNF-α, and TGF-β [55]. Macrophage-derived cytokines and chemokines, including CCL2, CCL3 and CCL5, induce endothelial cells to produce endothelins [56,57] which may further modulate the local endothelin concentrations in the tumour microenvironment.

The tumour microenvironment is diverse, even within one type of tumour, and the stimulation that gives rise to high endothelin concentrations and/or endothelin receptor expression is likely to vary between patients and adds a further degree of complexity and tumour-specificity to the relationship between the endothelin axis and tumour angiogenesis. An area that has yet received little attention, but will need to be addressed, is the actions of endothelins in combination with, for instance, cytokines present within the tumour. Our own observations suggest that not only do microenvironmental factors influence endothelin expression, but also the cells' response to both the endothelin and, for instance, the cytokine (unpublished observation).

Endothelins and HIF-1α

Transcriptional regulation of numerous hypoxia-responsive genes, including VEGF and ET-1, is via the critical mediator of hypoxia-induced transcription, HIF-1. HIF-1 is a dimer of HIF-1α and HIF-1β; HIF-1β is present in all cells and is stable under normoxia, but HIF-1α is rapidly ubiquitinated and degraded in the presence of oxygen. Hypoxia stabilises the HIF-1α monomer, leading to heterodimerisation and the formation of the HIF-1 complex that can then initiate transcription of genes whose promoter contains a hypoxia response element (HRE) [58].

Hypoxia induces endothelin transcription in several cell types including endothelial cells [59], and tumour cells [5,60]. There is a functioning proximal HRE in the anti-sense strand of the promoter of ET-1 [61,62] and induction of endothelin expression by hypoxia is via HIF-1 [63]. There are also essential roles for AP-1, GATA-2, and NF-1 in stabilizing the binding of HIF-1 and promoting recruitment of p300/CBP to the ET-1 HRE [64]. ET-2 is stimulated by hypoxia in cultured breast carcinoma cells, and in vivo endothelin expression co-localises with hypoxic areas of the tumour [5]. The upregulation of ET-2 bears the characteristics of being HIF-1-dependent (i.e. it is also induced by the iron chelators cobalt chloride and desferrioxamine, and hypoxic-induction is inhibited by the HIF-inhibitor diphenylene iodonium) but HIF-1α stabilisation and HIF/HRE binding has not yet been conclusively proven.

No HRE has yet been described in the promoter of either endothelin receptor but in certain cell types both endothelin receptors may be induced by hypoxia [5,65]. This may, however, be a secondary effect due to the increase in endothelin production seen under hypoxic conditions: endothelins themselves induce endothelin receptor production by breast carcinoma cells [25]. It is also possible that one or more of the cytokines induced by hypoxia stimulate receptor production.

4. Endothelins and Tumour Angiogenesis

Endothelins stimulate angiogenesis within solid tumours (table 6). Endothelins, by acting directly on endothelial cells via ET-RB, modulate different stages of neovascularisation, including proliferation, migration, invasion, protease production and morphogenesis, and also stimulates neovascularisation in vivo. Endothelins can also modulate tumour angiogenesis indirectly through the induction of VEGF expression by tumour and endothelial cells.

Direct Stimulation of Angiogenesis by Endothelins

The local concentration of endothelins in the vascular wall may be ≥100 fold that of the plasma level, stemming in part from the fact that 80% of ET-1 is secreted on the basal side of endothelial cells [2]. ET-1 is a potent mitogen for both endothelial cells and VSMCs. In normal blood vessels, endothelial cells express ET-RB, while VSMCs express ET-RA. Both ET-RA and ET-RB play varying roles in mediation of vasopressor actions depending on the species and vasculature involved.

Human umbilical vein endothelial cells (HUVECs) secrete ET-1 and express the B-type receptor and ET-1 production is stimulated via an autocrine positive feedback loop upon binding of the ET-1 peptide to ET-RB. HUVECs express lower levels of ET-RA. ET-1 promotes proliferation, migration, and invasion of endothelial cells derived from bovine adrenal capillaries and HUVECs in a dose-dependent manner [66]. In vitro, HUVECs cultured on matrigel in the presence of ET-1 migrate and align to form vascular cord-like structures [67]. Addition of the ET-RB antagonist BQ788 inhibits endothelin stimulation of HUVECs, whilst the ET-RA antagonist only partially blocks stimulation.

Table 6. Summary of data on the roles of endothelins in tumour angiogenesis.

Tumour	Angiogenic role of endothelins	Expression of receptors
Ovarian cancer	Stimulates neovascularisation. Stimulates VEGF via HIF1α. Expression correlates with vascularisation.	ET-RA in tumour cells and VSMCs. ET-RB only in endothelial cells.
Breast cancer	Expression correlates with VEGF expression and MVD. Induces VEGF via HIF1α. Induces bFGF expression by tumour cells. Stimulates TAMs to produce pro-angiogenic cytokines.	ET-RA & -RB produced by tumour cells, TAMs and endothelial cells. VEGF induction via ET-RA in tumour cells.
Bone metastases	Stimulates osteoblast proliferation and VEGF production.	ET-RA & -RB expressed by osteoblasts. VEGF induction via ET-RA.
Kaposi's sarcoma	Unknown.	Both receptors expressed by intratumoural vessels.
Lung cancer	Unknown.	Blood vessels and vascular stroma bind ET-1.
Astrocytoma	Expression correlates with vascularity.	

The pro-angiogenic effect of endothelins on HUVECs is even more marked when combined with VEGF; the effect of the endothelins and VEGF together is additive leading to a striking morphogenesis of vascular structures [67]. The mechanism by which endothelins and VEGF cooperate to produce an additive effect are presently unknown; one characteristic of the endothelins is the ability to amplify or modulate responses to apparently quite separate stimuli, such as chemokines [30] and cytokines [28], and it will be important that this question of mechanism is addressed in the future.

During the invasion of endothelial cells, various constituents of the interstitial stroma and basement membrane are degraded, and this involves the MMPs, particularly MMP-2, which is secreted when endothelial cell sprouting occurs. Another potentially pro-angiogenic affect of endothelins is that they induce production of active MMPs by endothelial cells, macrophages and tumour cells [30,34,67].

However, in vivo studies of the roles of endothelins in angiogenesis in normal (i.e. non-neoplastic) tissues have shown conflicting results. ET-1 was unable to stimulate blood vessel growth in the chick embryo chorioallantoic membrane (CAM), or in a rat sponge model [68,69]. In contrast, endothelins have been shown to have angiogenic activity in a matrigel plug implanted into mice [67]. ET-1 and ET-3 also displayed angiogenic activity in a rat cornea model and this was mediated via ET-RA [70].

In one study [71], Chinese hamster ovary (CHO) cells were stably transfected with ET-1 cell and grafted onto the CAM ectoderm. CHO-ET-1 cell aggregates formed highly vascularised nodules surrounded by radially rearranged vessels, with a strong angiogenic response. There was also an increase in endothelial cell proliferation in the CAM vasculature around CHO-ET-1 nodules. The specific involvement of ET-1 in the angiogenic effect mediated by CHO-ET-1 was demonstrated by the reduction or abolition of neovascularised CHO-ET-1 nodules by Bosentan (mixed antagonist of ET-RA/B), an ET-RA antagonist (Ru69986) and by phosporamidon, an inhibitor of ECE-1. VEGF is involved in CHO-ET-1-mediated angiogenesis, because a specific inhibitor of VEGF tyrosine kinase receptor activity abolished CHO-ET-1 nodule formation and CAM neovascularisation.

Indirect Modulation of Angiogenesis by Endothelins

Although endothelins have a direct angiogenic activity, they also indirectly stimulate angiogenesis, chiefly by modulating VEGF activity. VEGF stimulates angiogenesis and the regulation of its synthesis and activity is one of the important checkpoints regulating the formation of tumour vasculature.

ET-1 stimulates expression and secretion of VEGF by VSMC predominantly via ET-RA [72]. This, in turn, induces VEGF-mediated endothelial cell proliferation and invasion. The nodule formation by CHO-ET-1 in the CAM is VEGF-mediated as demonstrated by the inhibition of the CAM neovascularisation by a VEGF tyrosine receptor kinase inhibitor [71].

Endothelin-mediated stimulation of VEGF production by tumour cells is another mechanism by which endothelins give rise to angiogenesis in solid tumours. In ovarian carcinoma, endothelins induces VEGF production [36,72] and endothelin expression correlates with VEGF expression in IDC [42]. In OVCA 433 and HEY ovarian carcinoma cell lines, ET-1 treatment increases VEGF mRNA expression and induces VEGF protein levels in a time- and dose-dependent fashion, and does so to a greater extent under hypoxic conditions. Although hypoxia is the major factor that stabilises HIF-1α, other stimuli such as growth factors, hormones and nitric oxide may stabilise HIF-1α and induce transcription of HIF-1-dependent genes. One such factor that stabilises HIF-1α is, in fact, ET-1 which induces VEGF transcription in normoxic ovarian carcinoma cells in a HIF-1-dependent manner [36]. ET-1 stabilises the HIF-1α subunit leading to accumulation and activation of the HIF-1 transcription complex under both normoxic and hypoxic conditions, suggesting a role for HIF-1 in the induction of VEGF expression (figure 5). These effects are inhibited by the selective ET-RA antagonist, BQ123.

Inhibition of ET-RB, which may act as a clearance receptor and/or modulate the response to ET-RA ligand binding, induces expression of VEGF mRNA by melanoma cell lines [45].

Endothelins also stimulate VEGF expression and secretion by breast tumour cells (our unpublished data). The mechanism appears to be similar to that seen in ovarian carcinoma i.e. ligand-binding to ET-RA leads to stabilisation of HIF-1α and subsequent normoxic transcription of target genes including VEGF. Accumulation of the HIF-1α subunit is associated with breast cancer progression [73].

There have been many reports of hypoxia-responsive genes expressed by tumours, and many of these may be pro-angiogenic [74]. It is likely that endothelin-mediated stabilisation of HIF-1 will give rise to the induction of expression of many of these genes. Indeed, several of the genes described below as being induced by endothelins are also induced by hypoxia (e.g. IL-8 is induced by hypoxia in endothelial cells [75]) and it is likely that HIF-1 is also involved in the induction of these genes by endothelins.

Endothelins and other Angiogenic Cytokines

Angiogenesis is modulated by numerous factors, and the response elicited by any angiogenic factor is dependent on the presence or absence of further regulatory molecules. As well as inducing VEGF, endothelins may modulate the production of other pro-angiogenic cytokines by both tumour and stroma cells (table 7).

Table 7. Induction of potentially pro-angiogenic molecules by endothelins.

Gene	Angiogenic function	Cell type
VEGF	Mitogenic for endothelial cells and VSMCs.	Endothelial cells [53], ovarian tumour cells [37], breast tumour cells (our unpublished data), VSMCs [72].
TNF-α	TNF-α inhibits the growth of endothelial cells in vitro it is a potent promoter of angiogenesis in *vivo*.	Macrophages [96].
TGF-β	Although TGF-β inhibits the growth of endothelial cells it promote neovascularisation promote tumour development *in vivo*.	Breast tumour cells (our unpublished data).
IL-8	Macrophage-derived IL8 supports angiogenesis and may play a role in angiogenesis-dependent including tumour growth, and wound healing.	Endothelial cells [97]. Macrophages (our unpublished data).
bFGF	Chemotactic and mitogenic agent for endothelial cells, inducing production of factors involved in the breakdown of the basement membrane and the migration of capillary endothelial cells	Breast tumour cells (our unpublished data). VSMC [76].

One pro-angiogenic factor which may be widely regulated by endothelins is bFGF, a chemotactic and mitogenic agent for endothelial cells in vitro, inducing endothelial cell production of factors involved in the breakdown of the basement membrane and the migration of capillary endothelial cells into collagen matrices to form capillary-like tubes. These and other in vitro observations suggest that FGFs play a role in vivo in the modulation of such normal processes as angiogenesis, wound healing and tissue repair, embryonic development and differentiation, ET-1 can induce bFGF mRNA levels in rat aortic smooth muscle cells [76] and also by breast tumour cells (our unpublished data).

ET-1 induces human central nervous system-derived endothelial cells to produce and secrete the pro-angiogenic chemokine IL-8 via ET-RA, protein kinase C and protein tyrosine kinase pathways, and NF-κB [77,78]. Several further pro-angiogenic cytokines including

TNF-α and TGF-β may also be induced by endothelin stimulation of endothelial cells, tumour cells and macrophages (table 7).

As well as promoting production of pro-angiogenic molecules such as VEGF and bFGF, endothelins may also inhibit the production of anti-angiogenic molecules. ET-1 inhibits production of tissue inhibitor of matrix metalloproteinase (TIMP)-1 by ovarian carcinoma cells and by macrophages [34, and Hagemann et al. - submitted]. Expression of the anti-angiogenic cytokine IL-10 is decreased in macrophages by endothelins (our unpublished data).

Protection from Apoptosis by Endothelins

A further aspect of the actions of endothelins that may modulate tumour angiogenesis is that endothelins protect cells from apoptosis. ET-1, as well as being a mitogen, functions as an apoptosis survival factor for endothelial cells in an autocrine/paracrine manner via ET-RB [79]. When endothelial cells (obtained from the rat aorta) are serum starved, significant portions of cultured cells undergo apoptotic death. ET-1 dose-dependently suppresses the apoptosis induced by serum starvation. The ET-RB antagonist BQ788 and ET-RA/B antagonists PD142893 and PD145065, but not the ET-RA antagonist BQ123, block the protective effect of ET-1. The effect of ET-1 in suppressing apoptosis is unaffected by phospholipase C inhibition, a tyrosine kinase inhibitor, an MEK inhibitor, or phosphatidylinositol-3 kinase inhibitors [80].

ET-1 also inhibits nitric oxide- and serum deprivation-induced apoptosis of VSMCs via a MAPK pathway [81]. Both serum deprivation and NO donors (FK409 and SNAP) cause apoptosis of VSMCs, but ET-1 dose-dependently antagonises apoptosis. BQ123 and a non-selective receptor antagonist (TAK044), but not BQ788, inhibited the anti-apoptotic effect of ET-1, indicating that (unlike endothelial cells) the anti-apoptotic effect of ET-1 is mediated via ET-RA. ET-1 activates the MAPK pathway, and inhibition of MAPK activity with PD98059, a specific inhibitor of MAPKK-1, antagonises the anti-apoptotic effect of ET-1.

Further insight into ET-1's anti-apoptotic effects comes from studies of cardiac myocytes. ET-1 protects cardiac myocytes against CNP-induced apoptosis by influencing the cGMP-dependent pathway, and this effect is probably mediated through both a reduction of cGMP and antagonism of the CNP-induced reduction of intracellular ornithine decarboxylase expression [82].

5. Modulation of Blood Flow within Tumours by Endothelins

As well as modulating tumour neovascularisation - and hence delivery of both nutrients and therapeutic agents to the tumour cells - endothelins are thought to effect blood flow through the established tumour vasculature due to their vasoactive nature. However, as with many other aspects of the endothelin axis, the effect of endothelins on tumour blood flow appears to be tumour-specific.

Isolated tumour arterioles mounted in a pressure myograph have the ability, contrary to size-matched healthy arterioles, to contract in response to a transluminal pressure increase. This myogenic tone is dependent on the ET-1 pathway and is abolished by the ET-RA antagonist BQ123 [83]. Laser Doppler microprobes showed that administration of BQ123 led to an increase in tumour blood flow, whereas the perfusion in control healthy tissue was not altered. Acute administration of the ET-RA antagonist stimulates tumour oxygenation, as determined by electron paramagnetic resonance oximetry, and increases the efficacy of low-dose, clinically relevant fractionated radiotherapy. Thus, blocking the vascular ET-1/ET-RA pathway may potentially be used to induce vasorelaxation and this could, perhaps, be exploited to selectively increase tumour response to radiotherapy.

However, as noted previously, the effects of endothelins are tumour-dependent and the situation may be different in breast tumours. In one study [84], the systemic haemodynamics and regional circulatory effects of ET-1 in rats with breast tumours was examined. Tumour-bearing rats were treated with ET-1 and/or BQ788 and their cardiovascular parameters were measured using a radioactive microsphere technique, and blood perfusion to the breast tissue was also measured using a laser Doppler technique. ET-1 produced a significant increase in mean arterial pressure in normal and tumour-bearing rats. Blood flow to the tumour tissue increased significantly in response to ET-1 compared to breast tissue in normal rats. This response was accompanied by a concomitant decrease in vascular resistance in the tumour tissue. These results were confirmed by laser Doppler flowmetry, which showed a significant increase in blood perfusion to breast tumour compared to normal breast tissue. This increase in blood perfusion was attenuated by pre-treatment with BQ788, suggesting an ET-RB-mediated vasodilator action of ET-1 in rat breast tumour.

In another study, modulation of tissue blood flow and tissue vascular resistance by endothelins was examined in the female CBH rat, bearing a HSN fibrosarcoma [85]. Rats were treated with intravenous administration of ET-1 and blood flow was measured by the tissue uptake of ^{125}I-labelled-iodoantipyrine. ET-1 increased mean arterial blood pressure. Blood flow to the tumour was unaffected by ET-1 treatment, whereas blood flow to normal tissues was reduced (the exception being the heart and the brain in which flow was increased). Vascular resistance was increased in all tissues and the tumour by ET-1 indicating that the tumour vasculature was constricting. Tumour blood flow was significantly reduced by IRL 1620, an ET-RB agonist, while vascular resistance was significantly increased [86]. Pre-treatment of rats with BQ788 attenuated the tumour vascular response to IRL 1620.

The effects of endothelins and their antagonists on tumour blood flow is an area that merits further study. The tumour specificity of endothelin-mediated blood flow is an interesting conundrum itself, but also has implications for the therapy of solid tumours, either with traditional chemotherapeutic agents or with endothelin receptor antagonists. Particular care will have to be taken when designing pre-clinical and clinical trials involving the use of combined chemotherapy and anti-endothelin therapy, as drug delivery may be dramatically altered by inhibition of the endothelin axis.

6. Therapeutic Opportunities

The role of endothelins in vasoconstriction has led to the development of small molecule antagonists of the endothelin receptors, which are currently under investigation for the treatment of hypertension, heart failure and renal disease (table 3) [87]. These antagonists can be administered orally, are well tolerated and have few toxic side effects. Several of these antagonists have been used in pre-clinical or clinical trials for several types of cancer (table 8). Few of these studies have directly studied angiogenesis or angiogenic markers and so the data is still inconclusive regarding the efficacy of endothelin antagonists as an anti-angiogenic therapy. However, several studies have shown some therapeutic benefit (either in an experimental context or during clinical trials) and it is likely that the modulation of angiogenesis by these antagonists is, at least in part, responsible for the responses seen.

Table 8. Actions of endothelin receptor antagonists on tumour models and in clinical trials.

Tumour	Antagonist	Tumour response	Ref.
Prostate	Atrasentan	Improves time to progression in phase III clinical trials.	[98]
Ovarian	Atrasentan, BQ123, BQ788	Decreased xenograft growth associated with decreased VEGF expression and microvessel density.	[99]
Breast	BQ123, BQ788	Slowed tumour growth in a murine model by either antagonist, but apparently different mechanisms	[5]
Melanoma	BQ788	Slows melanoma xenograft growth in mice.	[44]
Kaposi's sarcoma	A-182086	Abolishes tumour xenograft growth in mice.	[47]
Ewing's sarcoma	BQ123	Inhibits cell line proliferation *in vitro*.	[88]
Neuroblastoma	BQ123	Inhibits cell line proliferation *in vitro*.	[88]
Cervical	Atrasentan	Inhibits growth and angiogenesis in xenografts.	[100]

Atrasentan, a highly selective ET-RA antagonist, has been given to cancer patients in phase II trials for prostate cancer and delayed time to clinical and PSA progression [21]. Phase III trials for hormone-refractory prostate cancer are underway.

In a small scale in vivo setting, we treated a murine model of breast carcinoma, HTH-K, with the commercially available modified peptide antagonists of the endothelin receptors, BQ123 [18] and BQ788 [20]. In this study, both antagonists showed a modest survival benefit by two apparently different mechanisms: both caused a delay in growth of the tumour yet BQ123 (ET-RA antagonist)-treated tumours did not show the increased necrosis associated with treatment with BQ788 (ET-RB antagonist) [5]. Whilst difficult to quantify by immunohistochemical methods, it appeared to us that treatment of the HTH-K tumour with BQ123 led to more disrupted and 'leaky' vessels than control tumours (our unpublished observation) indicating that endothelin receptor antagonists act on the vasculature in breast tumours as well as the tumour cells.

Endothelin receptor antagonists inhibit proliferation of Kaposi's sarcoma cells [46], Ewing's sarcoma and neuroblastoma cells [88], melanoma cells [44] and ovarian carcinoma cells [4]. In ovarian carcinoma xenografts, tumour growth is inhibited in Atrasentan-treated mice compared with control. Growth inhibition is associated with a reduction in microvessel density, expression of VEGF, and MMP-2, and increased apoptotic tumour cells. Combined treatment of Atrasentan with paclitaxel produced additive apoptotic and anti-angiogenic effects.

Endothelin receptor antagonists also hold the attractive possibility that they will 'hit' several different cell types and mechanisms of disease progression: the antagonists may potentially inhibit angiogenesis by inhibiting endothelial cell mitogenesis while simultaneously preventing macrophages from producing MMPs, and countering the anti-apoptotic effect of endothelins on the tumour cells themselves.

However, a caveat should be noted: the expression of endothelin receptors in solid tumours is dependent on the origin and location of the primary tumour, and thus modifying the endothelin axis may show unpredictable results at secondary sites. For instance, breast tumour cells (which express high levels of both ET-RA and ET-RB) often metastasise to the lungs yet primary tumours in the lung may have decreased ET-RA and hence it is difficult to predict the outcome of treatment with endothelin receptor antagonists on a breast cancer metastasis within the microenvironment of the lung. It is also true that the mechanistic details of endothelin-mediated tumour progression are yet to be elucidated and so the exact consequences of endothelin receptor inhibition cannot be predicted at this time. Only further research into the endothelin axis in breast cancer and pre-clinical trials of the receptor antagonists will provide an answer as to whether the endothelin receptors are a suitable therapeutic target for breast cancer.

7. Conclusion

The mechanism(s) by which endothelins induce angiogenesis are as yet incompletely described but potentially includes the interaction between the tumour cells, the stroma and the tumour microenvironment. This complex interaction leads to proliferation of endothelial cells, induction of MMP activity, cytokine expression, immune infiltrate activation, inhibition of apoptosis, and expression of the endothelins themselves. All these factors may cumulatively facilitate tumour angiogenesis. Small molecule inhibitors of the endothelin receptor already exist and the endothelin axis may be a suitable therapeutic target for the anti-angiogenic treatment of several cancers that can quickly be exploited.

Acknowledgements

M. Grimshaw was supported by an EU grant (QLK3-CT-2002-1980).

REFERENCES

[1] Nelson J, Bagnato A, Battistini B, Nisen P. The endothelin axis: emerging role in cancer. *Nat Rev Cancer* 2003;3;110-6.

[2] Kedzierski RM, Yanagisawa M. Endothelin system: the double-edged sword in health and disease. *Annu Rev Pharmacol Toxicol* 2001;41;851-76.

[3] Haendler B, Hechler U, Schleuning WD. Molecular cloning of human endothelin (ET) receptors ETA and ETB. *J Cardiovasc Pharmacol* 1992;20;S1-4.

[4] Bagnato A, Salani D, Di Castro V, et al. Expression of endothelin 1 and endothelin A receptor in ovarian carcinoma: evidence for an autocrine role in tumor growth. *Cancer Res* 1999;59;720-7.

[5] Grimshaw MJ, Naylor S, Balkwill FR. Endothelin-2 Is a Hypoxia-induced Autocrine Survival Factor for Breast Tumor Cells. *Mol Cancer Ther* 2002;1;1273-81.

[6] Itoh Y, Yanagisawa M, Ohkubo S, et al. Cloning and sequence analysis of cDNA encoding the precursor of a human endothelium-derived vasoconstrictor peptide, endothelin: identity of human and porcine endothelin. *FEBS Lett* 1988;231;440-4.

[7] Inoue A, Yanagisawa M, Kimura S, et al. The human endothelin family: three structurally and pharmacologically distinct isopeptides predicted by three separate genes. *Proc Natl Acad Sci U S A* 1989;86;2863-7.

[8] Saida K, Kometani N, Masuda H, Oka S, Uchide T. Structure of mouse preproendothelin-3 and phylogenetic analysis of the endothelins. *J Cardiovasc Pharmacol* 2000;36;S1-4.

[9] Saida K, Hashimoto M, Mitsui Y, Ishida N, Uchide T. The prepro vasoactive intestinal contractor (VIC)/endothelin-2 gene (EDN2): structure, evolution, production, and embryonic expression. *Genomics* 2000;64;51-61.

[10] Opgenorth TJ, Wu-Wong JR, Shiosaki K. Endothelin-converting enzymes. *Faseb J* 1992;6;2653-9.

[11] Lees DM, Khan NQ, Barker S, Corder R. Quantitative measurement of mRNA levels by RT-PCR. Studies of ECE-1 isoforms. *Methods Mol Biol* 2002;206;125-45.

[12] Corder R, Khan NQ, Harrison VJ, Wood EG, Lees DM, Barker S. Relationship between soluble intracellular endothelin-converting enzyme and endothelin-1 synthesis: effect of inhibitors of the secretory pathway. *J Cardiovasc Pharmacol* 2000;36;S19-21.

[13] Ehrenreich H, Anderson RW, Fox CH, et al. Endothelins, peptides with potent vasoactive properties, are produced by human macrophages. *J Exp Med* 1990;172;1741-8.

[14] Grimshaw MJ, Wilson JL, Balkwill FR. Endothelin-2 is a macrophage chemoattractant: implications for macrophage distribution in tumors. *Eur J Immunol* 2002;32;2393-400.

[15] Clozel M, Gray GA. Are there different ETB receptors mediating constriction and relaxation? *J Cardiovasc Pharmacol* 1995;26 Suppl 3;S262-4.

[16] Natarajan S, Hunt JT, Festin S, Serafino R, Zhang R, Moreland S. Endothelin analogs which distinguish vasoconstrictor and vasodilator ETB receptors. *Life Sci* 1995;56;1251-6.

[17] Masaki T, Miwa S, Sawamura T, Ninomiya H, Okamoto Y. Subcellular mechanisms of endothelin action in vascular system. *Eur J Pharmacol* 1999;375;133-8.

[18] Ihara M, Ishikawa K, Fukuroda T, et al. In vitro biological profile of a highly potent novel endothelin (ET) antagonist BQ-123 selective for the ETA receptor. *J Cardiovasc Pharmacol* 1992;20;S11-4.

[19] Ihara M, Noguchi K, Saeki T, et al. Biological profiles of highly potent novel endothelin antagonists selective for the ETA receptor. *Life Sci* 1992;50;247-55.

[20] Ishikawa K, Ihara M, Noguchi K, et al. Biochemical and pharmacological profile of a potent and selective endothelin B-receptor antagonist, BQ-788. *Proc Natl Acad Sci U S A* 1994;91;4892-6.

[21] Norman P. Atrasentan Abbott. *Curr Opin Investig Drugs* 2002;3;1240-8.

[22] Lassiter LK, Carducci MA. Endothelin receptor antagonists in the treatment of prostate cancer. *Semin Oncol* 2003;30;678-88.

[23] Ahmed SI, Thompson J, Coulson JM, Woll PJ. Studies on the expression of endothelin, its receptor subtypes, and converting enzymes in lung cancer and in human bronchial epithelium. *Am J Respir Cell Mol Biol* 2000;22;422-31.

[24] Nelson JB, Carducci MA. The role of endothelin-1 and endothelin receptor antagonists in prostate cancer. *BJU Int* 2000;85 Suppl 2;45-8.

[25] Grimshaw MJ, Hagemann T, Ayhan A, Gillett CE, Binder C, Balkwill FR. A Role for Endothelin-2 and Its Receptors in Breast Tumor Cell Invasion. *Cancer Res* 2004;64; 2461-2468.

[26] Bagnato A, Spinella F. Emerging role of endothelin-1 in tumor angiogenesis. *Trends Endocrinol Metab* 2002;14;44-50.

[27] Bell KM, Chaplin DJ. The effect of oxygen and carbon dioxide on tumor cell endothelin-1 production. *J Cardiovasc Pharmacol* 1998;31 Suppl 1;S537-40.

[28] Kopetz ES, Nelson JB, Carducci MA. Endothelin-1 as a target for therapeutic intervention in prostate cancer. *Invest New Drugs* 2002;20;173-82.

[29] Nelson JB, Lee WH, Nguyen SH, et al. Methylation of the 5' CpG island of the endothelin B receptor gene is common in human prostate cancer. *Cancer Res* 1997;57;35-7.

[30] Grimshaw MJ, Hagemann T, Ayhan A, Gillett CE, Binder C, Balkwill FR. A role for endothelin-2 and its receptors in breast tumor cell invasion. *Cancer Res* 2004;64;2461-8.

[31] Moraitis S, Langdon SP, Miller WR. Endothelin expression and responsiveness in human ovarian carcinoma cell lines. *Eur J Cancer* 1997;33;661-8.

[32] Bagnato A, Tecce R, Moretti C, Di Castro V, Spergel D, Catt KJ. Autocrine actions of endothelin-1 as a growth factor in human ovarian carcinoma cells. *Clin Cancer Res* 1995;1;1059-66.

[33] Moraitis S, Miller WR, Smyth JF, Langdon SP. Paracrine regulation of ovarian cancer by endothelin. *Eur J Cancer* 1999;35;1381-7.

[34] Rosano L, Varmi M, Salani D, et al. Endothelin-1 induces tumor proteinase activation and invasiveness of ovarian carcinoma cells. *Cancer Res* 2001;61;8340-6.

[35] Salani D, Di Castro V, Nicotra MR, et al. Role of endothelin-1 in neovascularization of ovarian carcinoma. *Am J Pathol* 2000;157;1537-47.

[36] Spinella F, Rosano L, Di Castro V, Natali PG, Bagnato A. Endothelin-1 induces vascular endothelial growth factor by increasing hypoxia-inducible factor-1alpha in ovarian carcinoma cells. *J Biol Chem* 2002;277;27850-5.

[37] Spinella F, Rosano L, Di Castro V, Natali PG, Bagnato A. Endothelin-1-induced prostaglandin E2-EP2,EP4-signaling regulates vascular endothelial growth factor production and ovarian carcinoma cell invasion. *J Biol Chem* 2004.

[38] Spinella F, Rosano L, Di Castro V, Nicotra MR, Natali PG, Bagnato A. Inhibition of cyclooxygenase-1 and -2 expression by targeting the endothelin a receptor in human ovarian carcinoma cells. *Clin Cancer Res* 2004;10;4670-9.

[39] Grimshaw MJ. Endothelins in breast tumour cell invasion. *Cancer Lett* 2005;222; 129-138.

[40] Alanen K, Deng DX, Chakrabarti S. Augmented expression of endothelin-1, endothelin-3 and the endothelin-B receptor in breast carcinoma. *Histopathology* 2000;36;161-7.

[41] Wulfing P, Diallo R, Kersting C, et al. Expression of endothelin-1, endothelin-A, and endothelin-B receptor in human breast cancer and correlation with long-term follow-up. *Clin Cancer Res* 2003;9;4125-31.

[42] Wulfing P, Kersting C, Tio J, et al. Endothelin-1-, endothelin-A-, and endothelin-B-receptor expression is correlated with vascular endothelial growth factor expression and angiogenesis in breast cancer. *Clin Cancer Res* 2004;10;2393-400.

[43] Guise TA, Yin JJ, Mohammad KS. Role of endothelin-1 in osteoblastic bone metastases. *Cancer* 2003;97;779-84.

[44] Lahav R, Heffner G, Patterson PH. An endothelin receptor B antagonist inhibits growth and induces cell death in human melanoma cells in vitro and in vivo. *Proc Natl Acad Sci U S A* 1999;96;11496-500.

[45] Lahav R, Suva ML, Rimoldi D, Patterson PH, Stamenkovic I. Endothelin receptor B inhibition triggers apoptosis and enhances angiogenesis in melanomas. *Cancer Res* 2004;64;8945-53.

[46] Bagnato A, Rosano L, Di Castro V, et al. Endothelin receptor blockade inhibits proliferation of Kaposi's sarcoma cells. *Am J Pathol* 2001;158;841-7.

[47] Rosano L, Spinella F, Di Castro V, et al. Endothelin receptor blockade inhibits molecular effectors of Kaposi's sarcoma cell invasion and tumor growth in vivo. *Am J Pathol* 2003;163;753-62.

[48] Leek RD, Harris AL. Tumor-associated macrophages in breast cancer. *J Mammary Gland Biol Neoplasia* 2002;7;177-89.

[49] Runkel S, Wischnik A, Teubner J, Kaven E, Gaa J, Melchert F. Oxygenation of mammary tumors as evaluated by ultrasound-guided computerized-pO2-histography. *Adv Exp Med Biol* 1994;345;451-8.

[50] Boudreau N, Myers C. Breast cancer-induced angiogenesis: multiple mechanisms and the role of the microenvironment. *Breast Cancer Res* 2003;5;140-6.

[51] Yu JL, Rak JW. Host microenvironment in breast cancer development: inflammatory and immune cells in tumour angiogenesis and arteriogenesis. *Breast Cancer Res* 2003;5;83-8.

[52] Goonewardene TI, Sowter HM, Harris AL. Hypoxia-induced pathways in breast cancer. *Microsc Res Tech* 2002;59;41-8.

[53] Matsuura A, Yamochi W, Hirata K, Kawashima S, Yokoyama M. Stimulatory interaction between vascular endothelial growth factor and endothelin-1 on each gene expression. *Hypertension* 1998;32;89-95.

[54] Matsuura A, Kawashima S, Yamochi W, et al. Vascular endothelial growth factor increases endothelin-converting enzyme expression in vascular endothelial cells. *Biochem Biophys Res Commun* 1997;235;713-6.

[55] Le Brun G, Aubin P, Soliman H, et al. Upregulation of endothelin 1 and its precursor by IL-1beta, TNF-alpha, and TGF-beta in the PC3 human prostate cancer cell line. *Cytokine* 1999;11;157-62.

[56] Molet S, Furukawa K, Maghazechi A, Hamid Q, Giaid A. Chemokine- and cytokine-induced expression of endothelin 1 and endothelin-converting enzyme 1 in endothelial cells. *J Allergy Clin Immunol* 2000;105;333-8.

[57] Simonson MS, Herman WH, Knauss TC, Schulak JA, Hricik DE. Macrophages--but not T-cell--derived cytokines stimulate endothelin-1 secretion by endothelial cells. *Transplant Proc* 1999;31;806-7.

[58] Wenger RH. Mammalian oxygen sensing, signalling and gene regulation. *J Exp Biol* 2000;203 Pt 8;1253-63.

[59] Kourembanas S, Marsden PA, McQuillan LP, Faller DV. Hypoxia induces endothelin gene expression and secretion in cultured human endothelium. *J Clin Invest* 1991;88;1054-7.

[60] Koong AC, Denko NC, Hudson KM, et al. Candidate genes for the hypoxic tumor phenotype. *Cancer Res* 2000;60;883-7.

[61] Aversa CR, Oparil S, Caro J, et al. Hypoxia stimulates human preproendothelin-1 promoter activity in transgenic mice. *Am J Physiol* 1997;273;L848-55.

[62] Hu J, Discher DJ, Bishopric NH, Webster KA. Hypoxia regulates expression of the endothelin-1 gene through a proximal hypoxia-inducible factor-1 binding site on the antisense strand. *Biochem Biophys Res Commun* 1998;245;894-9.

[63] Minchenko A, Caro J. Regulation of endothelin-1 gene expression in human microvascular endothelial cells by hypoxia and cobalt: role of hypoxia responsive element. *Mol Cell Biochem* 2000;208;53-62.

[64] Yamashita K, Discher DJ, Hu J, Bishopric NH, Webster KA. Molecular Regulation of the Endothelin-1 Gene by Hypoxia. Contributions of Hypoxia-Inducible factor-1, Activator Protein-1, Gata-2, and p300/CBP. *J Biol Chem* 2001;276;12645-53.

[65] Shibaguchi H, Himeno A, Shigematsu K, Kataoka Y, Niwa M. Transient hypoxia/hypoglycemia upregulates endothelin B receptors in cultured rat astrocytes. *Glia* 2000;31;91-4.

[66] Salani D, Taraboletti G, Rosano L, et al. Endothelin-1 induces an angiogenic phenotype in cultured endothelial cells and stimulates neovascularization In vivo [In Process Citation]. *Am J Pathol* 2000;157;1703-11.

[67] Salani D, Taraboletti G, Rosano L, et al. Endothelin-1 induces an angiogenic phenotype in cultured endothelial cells and stimulates neovascularization in vivo. *Am J Pathol* 2000;157;1703-11.

[68] Ribatti D, Presta M, Vacca A, et al. Human erythropoietin induces a pro-angiogenic phenotype in cultured endothelial cells and stimulates neovascularization in vivo. *Blood* 1999;93;2627-36.

[69] Hu DE, Hiley CR, Fan TP. Comparative studies of the angiogenic activity of vasoactive intestinal peptide, endothelins-1 and -3 and angiotensin II in a rat sponge model. *Br J Pharmacol* 1996;117;545-51.

[70] Bek EL, McMillen MA. Endothelins are angiogenic. *J Cardiovasc Pharmacol* 2000;36;S135-9.

[71] Cruz A, Parnot C, Ribatti D, Corvol P, Gasc JM. Endothelin-1, a regulator of angiogenesis in the chick chorioallantoic membrane. *J Vasc Res* 2001;38;536-45.

[72] Okuda Y, Tsurumaru K, Suzuki S, et al. Hypoxia and endothelin-1 induce VEGF production in human vascular smooth muscle cells. *Life Sci* 1998;63;477-84.

[73] Bos R, Zhong H, Hanrahan CF, et al. Levels of hypoxia-inducible factor-1 alpha during breast carcinogenesis. *J Natl Cancer Inst* 2001;93;309-14.

[74] Wykoff CC, Pugh CW, Harris AL, Maxwell PH, Ratcliffe PJ. The HIF pathway: implications for patterns of gene expression in cancer. *Novartis Found Symp* 2001;240;212-25; discussion 25-31.

[75] Karakurum M, Shreeniwas R, Chen J, et al. Hypoxic induction of interleukin-8 gene expression in human endothelial cells. *J-Clin-Invest* 1994;93;1564-70 issn: 0021-9738.

[76] Peifley KA, Winkles JA. Angiotensin II and endothelin-1 increase fibroblast growth factor-2 mRNA expression in vascular smooth muscle cells. *Biochem Biophys Res Commun* 1998;242;202-8.

[77] Hofman FM, Chen P, Jeyaseelan R, Incardona F, Fisher M, Zidovetzki R. Endothelin-1 induces production of the neutrophil chemotactic factor interleukin-8 by human brain-derived endothelial cells. *Blood* 1998;92;3064-72.

[78] Zidovetzki R, Chen P, Chen M, Hofman FM. Endothelin-1-induced interleukin-8 production in human brain-derived endothelial cells is mediated by the protein kinase C and protein tyrosine kinase pathways. *Blood* 1999;94;1291-9.

[79] Shichiri M, Kato H, Marumo F, Hirata Y. Endothelin-1 as an autocrine/paracrine apoptosis survival factor for endothelial cells. *Hypertension* 1997;30;1198-203.

[80] Shichiri M, Marumo F, Hirata Y. Endothelin-B receptor-mediated suppression of endothelial apoptosis. *J Cardiovasc Pharmacol* 1998;31 Suppl 1;S138-41.

[81] Shichiri M, Yokokura M, Marumo F, Hirata Y. Endothelin-1 inhibits apoptosis of vascular smooth muscle cells induced by nitric oxide and serum deprivation via MAP kinase pathway. *Arterioscler Thromb Vasc Biol* 2000;20;989-97.

[82] Han B, Fixler R, Beeri R, Wang Y, Bachrach U, Hasin Y. The opposing effects of endothelin-1 and C-type natriuretic peptide on apoptosis of neonatal rat cardiac myocytes. *Eur J Pharmacol* 2003;474;15-20.

[83] Sonveaux P, Dessy C, Martinive P, et al. Endothelin-1 is a critical mediator of myogenic tone in tumor arterioles: implications for cancer treatment. *Cancer Res* 2004;64;3209-14.

[84] Rai A, Gulati A. Evidence for the involvement of ET(B) receptors in ET-1-induced changes in blood flow to the rat breast tumor. *Cancer Chemother Pharmacol* 2003;51;21-8.

[85] Bell KM, Prise VE, Chaplin DJ, Tozer GM. Tumour blood flow modification by endothelin-related peptides in the rat HSN fibrosarcoma. *Br J Cancer Suppl* 1996;27;S161-3.

[86] Bell KM, Chaplin DJ, Poole BA, Prise VE, Tozer GM. Modification of blood flow in the HSN tumour and normal tissues of the rat by the endothelin ET(B) receptor agonist, IRL 1620. *Int J Cancer* 1999;80;295-302.

[87] Wessale JL, Adler AL, Novosad EI, et al. Pharmacology of endothelin receptor antagonists ABT-627, ABT-546, A-182086 and A-192621: ex vivo and in vivo studies. *Clin Sci (Lond)* 2002;103 Suppl 48;112S-7S.

[88] Berry P, Burchill S. Endothelins may modulate invasion and proliferation of Ewing's sarcoma and neuroblastoma. *Clin Sci (Lond)* 2002;103 Suppl 1;322S-6S.

[89] Gohji K, Kitazawa S, Tamada H, Katsuoka Y, Nakajima M. Expression of endothelin receptor a associated with prostate cancer progression. *J Urol* 2001;165;1033-6.

[90] Liu LY, Hu CL, Ma LJ, Zhang ZH, Mei YA. ET-1 inhibits B-16 murine melanoma cell migration by decreasing K(+) currents. *Cell Motil Cytoskeleton* 2004;58;127-36.

[91] Eberle J, Fecker LF, Orfanos CE, Geilen CC. Endothelin-1 decreases basic apoptotic rates in human melanoma cell lines. *J Invest Dermatol* 2002;119;549-55.

[92] Asham E, Shankar A, Loizidou M, et al. Increased endothelin-1 in colorectal cancer and reduction of tumour growth by ET(A) receptor antagonism. *Br J Cancer* 2001;85;1759-63.

[93] Lambert GL, Barker S, Lees DM, Corder R. Endothelin-2 synthesis is stimulated by the type-1 tumour necrosis factor receptor and cAMP: comparison with endothelin-converting enzyme-1 expression. *J Mol Endocrinol* 2000;24;273-83.

[94] Gonzalez W, Chen Z, Damon DH. Transforming growth factor-beta regulation of endothelin expression in rat vascular cell and organ cultures. *J Cardiovasc Pharmacol* 2001;37;219-26.

[95] Lee SD, Lee DS, Chun YG, et al. Transforming growth factor-beta1 induces endothelin-1 in a bovine pulmonary artery endothelial cell line and rat lungs via cAMP. *Pulm Pharmacol Ther* 2000;13;257-65.

[96] Ruetten H, Thiemermann C. Endothelin-1 stimulates the biosynthesis of tumour necrosis factor in macrophages: ET-receptors, signal transduction and inhibition by dexamethasone. *J Physiol Pharmacol* 1997;48;675-88.

[97] Hofman FM, Chen P, Jeyaseelan R, Incardona F, Fisher M, Zidovetzki R. Endothelin-1 induces production of the neutrophil chemotactic factor interleukin-8 by human brain-derived endothelial cells. *Blood* 1998;92;3064-72.

[98] Fisher M. The endothelin-1 antagonist, atrasentan, improves time to progression and quality of life in hormone-refractory prostate cancer. *Clin Prostate Cancer* 2002;1;79-80.

[99] Rosano L, Spinella F, Salani D, et al. Therapeutic targeting of the endothelin a receptor in human ovarian carcinoma. *Cancer Res* 2003;63;2447-53.

[100] Bagnato A, Cirilli A, Salani D, et al. Growth inhibition of cervix carcinoma cells in vivo by endothelin A receptor blockade. *Cancer Res* 2002;62;6381-4.

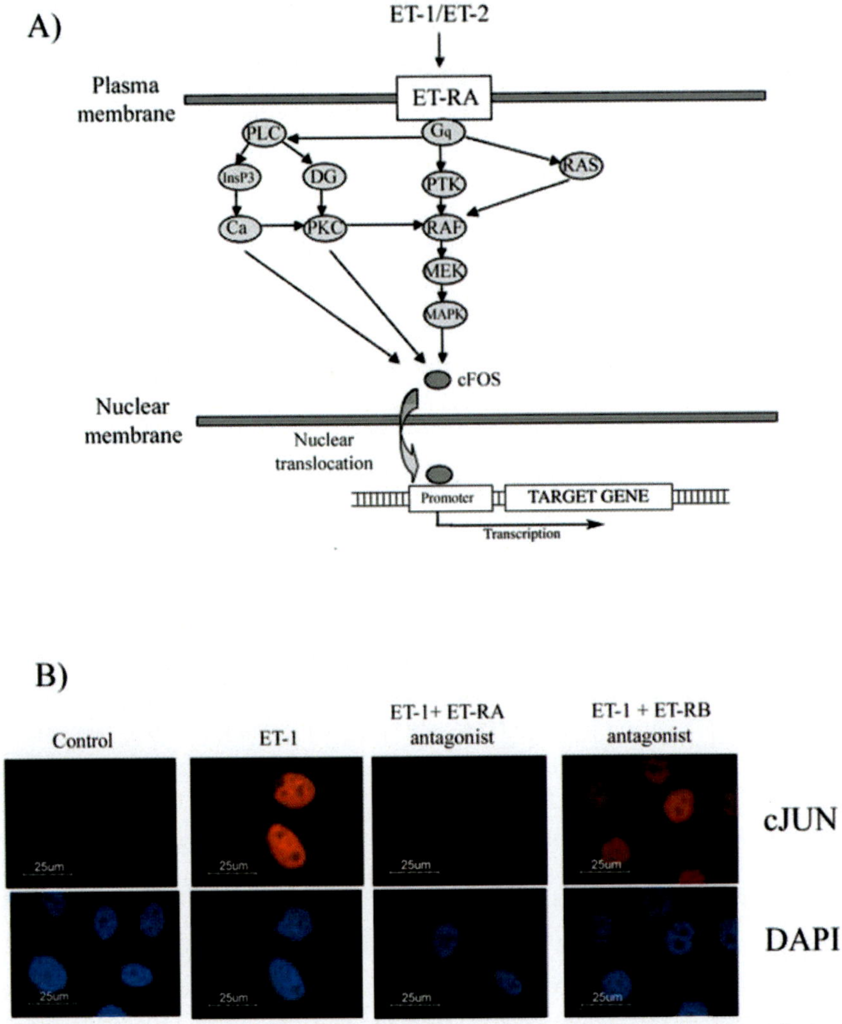

Figure 2. Endothelin/ET-RA induced signalling pathways. A) ET-1 or -2 bind to the G-protein coupled receptor ET-RA, which may trigger several different signal transduction pathways via G_q, a G-protein coupled to the intracellular domain of ET-RA. Activation of protein tyrosine kinases (PTK), phospholipase C (PLC) and RAS results in the activation of the RAF/MEK/MAPK pathway, while activation of PLC results in the mobilisation of intracellular calcium (Ca) via inositol 1,4,5 triphosphate (InsP3). PKC is also activated via PLC and diacylglycerol (DAG). The signal transduction pathways lead to nuclear translocation of transcription factors such as cFOS and cJUN and the expression of target genes. B) MCF-7 cells stimulated with ET-1 and immunohistochemically analysed for cJun nuclear localisation. ET-1 stimulates nuclear localisation and this can be inhibited by ET-RA antagonists. ET-RB antagonists have no effect on ET-1-stimulated nuclear localisation indicating that the effect is entirely ET-RA mediated.

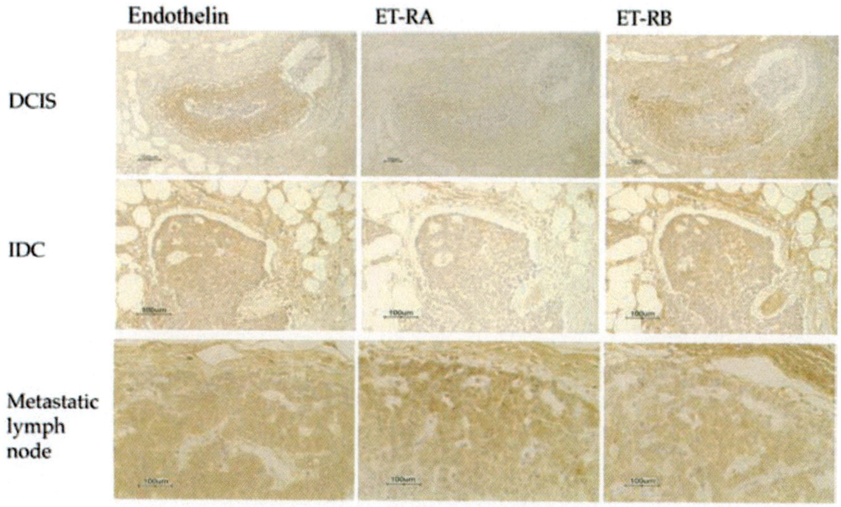

Figure 3. Expression of endothelins and receptors in breast cancer. Endothelins and receptors are expressed more widely by tumour cells in IDC of the breast compared to DCIS. Lymph node metastases show a greater degree of staining still. It is of note that tumour cells which express endothelins also show expression of one or both receptors. Endothelins and the receptors are expressed not only by the tumour cells but also by TAMs, fibroblasts and endothelial cells.

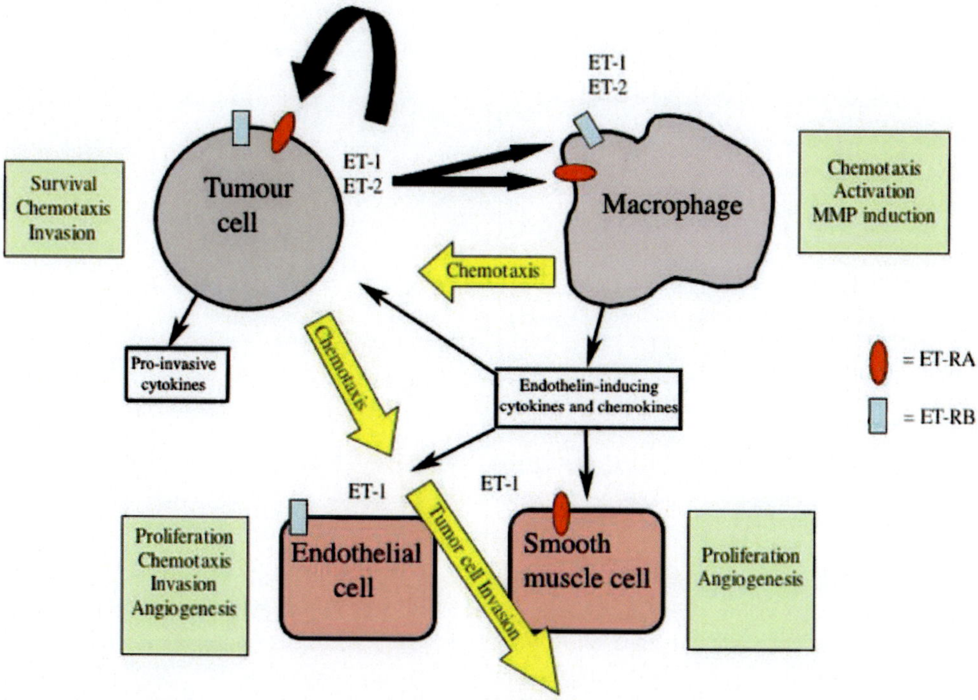

Figure 4. Putative roles of endothelins in breast tumours. TAMs express inflammatory cytokines that may induce endothelin expression by both tumour cells and macrophages, which release ET-1 and ET-2, and express both receptors. Microenvironmental factors, including hypoxia and the endothelins themselves, further stimulate the endothelin axis. Stimulation of tumour cells and macrophages with ET-1 or ET-2 leads to chemotaxis of these cells, induction of MMP activity and cytokine expression, and invasion of the tumour cells. ET-2 also protects tumour cells from apoptosis and activates macrophages. Endothelial cells and VSMCs express ET-RB and ET-RA respectively. Stimulation of endothelial cells and VSMCs with endothelins may stimulate angiogenesis.

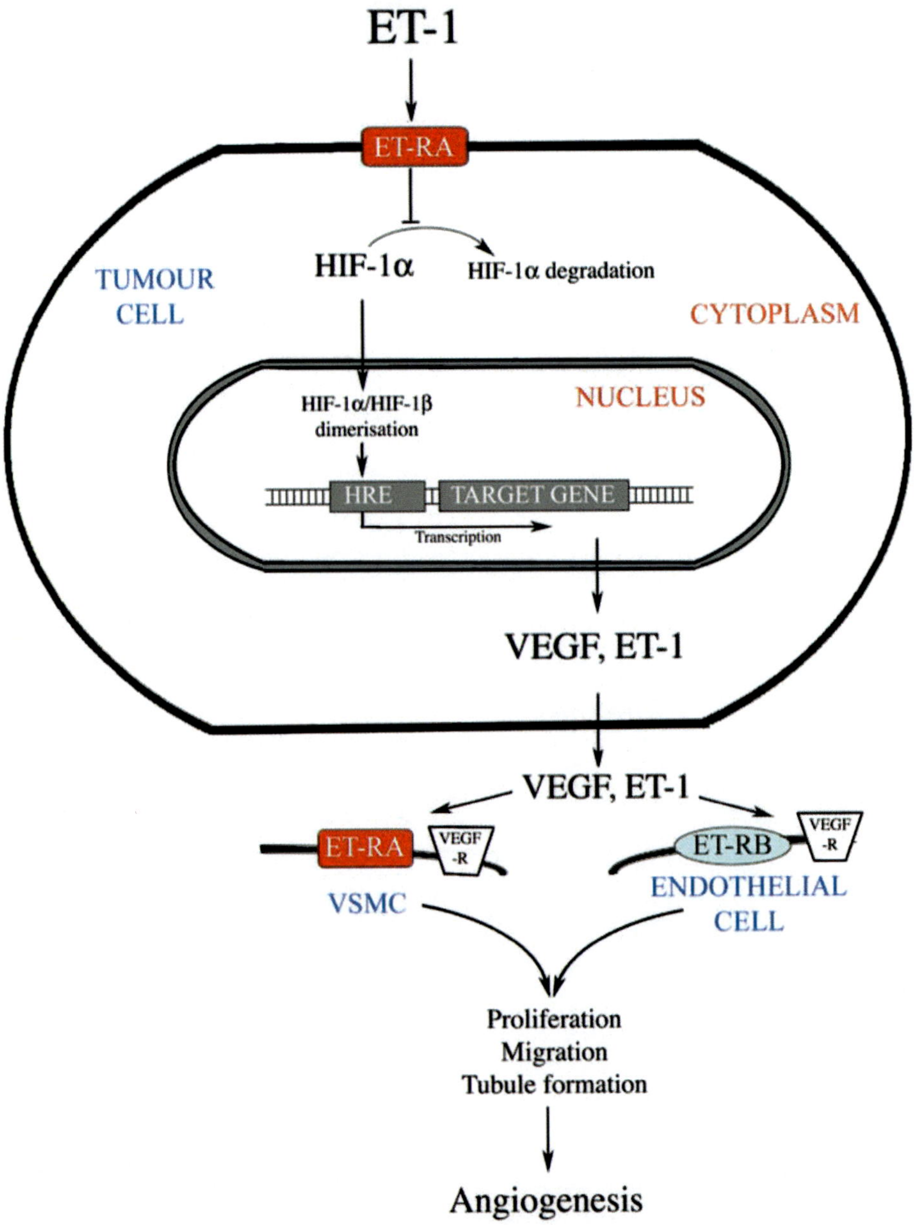

Figure 5. Indirect promotion of tumour angiogenesis by endothelins via HIF1 and VEGF. ET-1 (or ET-2) binds to ET-RA activating multiple signalling pathways. These pathways result in the stabilisation of HIF1α, even under normoxic situations, allowing the formation of the HIF1 complex in the nucleus. The HIF1 complex binds to the HRE in the promoter of 'hypoxia-responsive' genes such as VEGF and the endothelins themselves, and give rise to expression of the target gene. Protein products (e.g. VEGF and endothelins, and potentially several further pro-angiogenic genes which have an HRE in their promoter) act in an paracrine manner on VSMCs and endothelial cells and promote proliferation, migration of such cells and tubule formation resulting in neovascularisation of the tumour.

In: Trends in Angiogenesis Research
Editor: Roberta V. Zubar, pp. 183-209

ISBN 1-59454-452-2

Chapter VIII

Vascular Endothelial Growth Factor and Breast Cancer

Danila Coradini* and Maria Grazia Daidone

Tumor Biology and Experimental Therapy Unit, Department of Experimental Oncology and Laboratories, Istituto Nazionale per lo Studio e la Cura dei Tumori, Milan, Italy

Abstract

Angiogenesis is a complex multi-step process leading to the formation of new blood vessels from the existing vascular network. It is normally well regulated in the adult, where angiogenesis occurs transiently only during development, wound healing and in the female reproductive cycle. Otherwise, abnormal angiogenesis can occur during the pathogenesis of certain chronic diseases such as diabetes, rheumatoid arthritis, psoriasis and tumor, including breast cancer. The acquisition of the angiogenic phenotype occurs very early in the multistage process of solid tumor development. Beyond a critical volume, tumor cells cannot proliferate further in the absence of a sufficient nutrient and oxygen supplementation becoming angiogenesis activation an essential requirement for tumor growth, invasiveness and development of metastasis. Experimental and clinical findings have demonstrated that in breast cancer the most important angiogenesis promoter is vascular endothelial growth factor (VEGF) and that, in addition to the hypoxia-dependent activation via hypoxia-inducible factor (HIF)-1, VEGF synthesis can be also an estrogen-dependent process via estrogen receptor. In the present chapter, we first discuss the biological role of hypoxia- or estrogen-dependent angiogenesis on breast cancer development and the relationship between some angiogenesis-related biomarkers (HIF-1 and VEGF) with some other important pathobiologic characteristics of the tumor including histotype, hormone-responsiveness, cell proliferation and expression of pro- and anti-apoptotic factors. Then we focus on their clinical relevance in terms of patients outcome and responsiveness to radio-, endocrine- or chemotherapy.

* Correspondence concerning this article should be addressed to Danila Coradini, Department of Experimental Oncology and Laboratories, Unit #10, Istituto Nazionale Tumori, Via VEnezian, 1, Milan, 20133, Italy. Phone39-02-2390-3053; E-mail:danila.coradini@istitutotumori.mi.it

Key words: Breast cancer; Neoangiogenesis; VEGF; Clinical outcome

HYPOXIA, NEOANGIOGENESIS AND TUMOR GROWTH

The ability to maintain oxygen homeostasis is essential to the survival of all vertebrate species. Thus, a complex physiological structure, including lungs, heart and vasculature system, has evolved to ensure the optimal oxygen delivery to all cells of the organism. In addition, all nucleated cells sense oxygen concentration through specialized chemoreceptor and respond to reduced oxygen availability acutely and chronically: in the first case, through the activation of pre-existing proteins that, in concert, rapidly modulate pulmonary ventilation and blood circulation to optimize the supply of oxygen to tissues [1], in the second regulating gene transcription [2]. When such regulatory systems fail, a prolonged hypoxia can cause pathologic alterations that result in pulmonary hypertension, heart attack, stroke, and other significant acute fatal events.

At the cellular level, adaptation to hypoxia takes place very early (within few minutes) and occurs by decreasing energy-consuming processes and increasing the efficiency of energy-producing pathways, mainly switching from aerobic to anaerobic metabolism, and by promoting vascularization and enhancing the oxigen carrying capacity of the blood [3]. A consistent body of evidence indicates that a single transcription factor, termed hypoxia-inducible factor (HIF), is responsible for the several adaptive cellular responses regulating the transcription of a pool of about 40 genes involved in glucose delivery (glucose transporters glut1 and glut3), glycolytic metabolism (aldolase A and C, enolase 1, esokinase 1 and 3, lactate dehydrogenase A, phosphofructokinase L and 1), resistance to apoptosis and neo-angiogenesis [4]. HIF family includes till now three members, the most important of which is HIF-1 that functions as master switch to induce the expression of several pro-angiogenic factors, including vascular endothelial growth factor (VEGF), nitric oxide synthase (NOS) and platelet-derived growth factor (PDGF) [5,6].

HIF-1 is a heterodimeric transcription factor, consisting of an oxygen-dependent HIF-1α subunit and a constitutively expressed partner HIF-1β, which binds to specific hypoxia response element located in the promoter region of target genes. Whereas HIF-1β is present in excess, regardless of changes in oxygen availability, and is a common subunit for many other transcription factors, HIF-1α is unique for HIF-1 and the level of its expression is determinant for binding to DNA and transcriptional activity [5]. The predominant modality for HIF-1α regulation occurs post-transcriptionally. In fact, while HIF-1α mRNA level remains quite constant in normoxia and hypoxia, the corresponding protein is rapidly degraded in normoxia and accumulates in hypoxia. In fact, under normoxic conditions, HIF-1α protein is translated, but immediately ubiquitylated by the von Hippel-Lindau (VHL) tumor suppressor protein, a component of a multisubunit E3 ubiquitin ligase protein complex, which targets it for proteasome degradation [7,8]; the recognition of HIF-1α by VHL protein depends on the presence of hydroxylated proline residues localized within the oxygen-dependent degradation (ODD) domain of the protein which are hydroxylated by a family of prolyl hydroxylases in an oxygen-dependent manner and in the presence of co-factors that include oxoglutarate, iron and ascorbate [7,8]. Conversely, under hypoxic conditions, the activity of such prolyl hydroxylases is inhibited owing to the reduced availability of oxygen, the prolines within the ODD domain are not hydroxylated and the interaction between the VHL complex and HIF-1 does not occur with an accumulation of HIF-1α protein in the nucleus and the consequent induction of the HIF-1-inducible genes. This fine control of HIF-1α protein level can be disrupted also in normoxic condition as in the case of the inactivation of VHL protein, owing to deletions or missense mutations in the corresponding gene (like in von Hippel-Lindau cancer syndrome), which hamperes the binding to HIF-1α and leads to its constitutive expression [9]. Since hypoxic environment is a common feature of solid tumor cells, they adapt their metabolism to the low availability of oxygen by increasing HIF-1 activity which results in the over-expression of several target genes including VEGF [6,10].

The first suggestion that VEGF expression might be related to angiogenesis and regulated by oxygen came from studies of normal brain and brain tumors that demonstrated that VEGF mRNA is more expressed in the tumor cells localized near to necrotic areas of low-grade gliomas [11] and that high levels of Flk-1 mRNA, one of VEGF receptor types, are expressed in endothelial cells neighboring VEGF producing tumor cells [12]. Starting from these preliminary findings, the causal association between hypoxia, HIF-1, VEGF expression and tumor progression has becoming more and more evident: experimental and clinical models have provided findings of a spatial coexpression of HIF-1α and hypoxia (chemically evaluated using nitroimidazole - a compound able to identify the tumor hypoxic areas when injected in vivo - [13] or measured using an Eppendorf oxygen electrode [14]), and of a close temporal relation between hypoxia, expression of angiogenesis-related markers and neo-vascularization in tumors [15-19] as well as in other pathologic situations [20]. In fact, as postulated by Folkman in 1971 [21], the onset of tumor-associated angiogenesis was thought to go through two phases, the first of which defined "avascular" and corresponding to an occult lesion of not more than 1-2 mm in diameter which stay apparently dormant for a long time owing to a dynamic balance between proliferation and apoptosis; up to this size, tumor cells can obtain the necessary oxygen and nutrient supplies to grow and survive by simple passive diffusion from pre-existing capillaries.

The switch towards an angiogenic phenotype frequently occurs by a gradual increase of angiogenic potential. Indeed, the construction of a new vascular network requires different sequential steps: the release of proteases from activated endothelial cells with subsequent degradation of the basement membrane; migration of endothelial cells into the interstitial space; endothelial cells proliferation and differentiation into mature blood vessels. All these processes are mediated by a wide array of factors, including growth factors, chemokines, angiogenic enzymes, endothelial specific receptors and adhesion molecules [22-24]. Nevertheless, new tumor vessels are often structurally and functionally abnormal; in contrasts to normal vessels, tumor vasculature is highly disorganized, vessels are tortuous and dilated, tumor blood flow is chaotic and variable and leads to hypoxic and acidic areas with important consequence on tissue metabolism which results on the effectiveness of chemical and physical therapies [25-27].

In addition to hypoxia, many other microenvironment signals are able to trigger the angiogenic switch: metabolic stress (low pH, hypoglycemia); mechanical stress (pressure generated by proliferating cells); immune/inflammatory cells that infiltrate the tissue and can modulate the expression of cellular adhesion molecules and other surface markers on the endothelium; pro-angiogenic molecules produced by cancer cells, endothelial cells, stromal cells, and stored in extra-cellular matrix, which interplaying in a complex manner contribute to tumor development [28,29].

Among the pro-angiogenic factors, VEGF appears to have a predominant role [30]. VEGF is a secreted glycoprotein purified and cloned in the 1980s based on its activities as inducer of vascular permeability [31-33] and mitogen for endothelial cells [34]. Since then, it has become clear that VEGF plays a crucial role in the blood vessel growth during embryogenesis and tumor development, and that several other proteins are closely related in structure to VEGF and are involved in vascular development; all these proteins constitute the VEGF family [35]. Studies carried out over the past ten years have conclusively demonstrated that all the members of the VEGF family growth factors, originally defined on the basis of similarity of primary structure to VEGF, have a prominent role as extracellular signaling molecules in vascular development [36,37].

The VEGF family currently consists of VEGF (also known as VEGF-A) [34], VEGF-B [38], VEGF-C [39], VEGF-D [40], Orf virus VEGF (also known as VEGF-E) [41] and placenta growth factor (PIGF) [42]. All these glycoproteins are members of a structural superfamily of growth factors containing a cysteine knot motif which also includes platelet-growth factor BB (PDGF-BB) and transforming growth factor β2 (TGF-β2) [43]. Crystallographic studies of numerous cysteine growth factors, including VEGF, revealed that the six conserved cysteine residues of the motif contribute to a three-dimensional fold involving an unusual clustering of three cysteine bridges [44].

Also known as Vascular Permeability Factor, VEGF is an about 46kD homodimeric protein that dissociates under reductive condition into two apparently identical 23kD subunits linked together by two disulphide bridges. Alternative splicing of the VEGF mRNA transcript results in five different isoforms: $VEGF_{121}$, $VEGF_{145}$, $VEGF_{165}$, $VEGF_{189}$ and $VEGF_{206}$ [45,46]. Three of these isoforms ($VEGF_{121}$, $VEGF_{145}$ and $VEGF_{165}$) are secreted by a broad variety of cells, including vascular smooth muscle cells, monocytes, endothelial cells and megakaryocytes [47,48]. Secreted VEGF has multiple functions. During embryogenesis, VEGF deficiency impaired numerous steps of early vascular development and a lethal phenotype has been observed in embryos lacking a single VEGF allele [36,37]. In the adult, it can induce permeabilization of blood vessels, degradation of the vessel basement membrane, endothelial cell proliferation and migration through the surrounding matrix [49].

Four high affinity receptors for VEGF family have been identified, VEGFR-1 (also known as Flt1) [50], VEGFR-2 (also known as Flk1 and KDR in mouse and man, respectively) [51], VEGFR-3 (also known as Flt4) [39] and neuropilin-1 [52]. VEGFR-1 has several unique structural and functional characteristics: the VEGFR-1 gene encodes a full length membrane receptor and a soluble receptor, which is generated by alternative splicing of the VEGFR-1 mRNA and contains the extracellular ligand-binding domain but lacks the signaling tyrosine kinase domain; it is expressed in vascular endothelium and in several types of non-endothelial cells, including epithelial breast cells, and has more than 40-fold higher affinity than VEGFR-2 for VEGF [53]. VEGFR-2 is expressed on both the vascular and lymphatic endothelium, whereas VEGFR-3 is predominantly expressed on the lymphatic endothelium. All VEGF-A isoforms bind to both VEGFR-1 and VEGFR-2, whereas PIGF and VEGF-B are selective ligands for VEGFR-1, and VEGF-C and VEGF-D are selective for VEGFR-2 and VEGFR-3 [54].

In situ hybridization and immunohistochemistry have demonstrated that VEGF receptors are upregulated in tumor and correlate with the degree of vascularization in many experimental and clinical tumors, including breast cancer [55-57]. However, while VEGFR-2 is a positive angiogenic signal transducer, VEGFR-1, especially in its soluble form, is a negative regulator of VEGF availability and it is conceivable that, in agreement with the finding of a high concentration of soluble VEGFR-1 in biologic fluids from normal human subjects [58], normal breast tissue cells constitutively express soluble VEGFR-1 at levels sufficient to bind endogenous VEGF, thus preventing the induction of inappropriate angiogenesis and cell growth.

Angiogenesis and Breast Carcinogenesis

As in many other solid tumors, the relationship between hypoxia, angiogenesis and tumor progression, described in the previous paragraph, has been demonstrated also in breast carcinogenesis [59-61]. In fact, pre-invasive breast pathologies such as hyperplasia, atypical hyperplasia and carcinoma in situ have been shown to have an increased vascularity when compared with normal breast tissue [60] and in tumor specimens the amount of vascularity has been found correlated with the histological features associated with a malignant phenotype [61]. However, immunohistochemical studies have demonstrated that angiogenic factors, including VEGF, IGF-II and bFGF are present already in normal mammary gland, primarily in the epithelium, suggesting that the mere presence of angiogenic factors is not sufficient to determine an angiogenic phenotype even though the expression of many angiogenic agents increases considerably during tumor progression. VEGF, for example, is found upregulated at the transition from atypical hyperplasia to ductal carcinoma in situ and this elevated VEGF level is maintained in the invasive form of the tumor suggesting the formation of a carcinoma in situ as the critical point for breast carcinogenesis [62,63]. Unlike VEGF, which is primarily epithelial, bFGF and IGF-II level increase in nonepithelial components consistently with the fact that bFGF and IGF-II are both generally sequestered in the stroma [62].

But what about the vascularization in the normal human mammary gland? The mammary gland life cycle is constituted by massive physiologically changes in cell number, composition, architecture and functionality. In fact, breast tissue is highly responsive to changes in sex hormones concentration and it changes histologically, biochemically and in terms of cell proliferating pattern throughout each menstrual cycle [64]: pathologist experience documents large, rhytmic changes in the amount and distribution of blood flow, fat, connective and epithelial tissue within the breast during the menstrual cycle [65]. These rhythmic changes are drastically improved during pregnancy and lactation, which are characterized by the epithelium cells proliferation and vasculature expansion by sprouting angiogenesis [66]. In a recent study, Naccarato et al. [67] have demonstrated that the distribution and nature of microvascularization in normal breast ducts and lobules is quite different. In fact, whereas ducts are surrounded by a high number of microvessels with the appearance of typical small capillaries, lobules show fewer microvessels which are large and sinusoidal in shape. These different features probably result in dissimilar functions. The sinusoidal structure of the lobules may be related to their role as a hormone target within the breast parenchyma; large and tortuous capillaries would slow the blood flow favoring a prolonged contact of the hormones with the lobular elements, an hypothesis in agreement with the general observation that tumors arising from lobular structure are generally more frequently positive for estrogen receptor.

An in vivo study of transplanted breast tissues onto rabbit corneal assay found that 30% of hyperplastic breasts are angiogenic as compared to only 3% of normal breast tissue [68] demonstrating that the angiogenic switch occurs before that the typical morphological changes of cancer occur. In addition, strong evidence shows that hypoxia plays a fundamental role in promoting the dedifferentiated phenotype in ductal breast carcinoma in situ and that it is also associated with lost of polarization, increase of the nucleus/cytoplasm ratio, formation of necrotic areas and HIF-1α overexpression in the layer of cells surrounding the necrosis [69]. As regard HIF-1α, its overexpression has been reported to be associated to breast carcinogenesis [70]: HIF-1α expression has been detected neither in normal breast tissue nor in hyperplastic ductal lesions, but it has been found in higher stage tumors.

Since the occurrence of hypoxia within a pre-neoplastic lesion is believed to cause a higher genetic instability and oncogenes overexpression [71], a relation between oncogene products and induction of pro-angiogenic factors has been postulated and subsequently demonstrated. It is the case of the oncogene HER-2/neu, a member of the epidermal growth factor family of tyrosine kinase receptors, widely expressed in in situ carcinomas and overexpressed approximalety in 25-30% of invasive breast cancers, that has been found to upregulate the production of several angiogenic factors, including transforming growth factor (TGF)-β, angiopietin-1, plasminogen activator inhibitor (PAI)-1 and VEGF [72-74], and to increase the expression of VEGFR-2, the predominant receptor involved in VEGF-stimulated angiogenesis, in the adjacent breast tumor endothelial cells [63]. Furthermore, under hypoxic condition HER-2 has been shown to increase also the rate of HIF-1α protein synthesis by preventing its degradation [75].

Hormone Steroids, VEGF and Breast Cancer Development

As referred in the previous paragraph, normal breast tissue is highly responsive to changes in ovarian hormones concentration that induce a cyclic remodeling process involving epithelial, stromal and vascular components during each menstrual cycle [76,77]. Experimental and clinical evidences have clearly indicated that estrogens are involved in the physiological regulation of VEGF expression in the epithelial cells of the terminal ductal-lobular units [78] by binding to a functional estrogen response elements in the 5'-flanking promoter region of the gene coding for VEGF [79]; they decreased their effect on VEGF synthesis after menopause [80] and they are involved in VEGF synthesis in breast carcinoma [81-83].

However, the interrelation between the different pathways that may activate VEGF expression and induce the neoangiogenesis associated with breast cancer genesis and progression, mainly the hypoxia- and estrogen-dependent pathways, is not completely understood even though interesting information have been accumulated from in vitro experiments using breast cancer cell lines. In fact, when we investigated the direct effect of estradiol (the main endogenous estrogen) on HIF-1α and VEGF expression in two breast cancer cell lines, characterized by a different steroid receptor profile [84] we found that, as expected, already in normoxic conditions either MDA-MB231 (the hormone-independent and phenotipically estrogen receptor (ER)-negative cell line) or MCF7 (the hormone-dependent and phenotipically ER-positive cell line) constitutively expressed HIF-1α and VEGF even though in a quite different amount: with respect to MCF7 cells, MDA-MB231 cells showed a 2-fold increase in HIF-1α protein concentration associated with a 2-fold increase in mRNA VEGF expression and a 14-fold increase in total VEGF (intracellular plus secreted in the conditioned medium) protein concentration. This result is in agreement with clinical findings that indicate an inverse relationship between ER status and VEGF content (with ER-negative tumors more frequently VEGF-rich) and supports the hypothesis that tumor cells, characterized by a more aggressive phenotype (in this case represented by hormone-independence), can maintain high level of VEGF mRNA and protein via a hypoxia-mediated mechanism. In both cell lines, $VEGF_{165}$ represents the predominant isoform (57% and 77% of the total in MCF7 and MDA-MB231, respectively), more than 95% of which is secreted in he conditioned medium. The treatment with physiological concentration of estradiol (10 nM) induced a 3-fold increase in VEGF protein only in MCF7 cells, in keeping with the hypothesis that in estrogen-responsive cells VEGF synthesis is, at least in part, ER-mediated.

When hypoxic conditions were mimicked by adding cobalt chloride (which causes HIF-1α accumulation by occupying the von Hippel-Lindau domain of the HIF-1α protein and thereby preventing protein degradation and inducing expression of the downstream genes [85]) a 4-fold increase in VEGF total mRNA (without any specific isoform increase) and a 2-fold increase in $VEGF_{165}$ protein concentration in MCF7 cell line was found. Conversely, in MDA-MB231 cells both mRNA and protein levels were unaffected by the hypoxic stimulus probably due to the already very high basal content as suggested by the finding that hypoxia affected HIF-1α expression only in MCF7 cells, in which we found a 3-fold increase in mRNA level, a decrease in HIF-1α protein concentration (due to the activation of VEGF synthesis) and a concomitant increase in mRNA VEGF expression that was not further increased by the contemporarily presence of estradiol, indicating the hypoxic stimulus as more potent with respect to the hormonal stimulus [84].

These findings are in agreement with the results reported by other authors that, evaluating the effects of estrogen on the expression of VEGF mRNA (by RT-PCR) and protein (by Western blotting) in MCF7 cell line, demonstrated that estrogen induces VEGF overexpression both at mRNA and protein levels [79]. However, also progesterone and a number of synthetic progestins used as oral contraceptive, hormone replacement therapy and high-dose progestin treatment of breast cancer increase VEGF production in a progesterone receptor (PgR)-mediated manner [86]. In addition to these direct effects of estradiol on VEGF production, very recent findings [87] indicate that estrogens also exert a pro-angiogenic effect by inhibiting the expression of the soluble form of VEGFR-1 through an ER-mediated mechanism. This observation is of particular interest since only a minority of normal breast epithelial cells express detectable level of ER, whereas in breast tumors the majority of cells are ER-positive and therefore receptive to proliferative and angiogenic stimuli.

All these experimental findings provide a biological explanation for the clinical evidence that the menopausal status of a patient, i.e., the endogenous hormonal milieu, may play a relevant role on the outgrowth and progression of a breast tumor, having postmenopausal patients a better disease-free and overall survival than premenopausal women [88,89], probably due to the proliferative and pro-angiogenic effect of hormone steroids produced during premenopause. Accordingly, even if there is no consensus regarding VEGF concentration during the menstrual cycle [90,91], VEGF has been proposed as an indicator of the best time for surgery in premenopausal breast cancer patients [92].

Since changing the hormonal milieu at the time of surgery for breast cancer may have the ability to improve the prognosis for some patients with early breast cancer (being the luteal phase likely associated with a decreased risk of relapse [93-95]) the most convenient timing of surgery (in term of the phase of the menstrual cycle) for premenopausal women has been a debated issue for a long time. Thus, based on the findings that aggressiveness and invasion-related markers tend to be overexpressed in the primary tumor removed during the follicular phase and on the hypothesis that during specific times of the menstrual cycle upregulation of hormonally controlled genes might influence tumor cell shedding and survival [96], the role of serum and tissue VEGF content as indicator of the best time for breast cancer surgery in premenopausal women have been investigated by several authors [92,97]. In both cases (serum and tumor tissue) VEGF significantly lower in the luteal phase suggesting a possible decreased potential for micrometastases establishment in that phase. In particular, when we analyzed the fluctuation of intratumor VEGF concentration as a function of the patient menstrual cycle phase at time of removal of the primary lesion, in association with other biological variables involved in cell cycle and apoptosis regulation (p53, $p27^{kip1}$, Bcl-2, Bax) or hormone-related (ER and PgR) in a series of 629 breast cancer from premenopausal women [97], we found that intratumor VEGF concentration and PgR paralleled estradiol level fluctuation with an increase in the follicular phase with a peak around day 11 and a dramatic decrease during the luteal phase (Figure 1), probably due to the stimulatory effect of increasing plasma levels of estradiol which, after binding ER, induced the synthesis of the two estrogen-dependent proteins, and an inverse association with progesterone levels supporting the hypothesis of a more favourable outcome for women undergoing surgery during the second part of the menstrual cycle. Conversely, expression of $p27^{kip1}$, p53, bcl-2 and bax remained relatively stable in agreement with previous results [96]. These findings support one of the most accredited biological explanations for the benefit of surgical manipulation during the luteal phase of the menstrual cycle: the possibility that tumor eradication may minimize angiogenesis stimulation if scheduled when progesterone concentration is elevated, VEGF conversely is decreased and estradiol is insufficient to upregulate VEGFR-1 [58].

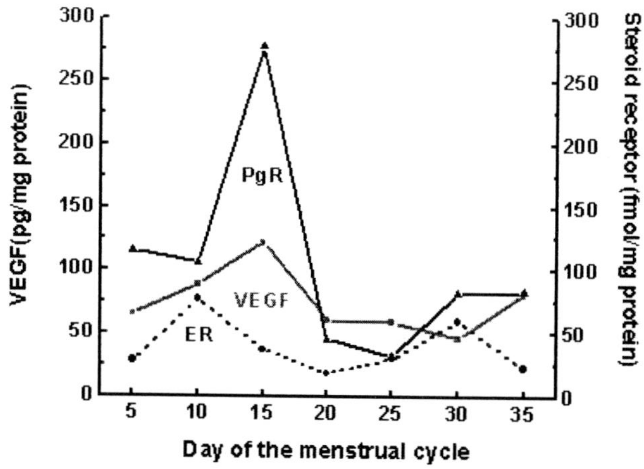

Figure 1. Fluctuation of intratumor estrogen receptors (ER), progesterone receptors (PgR) and vascular endothelial growth factor (VEGF) according to menstrual cycle phases. ER and PgR content was determined by a ligand binding assay and expressed as fmol/ mg of cytosol protein, and VEGF was measured by quantitative enzyme immunoassay and expressed as pg/mg of cytosol protein (for details see [97]).

VEGF and Tumor-Related Characteristics

Despite its unique origin at the terminal duct-lobular unit [98] carcinoma of the breast is a very heterogeneous disease due to the progressive gain and loss of functions accumulated during the expansion of the original transformed clone. In particular, infiltrating ductal (IDC) and lobular carcinomas (ILC) (thc most frequently observed varieties of invasive breast cancer, accounting for 70-75% and 10-14% of all invasive tumors, respectively) are characterized by differences in their histological structures and natural history [99]. In fact, even though following conservative surgery and radiation therapy patients with an ILC have an outcome similar to patients with IDC [100], they show a different metastatic pattern since bone marrow and peritoneum metastases are markedly more prevalent in patients with ILC than in those with IDC [101,102]. ILC and IDC appear to be quite different even in their biologic features. For instance, they differ in hormone receptor profile and proliferative activity - ILC being more frequently ER and PgR positive and slowly proliferating than IDC [103]. In addition, a more integrated analysis of the complex interrelations among the cellular mechanisms involved in breast tumor growth and progression [104] indicated that according to tumor histotype, ILC are more frequently VEGF-negative than IDC, probably related to the different angiogenic requirement of the ductal and lobule structures, and that a direct correlation between VEGF and tumor size, as well as an inverse relation between steroid receptors and VEGF level are present only in IDC.

Indeed, when we explored the interrelations among several biologic variables (consolidated or of a more recent acquisition) related to angiogenesis (VEGF and HIF-1α), hormone dependence (ER and PgR), proliferative activity and proliferation-related markers potential (S-phase cell fraction evaluated as thymidine labelling index [TLI], cyclin A), cell-cycle and apoptosis control ($p16^{ink4}$, $p27^{kip1}$, $p21^{waf1}$, p53 and bcl-2) in primary IDC (103 cases) and ILC (41 cases) without axillary lymph node involvement, matched for patient age (median age: 56 and 54 years for IDC and ILC, respectively) and tumor size (median diameter: 1.7 and 1.8 for IDC and ILC, respectively), we found that compared to IDC (Figure 2), ILC were more frequently ER+ (95% vs 75%, $P<0.01$), slowly proliferating (78% vs 57%, $P<0.02$), p53-negative (98% vs 77%, $P<0.005$) and VEGF-negative (71% vs 43%, $P<0.005$), with a statistically significant lower VEGF concentration (54 vs 71 pg/mg cytosolic protein, $P=0.005$) in agreement with data from literature [105]. Conversely, no difference was found between ILC and IDC considering the frequency distribution of PgR, $p16^{ink4}$, $p27^{kip1}$, $p21^{waf1}$, bcl-2 and HIF-1α protein expression, and a trend in favour of a lower median value of cyclin A-positive cells was observed in ILC than in IDC (3.2% vs 6.4%, $P=0.06$).

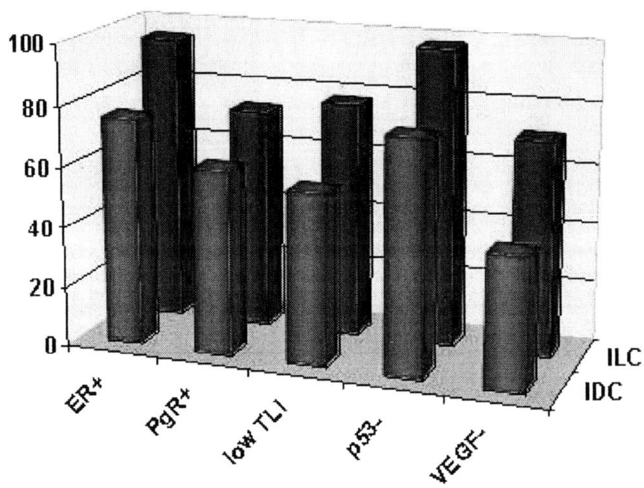

Figure 2. VEGF and other biomarkers (ER, PgR, TLI and p53 expression) as a function of tumor histotype. ER and PgR content was measured by ligand-binding assay and 10 and 25 fmol/mg of cytosol protein were used as cutoff values, respectively. Proliferative activity was evaluated as the fraction of ^{3}H-thymidine incorporating cells and expressed as ^{3}H-thymidine labeling index (TLI). The expression of p53 was evaluated by immunohistochemistry on formalin-fixed paraffin-embedded sections (cutoff value 5%). VEGF expression was measured by a quantitative enzyme immunoassay technique and median value was used as cutoff (for details see [104]).

In particular, when we analyzed the relationships between biologic variables according to histotype, a different profile of associations was observed. In fact, only the positive correlation between ER and PgR, between ER and bcl-2 expression, and between PgR and $p27^{kip1}$ expression (all statistically significant) were shared by the two histotypes. The results provide evidence that IDC and ILC are characterized by a different biological profile in which proteins related to angiogenesis, hormone responsiveness, cell-cycle control and apoptosis are differently integrated. In particular, considering the association among three of the four biological markers exhibiting the most different pattern of expression between the two histotype, namely steroid receptors, p53 and VEGF, ILC are characterized by the absence of p53 expression associated with very low VEGF levels in the majority of cases, regardless of hormone receptor status. Conversely, in IDC VEGF is expressed at high levels in about 50% of the cases, mainly in p53-negative tumors and regardless of hormone receptor status. Differently from IDC, in which tumor size was associated with VEGF or $p27^{kip1}$ expression, tumor growth in ILC seemed to be independent of VEGF but related to the expression of other factors. In fact, a direct relation between tumor size (considered as a surrogate marker of progression) and $p16^{ink4}$ or $p21^{waf1}$ was found, thereby suggesting a link between an aberrant accumulation of these proteins with concurrent loss of their function and activation of tumor proliferation [106]. Interestingly, as regards the angiogenesis-related proteins, a strong direct relation between VEGF content and IDC size and an inverse relation with both steroid receptors were observed. Conversely, in ILC, median VEGF concentration was very similar to that found in a series of normal breast tissues (about 40 pg/mg of cytosolic protein) suggesting that, in tumors arising in the lobular structure, angiogenesis activation, although essential for tumor growth and progression, does not need VEGF overexpression and the angiogenesis proced through pathways other than VEGF. Otherwise, the presence of antiangiogenic factors could be hypothesized, as recently demonstrated, in the myoepithelial cells surrounding lobular structures [107]. In ILC, VEGF expression and proliferation-related features seemed to be associated, in contrast to IDC.

Taking into account the link found in IDC between steroid receptors and p53 and VEGF expression, the observation that, in our case series, the p53+/VEGF+ phenotype is more frequently associated with a negative steroid receptor status confirms previous findings. Moreover, in ILC the lack of a relation between steroid receptors, p53 and VEGF expression is not surprising. Clinical studies have demonstrated a significant relation between p53 status and VEGF expression and their correlation with a poor prognosis [108,109]. The interrelations among hormonal control, p53 and angiogenesis activation could be explained by the presence in the VEGF promoter region [110] either of a specific cis-element recognized by p53 or of a specific estrogen-response element [79]. In addition, p53 protein, less frequently mutated in ILC than in IDC [111], is able to downregulate the promoter activity of VEGF in a dose-dependent manner [112] and to inactivate the HIF-1α protein [113]. Conversely, the higher incidence of p53+ IDC compared to ILC, associated with a higher VEGF concentration, is in keeping with a possible downregulation of angiogenesis by p53 tumor suppressor gene function through a block of HIF-1 activity, with the formation of a stable complex wild-type p53/HIF-1α [114] and the subsequent ubiquitination of HIF-1α. Mutation of the p53 gene and the generation of a nonfunctional protein that accumulates in the cell both inhibit the formation of the complex and result in the constitutive availability of the transcription factor and the subsequent transactivation of the VEGF gene [115].

VEGF and Clinical Outcome

Breast carcinoma is a heterogeneous disease with variations in clinical behavior, in terms of response to treatment, metastatic potential, and survival, even among patients with the same clinical or pathological stage. For instance, even though most of the patients with a node-negative breast cancer have a good prognosis, about 30% will develop recurrent disease within 10 years of initial therapy. Therefore, it is of great clinical interest to identify subgroups of patients at high risk for relapse to submit to systemic treatments and to design new therapeutic approaches to contrast progression-relevant molecular alterations.

Till now several endocrine, autocrine and genetic factors have been identified as important for tumor progression and metastatic spread [116] and more recently also angiogenesis has been included in this panel. In fact, many studies have shown a relationship between microvessel density (MVD, the extent of new blood vessel growth) within the invasive primary carcinoma and the risk of nodal/or distant metastasis and prognosis and the correlation of endothelial markers with survival [117-119] demonstrating that MVD is of prognostic value for identifying patients at high risk of recurrence, particularly in the node-negative subgroup [120-122]. Therefore, tumor vascularity has been for a long time investigated and measured by staining tissue sections with antibodies specific for antigens expressed by vascular endothelial cells such as factor VIII (von Willebrand factor), CD31 or CD34 and counting under high power, the number of highlighted vessels in so-called 'hotspots', i.e. localized areas where there are usually high numbers of vessels as first detected under lower power magnification.

However, since the identification of patients at an early stage of their disease is of primarily importance to guarantee an effective and timely treatment, MVD evaluation has been successively associated with intratumor or serum VEGF level determination. Many studies have been published and in most of them has emerged the independent role on prognosis of VEGF overexpression also when analyzed in a multivariate fashion with other consolidated pathobiologic features [123-128]. In particular, in a recent study [129] we investigated the adjunctive prognostic contribution of intratumor VEGF concentration to one of the most widely adopted prognostic classification: the Nottingham prognostic index (NPI), which is based on morphopathologic features such as lymph node stage, tumor size and histologic grading of malignancy and has been prospectively validated in several studies [130-132]. Although lymph node stage has a pivotal role in the NPI definition, NPI is a validated prognostic discriminator also in node-negative patients [133] and can be considered as a baseline reference for the evaluation of the additional prognostic role of biological variables. Therefore, when we evaluated the prognostic contribution of VEGF concentration to NPI, taking also into account the effect of steroid receptors and cell proliferation (two consolidated biological markers to classify breast cancer outcome) on a series of 226 node-negative primary breast cancer patients [129] we found a discriminatory effect of VEGF in identifying patients who differ in prognosis mainly in ER-poor tumors. For these patients, the estimated hazard ratio for disease, investigated by the Cox model, for high vs low VEGF was 1.79 (95% CL, 1.15-2.79). Conversely, in ER-rich tumors, VEGF was unable to segregate patients with different prognosis, and the HR was 1.18 (95% CL, 0.78-1.79). A possible explanation for this finding is that in ER-poor tumors the presence of high VEGF levels could indicate the activation of the angiogenic process, whereas in the ER-rich subset a functional hormone control could be yet able to counteract angiogenesis activation even though, as suggested by a previous study [134], a longer follow-up could be necessary to observe the disruption of the hormone-related growth control and angiogenesis balance. Therefore, in node-negative breast cancer patients, the expression of VEGF appeared to be related with the natural course of the disease and can provide additional prognostic information to select patients likely to receive an adjuvant treatment.

ANGIOGENESIS AND TUMOR DORMANCY

The concept that angiogenesis is required for the expansion of a tumor mass raises the question about the time of occurrence of neovascularization during tumor progression: is it simply a necessity to overcome size limitations or is it coupled to a specific stage in a tumor life? There is increasing evidence from a variety of human tumors and mouse models that angiogenesis can be switched on at different stages of tumor progression depending on the nature of the tumor itself and of the microenvironment. Human tumors (primary as well as metastasis), including breast cancer can remain dormant for years owing to a balance between cell proliferation and apoptosis. Dormant tumors have been discovered during autopsies of individual who died of causes other than cancer and it supports the notion that only a very small subset of dormant tumors enter to the second phase, i.e. the vascular phase, in which exponential tumor growth occurs. This same principle can be applied to tumor metastasis. Dormant metastases represent a critical problem as they can sometimes become activated by removal of the primary tumor [135]. Given the requirement of angiogenesis for growth and progression of dormant lesions it would be assumed that inhibition of the angiogenic switch could prevent progression of tumors and their metastases.

Already in 1959, Fisher and Fisher [136] provided experimental evidence of increased growth of dormant micrometastases in animal model and over the last decades questions have been raised regarding possible adverse effects of surgery on the outcome in cancer patients. Rapid acceleration of tumor growth following surgery for primary or secondary malignancy is a concern expressed by physicians probably as a consequence of the wounding tissue repair activated by surgical treatment. For many years, in fact, a role for wound healing in favouring local tumor recurrence has been debated, based on observations in clinical and experimental studies [137]. Surgery may accelerate the growth of residual disease not only by removal of anti-angiogenic factors produced by the primary, but also by the production of pro-angiogenic factors [138]. In fact, during oncologic surgical procedure, an accurate vascular clamping is routinely employed in order to safely and effectively resect malignant tumors. Such vascular inflow occlusion is accompanied by tissue hypoxia which may contribute to the induction of angiogenesis. In fact, as we have observed in two surgical samples from individual patients, obtained just after hepatic artery clamping, and subsequently 20 minutes after clamping, hypoxia induces a dramatic increase in HIF-1α mRNA level that corresponds to an increase in VEGF mRNA expression [17], and clinical studies support the concept that surgery-induced hypoxic stress unfavourably affects the prognosis of cancer patients by inducing angiogenesis [139]. Furthermore, one of the strongest indications supporting the opinion that surgery may enhance the outgrowth of micrometastases is offered by the identification of angiostatin and endostatin, both endogenous anti-angiogenic factors produced by the primary tumors [140,141]. These factors inhibit remote micrometastases from growing by suppressing the formation of their vascular supply. Their discovery was based on the observation that following the removal of a primary tumor, metastases appeared, developed new vessels and displayed an increased growth rate. By treating tumor-bearing mice with angiostatin or endostatin a state of dormancy is attained: tumor cells remain viable but do not progress [142,143]. Accelerated metastatic growth following the removal of the primary tumor has been observed also in patients after excision of primary breast cancer [144,145] suggesting that many of the locally produced pro-angiogenic factors are released into the systemic circulation and surgery may modulate the transition of quiescent tumor cells into rapidly growing one.

The production of these inhibitors may also change during the course of therapy. For example, radiation has been shown to increase the production of various anti-angiogenic molecules including tumor necrosis factor α, transforming growth factor β1 and endostatin [146] and when investigated in patients with breast cancer treated with adjuvant chemotherapy (CMF schedule), angiogenesis (evaluated as vascular index) appeared to be associated with the risk of recurrence [147]. In their study of the risk of recurrence, Gasparini et al. [147] observed that the hazard function of metastasis presented two peaks of incidence at 20 and 60 months after surgery, respectively, and that the risk of first recurrence was associated with vascular index. In addition, the authors found that at 5 years vascular index provided the highest prognostic contribution followed by the number of involved axillary lymph nodes supporting the clinical findings of the second peak of incidence of recurrence after 5 years and suggesting that a fraction of breast cancers may promote metastasis after a long period of tumor dormancy.

VEGF and Response to Therapy

An increasing body of evidence indicates that in addition to their prognostic value in node-negative patients, angiogenesis-related factors could be promising indicators also in predicting the response to radio-chemical treatments. It is the case of HIF-1 which has provided to be specifically related with resistance to radiotherapy (RT). For instance, in patients with oropharyngeal cancer, overexpression of HIF-1α in tumor biopsy is associated with an increased risk of failure to achieve complete remission after RT [26]. Similarly, VEGF content predicts for a reduced efficacy of postoperative RT as part of breast-conserving therapy in node-negative breast cancer patients [148]. This finding is in agreement with previously discussed role of HIF-1 in VEGF synthesis [17]. Hypoxia triggers tumor to produce VEGF, which in turn stimulates endothelial cells radioresistance as suggested by Gorski et al. [149] who demonstrated that tumor actively protects itself from secondary radiation damage by promoting endothelial cells radioresistance and pointed out the attention on the sensitivity of tumor vasculature to radiation that could be a relevant determinant in the response to RT [150].

As regards systemic therapy, VEGF levels have been found an independent prognostic factor of survival in primary node-positive breast cancer and a useful outcome predictor after adjuvant endocrine therapy whereas there is no consensus in the literature about the role of VEGF content after polychemiotherapy [151-153]. The relation between VEGF levels and patients outcome is particularly evident in node-positive ER-positive postmenopausal women who, accordingly to the recently revised guidelines for early breast cancer, receive adjuvant hormone therapy [154]. Although expected to respond to the treatment because of their ER positive status, some of them fail and become resistant to endocrine therapy. Among the hypotheses proposed to explain treatment failure there is overexpression and/or dysregulation of VEGF. In accordance with this hypothesis, in a recent study [155] we observed that in postmenopausal women with primary resectable invasive breast cancer, histologically classified as node-positive and who received adjuvant tamoxifen for at least 2 years because ER-positive, the risk of 6-year relapse increased with increasing values of intratumoral VEGF and that this finding was primarily evident in patients whose tumors had a low/intermediate ER content. In fact, the VEGF level did not show prognostic effect in patients whose tumors had a high ER content (Figure 3). These findings suggest that in tumors characterized by a low ER concentration, tamoxifen failed to inhibit tumor progression activated or sustained by high VEGF levels, while in those with high ER concentration and therefore more likely to be hormonally regulated, tumor progression, activated or sustained by VEGF, may be counteracted by the protective effect of endocrine therapy.

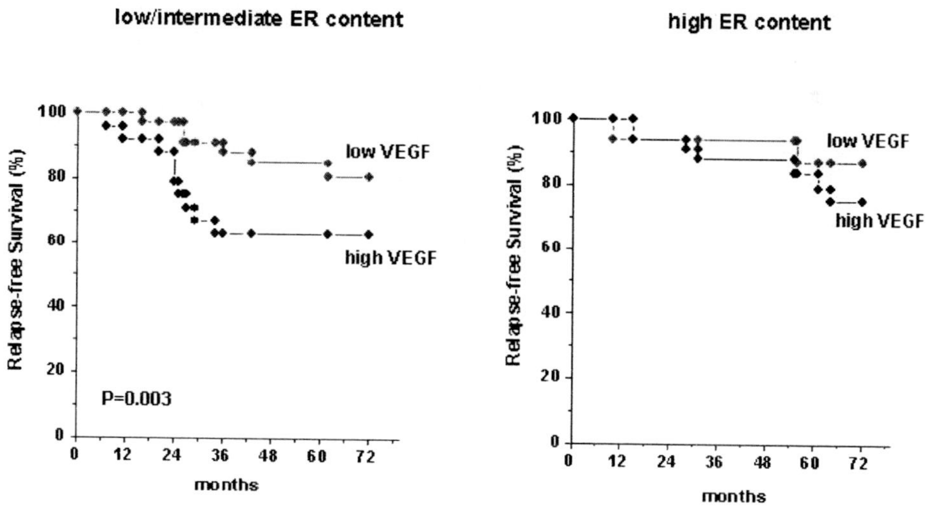

Figure 3. Relapse-free survival curves for 212 postmenopausal women with node-positive primary breast cancer treated with adjuvant tamoxifen because ER-positive. VEGF content was predictor of relapse in patients with a low/intermediate tumor ER content (less than or equal to 70 fmol/mg cytosol protein, left panel) but not in patients with a high tumor ER content (more than or equal to 220 fmol/mg cytosolic protein (for details see [155]).

These results are an indirect evidence that the patients with highly vascularized breast cancer may have poor benefit of adjuvant tamoxifen, unable to contrast the tumor's metastatic potential, and are in agreement with that of Gasparini et al. [151] who correlated the degree of vascularization of the primary tumors (by CD31 staining and microvessels count) with the risk of recurrence in node-positive patients treated with adjuvant tamoxifen for three years. They found that the risk of first recurrence was strictly associated with vascular index having the patients with the highest microvessel counts the highest risk of metastasis which differed according to receptor status: in the subgroup of patients with ER-positive tumors the hazard of metastasis was almost constant in time, while in that with ER-negative tumors it increased rapidly up to 20 months and thereafter decreased sharply according to the previously reported theory of tumor dormancy.

As already discussed in a previous paragraph of this chapter, also soluble VEGFR-1 expression, a negative regulator of VEGF availability, could represent a good marker to predict patient responsiveness to an antiestrogenic therapy. In fact, as demonstrated by Elkin et al. [87] the incubation of ER-positive breast cancer cell lines with a pure antiestrogen result in an increase of VEGFR-1 expression and in a concomitant decrease of angiogenesis.

To explain the role of VEGF expression in tamoxifen failure we investigated the effect of this conventional antiestrogenic agent, known to exert both agonist and antagonist activities, and that of a pure antiestrogen (ICI 182,780) on MCF7, an estrogen-dependent cell line both under normoxic and hypoxic condition [84]. The findings indicated that the pure antiestrogen ICI 182,780 completely counteracted estradiol-induced VEGF synthesis but only in normoxia, suggesting, once again, the hypoxic stimulation as the most potent and arising the hypothesis that hypoxia could be the possible cause for the failure of the adjuvant treatment with tamoxifen observed in patients with ER-positive tumors but with very high intratumor VEGF level.

Also the prognostic role of tumor angiogenesis in node-positive breast cancer patients treated with adjuvant chemotherapy has been investigated but the results are contrasting and not conclusive. In fact, some studies indicate that anthracycline-based adjuvant chemotherapy is more effective than CMF schedule in terms of relapse prevention [156]. However, some authors suggested that the assessment of angiogenesis (in terms of microvessel density), even if related to tumor progression and decreased disease-free or overall survival, does not provide useful information regarding prognosis in node-positive breast cancer patients treated with adjuvant cyclophosphamide doxorubicin and fluorouracil [157]. In contrast, other authors [151] have found that high levels of thymidine phosphorylase (the target enzyme for cytotoxicity of 5-fluorouracil and methotrexate) and low levels of VEGF characterize the patients with node-positive breast cancer treated with adjuvant CMF who have the highest likelihood of favorable outcome.

Interestingly, the results of a randomized clinical trial aimed to assess the impact of neoadjuvant versus adjuvant chemoendocrine therapy for operable breast cancer patients [158] suggested that neoadjuvant therapy causes a reduction in microvessel density in primary breast carcinomas which could be secondary to tumor regression or due to a direct effect on angiogenesis.

Conclusion

In this chapter, we discussed the very close biological relationship between breast cancer progression and angiogenesis activation triggered by microenvironment stimuli such as hypoxia or the presence of hormone steroids. Moreover, we illustrated the clinical role of some of the most important tumor angiogenesis-related markers (HIF-1 and VEGF) in predicting patients outcome and responsiveness to radio-, endocrine- and chemotherapy. However, these stimuli can act also on other than epithelial cells; in fact, stromal cells can actively contribute to increase the production of VEGF and other angiogenic factors, including bFGF and PDGF, as demonstrated by the finding that breast tumors implanted in animals into different tissue sites show differences in the extent and nature of the angiogenic response [159] and suggests that local stromal conditions and immune reactions can play a critical role.

In this regard, also breast cancer therapeutic strategies should be revised and the endothelial cell compartment of a tumor mass might receive a greater therapeutic attention than in the past. In fact, the process of disease formation in breast tissue is both morphologically and genetically complex and the regulation of vascularity multifactorial. Thus, the concept of treating solid tumors by inhibiting only tumor angiogenesis should be changed and new targets or anti-cancer strategies should now consider also the endothelial cells of tumor vessels, by improving the use of anti-vascular targeting strategies combined with conventional cytotoxic drugs as suggested by preclinical evidence [160]. These drugs kill endothelial cells of newly formed blood vessels by different mechanisms causing a vascular collapse and the subsequent death of much larger number of tumor cells. In this perspective, some clinical trials have been activated to evaluate the effectiveness of a such anti-angiogenic approach and the near future will tell us whether the combination of a cytotoxic agent with an angiogenesis inhibitor is a winning strategy against tumor progression.

References

[1] Zhu H, Bunn HF. Oxygen sensing and signaling: impact on the regulation of physiologically important genes. *Respiration Physiol 115*:239-247,1999.

[2] Boutilier RG. Mechanisms of cell survival in hypoxia and hypothermia. *J Exp Biol 204:*3171-3181,2001.

[3] Bunn HF, Poyton RO. Oxygen sensing and molecular adaptation to hypoxia. *Physiol Rev 76*:839-845,1996.

[4] Carmeliet P, Dor Y, Harbert JM, *et al.* Role of HIF-1a in hypoxia-mediated apoptosis, cell proliferation and tumor angiogenesis. *Nature 394*:485-490,1998.

[5] Semenza G. Expression of hypoxia-inducible factor 1: mechanisms and consequences. *Biochem Pharmacol 59*:47-53,2000.

[6] Harris AL. Hypoxia - a key regulatory factor in tumour growth. *Nat Rev Cancer 2*:38-47,2002.

[7] Ivan M, Kondo K, Yang H, *et al.* HIFα targeted for VHL-mediated destruction by proline hydroxylation: implications for O_2 sensing. *Science 292*:464-467,2001.

[8] Jaakkola P, Mole DR, Tian YM, *et al.* Targeting of HIF-1α to the von Hippel-Lindau ubiquitylation complex by O_2-regulated prolyl hydroxylation. *Science 292*:468-472,2001.

[9] Sutter CH, Laughner E, Semenza GL. Hypoxia-inducible factor 1α protein expression is controlled by oxygen-regulated ubiquitination that is disrupted by deletions and missense mutations. *Proc Natl Acad Sci USA 97*:4748-4753,2000.

[10] Semenza GL. Hypoxia, clonal selection and the role of HIF-1 in tumor progression. *Crit Rev Biochem Mol Biol 35*:71-103,2000.

[11] Shweiki D, Itin A, Soffer D, Keshet E. Vascular endothelial growth factor induced by hypoxia may mediate hypoxia-initiated angiogenesis. *Nature 359*:843-845,1992.

[12] Plate KH, Breier G, Weich HA, Risau W. Vascular endothelial growth factor in human gliomas in vivo. *Nature 359*:845-848,1992.

[13] Vukovic V, Haugland HK, Nicklee T, *et al.* Hypoxia-inducible factor-1alpha is an intrinsic marker fo hypoxia in cervical cancer xenografts. *Cancer Res 61*:7394-7398,2001.

[14] Haugland HK, Vukovic V, Pintilie M, *et al.* Expression of hypoxia-inducible factor-1 alpha in cervical carcinomas: correlation with tumor oxygenation. *Int J Radiat Oncol Biol Phys 53*:854-861,2002.

[15] Jewell UR, Kvietikova I, Scheid A, *et al.* Induction of HIF-1 in response to hypoxia is istantaneous. *FASEB J 15*:1312-1314,2001.

[16] Dupuy E, Hainaud P, Villemain A, *et al.* Tumoral angiogenesis and tissue factor expression during hepatocellular carcinoma progression in a transgenic mouse model. *J Hepatol 38*:793-802,2003.

[17] Coradini D, Costa A, Pellizzaro C, *et al.* Instantaneous response to surgically induced hypoxia of hepatocellular carcinoma. *J Hepatol 40*:563-564,2004.

[18] Talks KL, Turley H, Gatter KC, *et al.* The expression and distribution of the hypoxia-inducible factors HIF-1α and HIF-2α in normal human tissues, cancers, and tumor-associated macrophages. *Am J Pathol 157*:411-421,2000.

[19] Zhong H, De Marzo AM, Laughner E, *et al.* Overexpression of hypoxia-inducible factor 1α in common human cancers and their metastases. *Cancer Res 59*:5830-5835,1999.

[20] Marti HJH, Bernaudin M, Bellail A, *et al.* Hypoxia-induced vascular endothelial growth factor expression precedes neovascularization after cerebral ischemia. *Am J Pathol 156*:965-976,2000.

[21] Folkman J. Tumor angiogenesis: therapeutic implications. *N Engl J Med 285*:1182-1186,1971.

[22] St. Croix BM, Rago C, Velculescu V, *et al.* Gene expressed in human tumor endothelium. *Science 289*:1197-1202,2000.

[23] Kuzu I, Bicknell R, Fletcher CD, Gatter KC. Expression of adhesion molecules on the endothelium of normal tissue vessels and vascular tumors. *Lab Invest 69*:322-328,1993.

[24] Elicieri BP, Cheresh DA. The role of $alpha_v$ integrins during angiogenesis: insights into potential mechanisms of action and clinical development. *J Clin Invest 103*:1227-1230,1999.

[25] Hockel M, Schlenger K, Mitze M, *et al.* Hypoxia and radiation response in human tumours. *Semin Radiat Oncol 6*:3-9,1996.

[26] Aebersold DM, Burri P, Beer DT, *et al.* Expression of hypoxia-inducible factors-1α: a novel predictive and prognostic parameter in the radiotherapy of oropharyngeal cancer. *Cancer Res 61*:2911-2916,2001.

[27] Koukourakis MI, Giatromanolaki A, Skarlatos J, *et al.* Hypoxia inducible factor (HIF-1a and HIF-2a) expression in early esophageal cancer and response to photodynamic therapy and radiotherapy. *Cancer Res 61*:1830-1832,2001.

[28] Hanahan D, Folkman J. Patterns and emerging mechanisms of the angiogenic switch during tumorigenesis. *Cell 86*:353-364,1996.

[29] Folkman J. Role of angiogenesis in tumor growth and metastasis. *Sem Oncol 29*:15-18,2002.

[30] Siemeister G, Martiny-Baron G, Marmé D. The pivotal role of VEGF in tumor angiogenesis: Molecular facts and therapeutic opportunities. *Cancer Metastasis Rev 17*:241-248,1998.

[31] Senger DR, Galli SJ, Dvorak AM, *et al.* Tumor cells secrete a vascular permeability factor that promotes accumulation of ascites fluid. *Science 219*:983-985,1983.

[32] Connolly DT, Olander JV, Heuvelman D, *et al.* Human vascular permeability factor. Isolation from U937 cells. *J Biol Chem 264*:20017-20024,1989.

[33] Keck PJ, Hauser SD, Krivi G, *et al.* Vascular permeability factor, and endothelial cell mitogen related to PDGF. *Science 246*:1309-1312,1989.

[34] Leung DW, Cachianes G, Kuang WJ, *et al.* Vascular endothelial growth factor is a secreted angiogenic mitogen. *Science 246*:1306-1309,1989.

[35] Achen MG, Stacker SA. The vascular endothelial growth factor family: proteins which guide the development of the vasculature. *Int J Exp Path 79*:255-265,1998.

[36] Carmeliet P, Ferreira V, Breier G, *et al.* Abnormal blood vessel development and lethality in embryos lacking a single VEGF allele. *Nature 380*:435-439,1996.

[37] Ferrara N, Carver-Moore K, Chen H, *et al.* Heterozygous embryonic lethality induced by targeted inactivation of the VEGF gene. *Nature 380*:439-443,1996.

[38] Olofsson B, Pajusola K, Kaipainen A, *et al.* Vascular endothelial growth factor B, a novel growth factor for endothelial cells. *Proc Natl Acad Sci USA 93*:2576-2581,1996.

[39] Joukov V, Pajusola K, Kaipainen A, *et al.* A novel vascular endothelial growth factor VEGF-C is a ligand for the Flt-4 (VEGF-R3) and KDR (VEGFR-2) receptor tyrosine kinases. *EMBO J 15*:290-298,1996.

[40] Achen MG, Jeltsch M, Kukk E, *et al.* Vascular endothelial growth factor D (VEGF-D) is a ligand for the tyrosine kinases VEGF receptor 2 (Flk-1) and VEGF receptor 3 (Flt-4). *Proc Natl Acad Sci USA 95*:548-553,1998.

[41] Meyer M, Clauss M, Lepple-Wienhues A, *et al.* A novel vascular endothelial growth factor encoded by Orf virus, VEGF-E, mediates angiogenesis via signaling through VEGFR-2 (KDR) but not VEGFR-1 (Flt-1)receptor tyrosine kinases. *EMBO J 18*:363-374,1999.

[42] Maglione D, Guerriero V, Viglietto G, *et al.* Two alternative mRNAs coding for the angiogenic factor placenta growth factor (PIGF) are transcribed from a single gene of chromosome 14. *Oncogene 8:*925-931,1993.

[43] McDonald ND, Hendrickson WA. A structural superfamily of growth factors containing a cysteine knot motif. *Cells 73*:421-424,1993.

[44] Muller YA, Li B, Christinger HW, *et al.* Vascular endothelial growth factor: crystal structure and functional mapping of the kinase domain receptor binding site. *Proc Natl Acad Sci USA 94*:7192-7197,1997.

[45] Houck KA, Ferrara N, Winer J, *et al.* The vascular endothelial growth factor family: identification of a fourth molecular species and characterization of alternative silencing RNA. *Mol Endocrinol 5*:1806-1814,1991.

[46] Neufeld G, Cohen T, Gengrinovitch S, Poltorak Z. Vascular endothelial growth factor (VEGF) and its receptors. *FASEB J 13*: 9-22, 1999.

[47] Mohle R, Green D, Moore MA, *et al.* Constitutive production and thrombin-induced release of vascular endothelial growth factor by human megakaryocytes and platelets. *Proc Natl Acad Sci 94*:663-668,1997.

[48] Robinson CJ, Stringer SE. The splice variants of vascular endothelial growth factor (VEGF) and their receptors. *J Cell Sci 114*:853-865,2001.

[49] Park JE, Keller GA, Ferrara N. The vascular endothelial growth factor (VEGF) isoforms: differential deposition into the subepithelial extracellular matrix and bioactivity of extracellular matrix-bound VEGF. *Mol Biol Cell 4*:1317-1326,1993.

[50] De Vries C, Escobedo JA, Ueno H, *et al.* The fms-like tyrosine kinase, a receptor for vascular endothelial growth factor. *Science 255*:989-991,1992.

[51] Quinn TP, Peters KG, De Vries C, *et al.* Fetal liver kinase 1 is a receptor for vascular endothelial growth factor and is selectively expressed in vascular endothelium. *Proc Natl Acad Sci USA 90*:7533-7537,1993.

[52] Soker S, Takashima S, Miao HQ, *et al.* Neuropilin-1 is expressed by endothelial and tumor cells as an isoform-specific receptor for vascular endothelial growth factor. *Cell 92*:735-745,1998.

[53] Shibuya M. Structure and dual function of vascular endothelial growth factor receptor-1 (Flt-1). *Int J Biochem Cell Biol 33*:409-420,2001.

[54] Cross MJ, Dixelius J, Matsumoto T, Claesson-Welsh L. VEGF-receptor signal transduction. *Trends in Biochem Sci 28*:488-494,2003.

[55] Brown LF, Berse B, Jackman RW, *et al.* Expression of vascular permeability factor/vascular endothelial growth factor and its receptors in breast cancer. *Human Pathol 26:*86-91,1995.

[56] Yoshiji H, Gomez DE, Shibuya M, Thorgeirsson UP. Expression of vascular endothelial growth factor its receptor and other angiogenic factors in human breast cancer. *Cancer Res 56*:2013-2016,1996.

[57] Valtola R, Salven P, Heillila P, *et al.* VEGFR-3 and its ligand VEGF-C are associated with angiogenesis in breast cancer. *Am J Pathol 154*:1381-1390,1999.

[58] Barleon B, Reusch P, Totzke F, *et al.* Soluble VEGFR-1 secreted by endothelial cells and monocytes is present in human serum and plasma from healthy donors. *Angiogenesis 4*:43-54,2001.

[59] Contrino J, Hair G, Kreutzer DL, Rickles FR. In situ detection of tissue factor in vascular endothelial cells: correlation with the malignant phenotype of human breast disease. *Nat Med 2*:209-215,1996.

[60] Heffelfinger SC, Yassin E, Miller MA, Lower E. Vascularity of proliferative breast disease and carcinoma in situ correlates with histologic features. *Clin Cancer Res 2*:1873-1878,1996.

[61] Weidner N, Semple JP, Welch WR, Folkman J. Tumor angiogenesis and metastasis – correlation in invasive breast carcinoma. *New Engl J Med 324*:9-19,1991.

[62] Heffelfinger SC, Miller MA, Yassin R, Gear R. Angiogenic growth factors in preinvasive breast disease. *Clin Cancer Res 5*:2867-2876,1999.

[63] Guidi AJ, Schnitt SJ, Fischer L, *et al.* Vascular permeability factor (vascular endothelial growth factor) expression and angiogenesis in patients with ductal carcinoma in situ of the breast. *Cancer 80*:1945-1953,1997.

[64] Potten C, Watson RJ, Williams GT, *et al.* The effect of age and menstrual cycle upon proliferative activity of the normal human breast. *Br J Cancer 58*:163-170,1988.

[65] Anderson T. Mitotic activity in breast. *J Obstet Gynecol 4*:S114-S118,1984.

[66] Djonov V, Andres AC, Ziemicki A. Vascular remodeling during the normal and malignant life cycle of the mammary gland. *Microsc Res Tech 52*:182-189,2001.

[67] Naccarato AG, Viacava P, Bocci G, *et al.* Definition of the microvascular pattern of the normal human adult mammary gland. *J Anat 203*:599-603,2003.

[68] Brem SS, Jensen HM, Gullino PM. Angiogenesis as a marker of preneoplastic lesions of the human breast. *Cancer 41*:239-244,1978.

[69] Helczynska K, Kronblad A, Jogi A, *et al.* Hypoxia promotes a dedifferentiated phenotype in ductal breast carcinoma in situ. *Cancer Res 63:*1441-1444,2003.

[70] Bos R, Zhong H, Hanrahan CF, *et al.* Levels of hypoxia-inducible factor-1α during breast carcinogenesis. *J Natl Cancer Inst 93:*309-314,2001.

[71] Reynolds TY, Rockwell S, Glazer PM. Genetic instability induced by tumor microenvironment. *Cancer Res 56*:5754-5757,1996.

[72] Petit AM, Rak J, Hung MC, *et al.* Neutralizing antibodies against EGF and ErbB-2/neu receptor tyrosine kinase down-regulate VEGF production by tumor cells in vitro and in vivo: angiogenic implications for signal transduction therapy of solid tumors. *Am J Pathol 151*:1523-1530,1997.

[73] Brown LF, Guidi AJ, Schnitt SJ, *et al.* Vascular stroma formation in carcinoma in situ invasive carcinoma and metastatic carcinoma of the breast. *Clin Cancer Res 5*:1041-1056,1999.

[74] Yen L, You XL, Moustafa AE, *et al.* Heregulin selectively upregulates vascular endothelial growth factor secretion in cancer cells and stimulates angiogenesis. *Oncogene 19:*3460-3469,2000.

[75] Laughner E, Taghavi P, Chiles K, *et al.* HER2 (neu) signaling increases the rate of hypoxia-inducible factor 1alpha (HIF-1alpha) synthesis: novel mechanism for HIF-1-mediated vascular endothelial growth factor expression. *Mol Cell Biol 21*:3995-4004,2001.

[76] Losordo DW, Isner JM. Estrogen and angiogenesis: a review. *Arterioscler Thromb Vasc Biol 21*:6-12,2001.

[77] Vogel PM, Georgiade NG, Fetter BF, *et al.* The correlation of histologic changes in human breast with the menstrual cycle. *Am J Pathol 104*:23-34,1981.

[78] Nakamura J, Lu Q, Aberdeen G, *et al.* The effect of estrogen on aromatase and vascular endothelial growth factor messenger ribonucleic acid in the normal nonhuman primate mammary gland. *J Clin Endocrinol Metab 84*:1432-1437,1999.

[79] Hyder SM, Nawaz Z, Chiappetta C, Stancel GM. Identification of functional response elements in the gene coding for the potent angiogenic factor vascular endothelial growth factor. *Cancer Res 60*:3183-3190,2000.

[80] Greb RR, Maier I, Wallwiener D, Kissel L. Vascular endothelial growth factor a (Vegf-a) mRNA expression levels decrease after monopause in normal breast tissue but not in breast cancer lesions. *Br J Cancer 81*:225-231,1999.

[81] Haran EF, Maretzek AF, Goldberg I, Horowitz A, Degani H. Tamoxifen enhances cell death in implanted MCF7 breast cancer by inhibiting endothelium growth. *Cancer Res 54*:5511-5514, 1994.

[82] Ruohola JK, Valve EM, Karkkainen MJ, *et al.* Vascular endothelial growth factors are differentially regulated by steroid hormones and antiestrogens in breast cancer cells. *Mol Cell Endocrinol 129:*29-40, 1999.

[83] Hyder SM, Huang JC, Nawaz Z, *et al.* Regulation of vascular endothelial growth factor expression by estrogens and progestins. *Environ Health Perspect 108*:785-790,2000.

[84] Coradini D, Pellizzaro C, Speranza A, Daidone MG. Hypoxia and estrogen receptor profile influence the responsiveness of human breast cancer cells to estradiol and antiestrogens. *Cell Mol Life Sci 61*:76-82,2004.

[85] Yuan Y, Hulliard G, Ferguson T, Millhorn D.E. Cobalt inhibits the interaction between hypoxia-inducible factor-α and von Hippel-Lindau protein by direct binding to hypoxia-inducible factor-α. *J Biol Chem 278*:15911-15916,2003.

[86] Hyder SM, Murthy L, Stancel GM. Progestin regulation of vascular endothelium growth factor in human breast cancer cells. *Cancer Res 58*:392-395,1998.

[87] Elkin M, Orgel A, Kleinman HK. An angiogenic switch in breast cancer involves estrogen and soluble vascular endothelial growth factor receptor 1. *J Natl Cancer Inst 96*:875-878,2004.

[88] Retsky M, Demicheli R, Hrushesky W. Premenopausal status accelerates relapse in node positive breast cancer: hypothesis links angiogenesis, screening controversy. *Breast Cancer Res Treat 65*:217-224,2001.

[89] Daidone MG, Coradini D, Martelli G, Veneroni S. Primary breast cancer in elderly women: biological profile and relation with clinical outcome. *Crit Rev Oncol Hematol 45*:313-325,2003.

[90] Agrawal R, Conway GS, Sladkevicius P, *et al.* Serum vascular endothelial growth factor (VEGF) in the normal menstrual cycle: association with changes in ovarian and uterine Doppler blood flow. *Clin Endocrinol 50*:101-106,1999.

[91] Benoy I, Vermeulen P, Wuyts H, Dirix L. Vascular endothelial cell growth factor (VEGF) serum concentrations change according to the phase of the menstrual cycle. *Eur J Cancer 34*:1298-1299,1998.

[92] Heer K, Kumar H, Speirs V, *et al.* Vascular endothelial growth factor in premenopausal women – indicator of the best time for breast cancer surgery? *Br J Cancer 78*:1203-1207,1998.

[93] Fentiman IS. Timing of surgery for breast cancer. *Int J Clin Pract* 56:188-190,2002.

[94] Zurrida S, Galimberti V, Gibelli B, *et al.* Timing of breast cancer surgery in relation to the menstrual cycle: an update of developments. *Crit Rev Oncol Hematol 38*:223-230,2001.

[95] Goldhirsch A, Gelber RD, Castiglione M, *et al.* Menstrual cycle and timing of breast surgery in premenopausal node-positive breast cancer: results of the International Breast Cancer Study Group (IBCSG) Trial VI. *Ann Oncol 8*:751-756,1997.

[96] Balsari A, Casalini P, Tagliabue E, *et al.* Fluctuation of HER2 expression in breast carcinomas during the menstrual cycle. *Am J Pathol 155*:1543-1547,1999.

[97] Coradini D, Veneroni S, Pellizzaro C, Daidone MG. Fluctuation of intratumor biological variables as a function of menstrual timing of surgery for breast cancer in premenopausal patients. *Ann Oncol 14:*962-964,2003.

[98] Lakhani SR, Chaggar R, Davies S, *et al.* Genetic alterations in 'normal' luminal and myoepithelial cells of the breast. *J Pathol 189*:496-503,1999.

[99] Harris JR, Lippman ME, Veronesi U, Willett W. Breast Cancer (1). *New Engl J Med 327:*319-328,1992.

[100] Peiro G, Bornstein BA, Connolly JL, *et al.* The influence of infiltrating lobular carcinoma on the outcome of patients treated with breast-conserving surgery and radiation therapy. *Breast Cancer Res Treat 59:*49-54,2000.

[101] Borst MJ and Ingold JA. Metastatic patterns of invasive lobular versus invasive ductal carcinoma of the breast. *Surgery 114*:637-641,1993.

[102] Jain S, Fisher C, Smith P, *et al.* Patterns of metastatic breast cancer in relation to histological type. *Eur J Cancer 29*:2155-2157,1993.

[103] Kruger S, Fahrenkrog T, Muller H. Proliferative and apoptotic activity in lobular breast carcinoma. *Int J Mol Med 4*:171-174,1999.

[104] Coradini D, Pellizzaro C, Veneroni S, *et al.* Infiltrating ductal and lobular breast carcinomas are characterised by different interrelationships among markers related to angiogenesis and hormone dependence *Br J Cancer 87*:1105-1111,2002.

[105] Lee AHS, Dublin EA, Bobrow LG, Poulsom R. Invasive lobular and invasive ductal carcinoma of the breast show distinct patterns of vascular endothelial growth factor expression and angiogenesis. *J Pathol 185*:394-401,1998.

[106] Emig R, Magener A, Ehemann V, *et al.* Aberrant cytoplasmic expression of the p16 protein in breast cancer is associated with accelerated tumor proliferation. *Br J Cancer 78*:1661-1668,1998.

[107] Nguyen M, Lee MC, Wang JL, *et al.* The human myoepithelial cell displays a multifaceted anti-angiogenic phenotype. *Oncogene 20*:3449-3459,2000.

[108] Linderholm B, Lindh B, Tavelin B, *et al.* P53 and vascular endothelial growth factor (VEGF) expression predicts outcome in 833 patients with primary breast carcinoma. *Int J Cancer 89*:51-62,2000.

[109] Linderholm BK, Lindhal T, Holmberg L, *et al.* The expression of vascular endothelial growth factor correlates with mutant p53 and poor prognosis in human breast cancer. *Cancer Res 61*:2256-2260,2001.

[110] Zhang L, Yu D, Hu M, *et al.* Wild-type p53 suppresses angiogenesis in human leiomyosarcoma and synovial sarcoma by transcriptional suppression of vascular endothelial growth factor expression. *Cancer Res 60*:3655-3661,2000.

[111] Marchetti A, Buttitta F, Pellegrini S, *et al.* P53 mutation and histological type of invasive breast carcinoma. *Cancer Res 53*:4665-4669,1993.

[112] Mukhopadhyay D, Tsiokas L, Sukhatme VP. Wild-type p53 and v-Src exert opposing influences on human vascular endothelial growth factor gene expression. *Cancer Res 55:*6161-6165,1995.

[113] Blagosklonny MV, An WG, Romanova LY, *et al.* P53 inhibits hypoxia-inducible factor-stimulated transcription. *J Biol Chem 73*:11995-11998,1998.

[114] An WG, Kanekal M, Simon MC, *et al.* Stabilization of wild-type p53 by hypoxia-inducible factor 1α. *Nature 392*:405-409,1998.

[115] Ravi R, Mookerjee B, Bhujwalla ZM, *et al.* Regulation of tumor angiogenesis by p53-induced degradation of hypoxia-inducible factor 1 alpha. *Genes Dev 14*:34-44,2000.

[116] Marx J. Cellular changes on the route to metastasis. *Science 259:*626-629,1993.

[117] Gasparini G, Weidner N, Bevilacqua P, *et al.* Tumor microvessel density, p53 expression, tumor size and peritumoral lymphatic vessel invasion are relevant prognostic markers in node-negative breast carcinoma. *J Clin Oncol 12*:454-466,1994.

[118] Toi M, Insada K, Suzuki H, Tominaga T. Tumor angiogenesis in breast cancer: its importance as a prognostic indicator and the association with vascular endothelial growth factor expression. *Breast Cancer Res Treat 36:*193-204,1995.

[119] Obermair A, Kurz C, Czerwenka K, *et al.* Microvessel density and vessel invasion in lymph-node-negative breast cancer. Effect on recurrence-free survival. *Int J Cancer 62*:126-131,1995.

[120] Bevilacqua P, Barbareschi M, Verderio P, *et al.* Prognostic value of intratumoral micrivessel density, a measure of tumor angiogenesis in node-negative breast carcinoma. *Breast Cancer Res Treat 36*:205-217,1995.

[121] Heimann R, Ferguson D, Powers C, *et al.* Angiogenesis as predictor of long-term survival for patients with node-negative breast cancer. *J Natl Cancer Inst 88:* 1764-1769,1996.

[122] Arona R, Joshi K, Nijhawan R, *et al.* Angiogenesis as an independent prognostic indicator in node-negative breast cancer. *Anal Quant Cytol Histol 24*:228-233,2002.

[123] Toi M, Insada K, Hoshina S, *et al.* Vascular endothelial growth factor and platelet-derived endothelial cell growth factor are frequently coexpressed in highly vascularized human breast cancer. *Clin Cancer Res 1*:961-964,1995.

[124] Tanaka M, Torisu. Vascular endothelial growth factor and platelet-derived growth factor are potential angiogenic and metastatic factors in human breast cancer. *Surgery 119*:333-339,1996.

[125] Obermair A, Kucera E, Mayerhofer K, *et al.* Vascular endothelial growth factor (VEGF) in human breast cancer. Correlation with disease-free survival. *Int J Cancer 74*:455-458,1997.

[126] Manders P, Beex LVAM, Tjan-Heijnen, *et al.* The prognostic value of vascular endothelial growth factor in 574 node-negative breast cancer patients who did not receive adjuvant systemic therapy. *Br J Cancer 87*:772-778,2002.

[127] Gasparini G, Toi M Gion M, *et al.* Prognostic significance of vascular endothelial growth factor in node-negative breast carcinoma. *J Natl Cancer Inst 89*:139-147,1997.

[128] Linderholm B, Tavelin B, Grankvist K, Henriksson R. Vascular endothelial growth factor is of high prognostic value in node-negative breast carcinoma. *J Clin Oncol 16:*3121-3128,1998.

[129] Coradini D, Boracchi P, Daidone MG, *et al.* Contribution of vascular endothelial growth factor to the Nottingham prognostic index in node-negative breast cancer. *Br J Cancer 85*:795-797,2001.

[130] Haybittle JL, Blamey RW, Elson CW, *et al.* A prognostic index in primary breast cancer. *Br J Cancer 45*: 361-366,1982.

[131] Galea MH, Blamey RW, Elston CE, Ellis IO. The Nottingham Prognostic Index in primary breast cancer. *Breast Cancer Res Treat 22*: 207-219,1992.

[132] Balslev I, Axelsson CK, Zedeler K, *et al.* The Nottingham Prognostic Index applied to 9149 patients from the studies of the Danish breast cancer cooperative group (DBCG). *Breast Cancer Res Treat 32*: 281-290,1994.

[133] Saurbrei W, Hubner K, Schmoor C, Schumacher M. Validation of existing and development of new prognostic classification schemes in node-negative breast cancer: German breast cancer study group. *Breast Cancer Res Treat 42*: 149-163,1997.

[134] Coradini D, Daidone MG, Boracchi P, *et al.* Time-dependent relevance of steroid receptors in breast cancer. *J Clin Oncol 18*: 2702-2709,2000.

[135] Homgren L, O'Reilly MS, Folkman J. Dormancy of micrometastases: balanced proliferation and apoptosis in the presence of angiogenesis suppression. *Nat Med 1*:149-153,1995.

[136] Fisher B, Fisher ER. Experimental evidence in support of the dormant tumor cells. *Science 130*:918-919,1959.

[137] Hofer SO, Molema G, Hermens HJ *et al.* The effect of surgical wounding on tumor development. *Eur J Surg Oncol 25*:231-243,1999.

[138] McNamara DA, Harmey JH, Walsh TN, *et al.* Significance of angiogenesis in cance therapy. *Br J Surg 85*:1044-1055,1998.

[139] Elias D, Cavalcanti de Albuquerque A, Eggenspieler P, *et al.* Resection of liver metastases from a noncolorectal primary: indications and results based on 147 monocentric patients. *J Am Coll Surg 187*:487-493,1998.

[140] O'Reilly MS, Holmgren L, Shing Y *et al.* Angiostatin: a novel angiogenesis inhibitor that mediates the suppression of metastases by Lewis lung carcinoma. *Cell 79:*315-328,1994.

[141] O'Reilly MS, Boehm T, Shing Y, *et al.* Endostatin: an endogenous inhibitor of angiogenesis and tumor growth *Cell 88*:277-285,1997.

[142] Holmgren L, O'Reilly MS, Folkman J. Dormancy of micrometastases: balanced proliferation and apoptosis in the presence of angiogenesis suppression. *Nat Med 1*:149-153,1995.

[143] O'Reilly MS, Holmgren L, Chen C, Folkman J. Angiostatin induces and sustains dormancy of human primary tumors in mice. *Nat Med 2*:689-692,1996.

[144] Demicheli R, Valagussa P, Bonadonna G. Does surgery modify growth kinetics of breast cancer micrometastases? *Br J Cancer 85:*490-492,2001.

[145] Demicheli R, Bonadonna G, Hrushesky WJ, *et al.* Menopausal status dependence of early mortality reduction due to diagnosis of smaller breast cancers (T1 v T2-T3): relevance to screening. *J Clin Oncol 22:*102-107,2004.

[146] Hartford AC, Gohongi T, Fukumura D, Jain RK. Irradiation of a primary tumor unlike surgical removal enhances angiogenesis suppression at a distal site: potential role of host-tumor interaction. *Cancer Res 60*:2128-2131,2000.

[147] Gasparini G, Biganzoli E, Bonoldi E, *et al.* Angiogenesis sustains dormancy in patients with breast cancer treated with adjuvant chemotherapy. *Breast Cancer Res Treat 65*:71-77,2001.

[148] Manders P, Sweep FC, Tjan-Heijnen VC, *et al.* Vascular endothelial growth factor independently predicts the efficacy of postoperative radiotherapy in node-negative breast cancer patients. *Clin Cancer Res 9:*6363-6370,2003.

[149] Gorski DH, Beckett MA, Jaskowiak NT, *et al.* Blockage of the vascualr endothelial growth facto stress response increases the antitumor effects of ionizing radiation. *Cancer Res 59*:3374-3378,1999.

[150] Denekamp J. Review article: angiogenesis, neovascular proliferation and vascular pathophysiology as target for cancer therapy. *Br J Radiol 66*:181-196,1993.

[151] Gasparini G, Toi M, Miceli R, *et al.* Clinical relevance of vascular endothelial growth factor and thymidine phosphorylase in patients with node-positive breast cancer treated with either adjuvant chemotherapy or hormone therapy. *Cancer J Sci Am 5*:101-119,1999.

[152] Linderholm B, Grankvist K, Wilking N, *et al.* Correlation of vascular endothelial growth factor content with recurrences, survival, and first relapse site in primary node-positive breast carcinoma after adjuvant treatment. *J Clin Oncol 18*:1423-1431,2000.

[153] Foekens JA, Peters HA, Grebenchtchikov N, *et al.* High tumor levels of vascular endothelial growth factor predict poor response to systemic therapy in advanced breast cancer. *Cancer Res 61*:5407-5414,2001.

[154] Goldhirsch A, Glick JH, Gelber RD, *et al.* Meeting Highlights: International Consensus Panel on the Treatment of Primary Breast Cancer. *J Clin Oncol 19*:3817-3827,2001.

[155] Coradini D, Biganzoli E, Pellizzaro C, *et al.* Vascular endothelial growth factor in node-positive breast cancer patients treated with adjuvant tamoxifen. *Br J Cancer 89*:268-270,2003.

[156] Gunel N, Akcali Z, Coskun U, *et al.* Prognostic importance of tumor angiogenesis in breast carcinoma with adjuvant chemotherapy. *Pathol Res Pract 198*:7-12,2002.

[157] Guidi AJ, Berry DA, Broadwater G, *et al.* Assotiation of angiogenesis and disease outcome in node-positive breast cancer patients treated with adjuvant cyclophosphamide doxorubicin and fluorouracil: a Cancer and Leukemia Group B correlative science study from protocol 8541*8869. *J Clin Oncol 20*:732-42,2002.

[158] Makris A, Powles TJ, Kakolyris S, *et al.* Reduction in angiogenesis after neoadjuvant chemoendocrine therapy in patients with operable breast carcinoma. *Cancer 85*:1996-2000,1999.

[159] Boudreau N, Myers C. Breast cancer-induced angiogenesis: multiple mechanisms and the role of the microenvironment. *Breast Cancer Res 5*:140-146,2003.

[160] Teicher BA. *Potentiation of cytotoxic cancer therapies by antiangiogenic agents.* In: Teicher BA (ed.) Antiangiogenic agents in cancer therapy, Humana Press Inc., Totowa NJ pp.277-316,1999.

In: Trends in Angiogenesis Research
Editor: Roberta V. Zubar, pp. 211-242

ISBN 1-59454-452-2

Chapter IX

Involvement of Erythropoietin in Angiogenesis of Normal and Malignant Tissues of Female Reproductive Organs

*Yoshiko Yasuda**
Department of Anatomy, Division 1, Kinki University School of Medicine, Osaka, Japan

Abstract

There is increasing evidence that the glycoprotein erythropoietin plays a role other than in erythropoiesis. We have found that erythropoietin and its receptor are expressed in human malignancies and that the signaling promotes not only tumorigenesis but also angiogenesis. In this chapter, the following four items are described to analyze the role of erythropoietin in normal and malignant ovarian and uterine tissues with special reference to the vascular formation.

1. Role of erythropoietin in normal uterine and ovarian tissues. In the normal ovarian and uterine endometrial tissues erythropoietin responsive sites are detectable in cells undergoing cyclic changes and capillary endothelial cells, which also expressed the estrogen receptor α. The components of the uterine and ovarian tissues differed in vascular density, implicating the involvement of angiogenesis in the characteristic cyclic changes of the reproductive organs.

2. Blockade of the erythropoietin signal destroys the vascularities in ovarian and uterine cancers in vitro. Injection of antibody to erythropoietin or soluble erythropoietin receptor that is an extracellular domain of the receptor, capable of binding to its ligand decreased significantly the number of living tumor cells and the capillary endothelial cells leading to destruction of the tumor masses.

3. Deprivation of the erythropoietin signal destroys xenografts of ovarian and uterine cancers in nude mice. Blocks of resected malignant ovarian and uterine cancer tissues were transplanted into nude mice. After the transplanted tumor grew larger, three or

* Correspondence concerning this article should be addressed to Dr. Yoshiko Yasuda, Department of Anatomy, Division 1, Kinki University School of Medicine, Osakasayama, Osaka, 589-8511, Japan. Tel : 81-72-366-0221; Fax : 81-72-366-0206; E-mail : y1126yas@med.kindai.ac.jp.

more, than initial growth, antibody to erythropoietin or soluble erythropoietin receptor were injected locally. Some xenografts died, and others showed severe necrotic regions in which margins, tremendous recruitment of macrophages, neutrophil leucocytes, and fibroblasts were detected concomitant with fibrous tissues.
4. Endogenous soluble erythropoietin receptor destroys angiogenesis in xenografts of Hela cell line. The Hela cell line transfected with cDNA of soluble erythropoietin receptor was transplanted into nude mice and allowed to grow to see the effects of endogenous sEpoR on tumorigenesis. Xenografts from transfected-cell line showed larger dead areas and less vascularity than those of the non-transfected cell line. The results of this study implies that an erythropoietin signal is involved in the survival and angiogenesis of the original tumor, uterine adenocarcinoma, in vivo. In conclusion, erythropoietin signal transduction operates in normal and malignant female reproductive organs to regulate angiogenesis to perform its physiological functions, especially in normal cyclic changes, and in malignancies to stimulate tumor growth and angiogenesis.

Color graphics are presented at the end of the chapter.

Key words: ovary, uterus, erythropoietin signal, functions

Introduction

Erythropoietin (Epo) is a secreting glycoprotein involved in red blood cell production, erythropoiesis. By preventing Epo-responsive erythroid precursor cells from apoptotic death, Epo stimulates their proliferation and differentiation [1,2,3]. In the fetus, Epo is produced in the liver and contributes to the fetal erythropoiesis, primitive and definitive erythropoiesis. In the adult, Epo is primarily produced in the kidney and kidney-derived Epo is responsible for stimulation of adult erythropoiesis [1,2]; Epo binds to its receptor (EpoR) on erythroid precursor cells and induces the receptor homodimerization, following autophosphorylation of tyrosine residues in JAK2 that associate with the intracellular domain of EpoR [3,4]. Phosphorylation of JAK2 activates JAK2, and the activated JAK2 then phosphorylates itself, the receptor, and cellular substrates recruited to the receptor complex. One of the substrates, phosphorylation of a transcriptional factor STAT5 is thought to be responsible for the mitosis of erythroid precursor cells.

EpoR is expressed in endothelial cells and Epo exhibits angiogenic activity on these cells in vitro [5,6,7,8,9]. Epo signaling in endothelial cells is conducted via tyrosine phosphorylation of proteins including phosphorylation of transcriptional factor STAT5, which is similar to that in erythroid cells [9]. However, it has been unclear whether endothelial EpoR is physiologically functional or is only a remnant reflecting a common developmental origin between endothelial cells and hematopoietic cells [10]. We have shown that Epo takes part in cyclical angiogenesis in an estradiol-17β (E_2)- dependent manner in the uterine endometrium. Thus far EpoR expressed in the capillary endothelium, has functional activity at least in the uterine endometrium.

Recently there is increasing evidence that non-hematopoietic sites produce Epo and express EpoR. Non-hematopoietic Epo production sites are brain [11,12,13,14,15], uterus [16], placental trophoblasts [17], embryos including the developing nervous system [18,19], yolk sac [20], spleen and lungs [21], ovaries [22], epididymis [23], macrophages [24,25] early colony-forming cells [26], embryonal stem cells and embryonal carcinoma cells [27]. While EpoR expression sites include Leydig cells [28], fetal liver stromal cells [29], embryonal stem cells [30], various sites in the embryo including the developing nervous system [18, 19, 31], placental trophoblast cells [32] vascular smooth muscle cells [33] and epididymis [23]. The physiological significance of these Epo production and EpoR expression sites in normal organ or tissues remains unknown except for two sites, brain and uterus. In the brain, there is paracrine Epo-EpoR system [11,12,13,15,34]; neuron produce EpoR [35,36] and astrocytes produce Epo [34]. Epo is hypoxia inducible in the brain and protects neurons from ischemia [35,36] and death caused by neurotoxic substances [14]. In the uterus, Epo is estrogen-inducible but not hypoxia inducible; Epo mRNA is hypoxia inducible only in the presence of E_2 [16,37]. Moreover Epo takes part in angiogenesis through EpoR that is expressed in the endothelial cells of uterine endometrium [16]. These facts suggest that Epo-EpoR signaling plays a tissue-specific role. The various expression sites implicate tissue- specific functions as seen in the brain and uterus in our body.

Expression of Epo in malignant cerebellar hemangioma [38] and meningioma [39] has been reported to cause secondary polycytemia in the patients, but until the present, involvement of Epo in these malignancies has never been studied. There is increasing evidence that Epo is related to the growth of malignant tumors and in their angiogenesis.

In this chapter, I address the expression of Epo and EpoR mRNA in normal and malignant ovarian and uterine tissues. In normal tissues the Epo signal participates in cyclic cellular alteration or change that are characteristic phenomena in female reproductive organs. In malignant tumors, we clarified that the Epo signal promotes the tumor growth and their angiogenesis through deprivation of Epo signal via Epo antibody or soluble form of EpoR (sEpoR) in vitro and in vivo system. Moreover, the xenografts of the cell line derived from uterine adenocarcinoma, Hela, transfected with cDNA of sEpoR in nude mice were created, and the resultant xenografts were analyzed to confirm the role of Epo in the malignant tumors.

MATERIALS AND METHODS

Materials sampled: According to the guidelines of the Research Ethical Committee of Kinki University School of Medicine, the patients' informed consent was obtained for their specimens to be used in the experiments. We put the resected tissues into liquid nitrogen, in Zamboni solution for fixation or put into α-MEM (Gibco BRL, Gainsburg, MD) containing streptomycin (100 μl / ml) and penicillin (100 IU / ml) for organ culture. Until the beginning of the respective experiment, the samples were stored at –80 °C or 4 °C. The frozen materials were used for the extraction of total RNA and protein, and the fixed materials, for immunostaining.

Immunohistochemistry: After 5 hours of fixation in Zamboni solution, samples were processed for light microscopic immunohistochemistry. The methods have been described previously [18]. The following antibodies were used as primary antibodies: anti-EpoR (1 : 250; [18]), anti-FactorVIII (FVIII) (DAKO 1 : 200), anti-JAK2 (1 : 250, Upstate

Biotechnology, Lake Placid NY), anti-phosphotyrosine (PY) (1 : 500, Upstate Biotechnology), anti-STAT5 (1 : 25, Transduction) and anti-estrogen receptor α (1 : 20, Chemicon). With a standard procedure using ABC complex (Vector), we detected the color reaction with diaminobenzidine (Dojin, Wako, Osaka, Japan). No antigens for JAK2, STAT5 and EstRα were available, so normal rabbit IgG and mouse IgG were used. The expression of EpoR on the capillary endothelial cells was confirmed by double staining with anti-EpoR (1 : 10 Genzyme) and anti-FVIII. Furthermore, the signal transduction of Epo and EpoR was detected by double staining with anti-JAK2 and anti-phosphotyrosine antibodies or with anti-EpoR and anti-STAT5 antibodies in the same cryosections on the glass slide incubated with either a mixture of rabbit antiserum against JAK2 (1 : 2000) and mouse IgG against PY (1 μg / ml) or a mixture of anti-EpoR (1:2000) and mouse IgG against STAT5 (1 μg / ml). After 8 to 12 hours at room temperature, the slides were washed twice with PBS containing 1 % Triton X-100, covered with biotinylated anti-mouse IgG (10 μg / ml) for 1 hour at room temperature, washed twice and then incubated with Texas Red Avidin D (5 μg / ml; Vector), FITC-labeled goat antibody against rabbit IgG (10 μg / ml) and 10 % normal rabbit serum for 6 hours.

Immunoblot: Samples were lysed in 500 μl lysis buffer (60 mM Tris-HCl, pH 6.8, 1 mM sodium vanadate, 10 % glycerol, 1 % Triton X-100) containing a Protease Inhibitor Cocktail (Roche Diagnosis). The insoluble materials were discarded by centrifugation. The lysates, 50 μg protein / 10μl, were electrophoresed in SDS-10 % polyacrylamide gels (PAGEL, Atto), and western blotting analysis was performed with each antibody. Signals were detected with an enhanced chemiluminescence detection system (Amersham).

RT-PCR: Total RNA was prepared with total RNA isolation kit (Trizol, Gibco BRL). cDNA was synthesized from 1 μg of the total RNA with 5 units of an avian myeloblastosis virus (AMV) reverse transcriptase, random nanomer primer and 3 μg of each RNA in a volume of 20μl with the use of a Takara RNA LAPCR^{TM} kit (AMV) Ver. 1·1. PCR primer for Epo, EpoR [20] and β-actin [34] were described previously. PCR cycles and conditions for denaturation, annealing, and elongation were 38 cycles, 30 sec at 94 °C, 30 sec at 65 °C and 30 sec at 72 °C of Epo; 38 cycles, 30 sec at 94 °C, 30 sec at 60 °C and 30 sec at 72 °C of EpoR and β-actin. The amplified DNA was fractioned by electrophoresis and stained with ethidium bromide.

The contents of Epo mRNA in xenografts of cell lines with or without transfection of cDNA of sEpoR, were compared by measuring Epo mRNA expression by real-time quantitative PCR with an ABI PRISM 7700 sequence detection system (Applied Biosystems). All PCR reactions were performed with the Quantitative PCR Supermix-UDG (Invitrogen) in a final volume of 25 μl, Epo and 18S rRNA primers and probes were supplied by Applied Biosystems as Assays-on-Demand Gene Expression Products and Taq Man Ribosomal RNA Control Reagents. Ten-fold serially diluted plasmid solution containing Epo (10^6 – 10^1 copies / μl) and 18S rRNA (10^9 – 10^4 copies / μl) cDNA were used to construct standard curves. The thermal cycling conditions were composed of an initial denaturation step at 50 °C for 2 minutes and at 95 °C for 10 minutes followed by 40 cycles consisting of denaturation for 15 seconds at 95 °C and hybridization and extension for 1 minute at 60 °C.

Southern hybridization: Ten μl of each PCR products was loaded on 1 % agarose gel electrophoresis and transferred to Hybond-N filter (Amersham). Hybridization was performed with a ^{32}P labeled 440 bp fragment of human Epo cDNA used as a probe. Human cDNA probe was prepared by PCR, sense (HEP351F, 5'-CTGAACACTGCAGCTTGAAT-3') and antisense (HEP790R, 5'TGGATAGCCCAGGTGGACA-3') as primers, and human Epo cDNA [40] as a template. A multiprime DNA labeling system for preparation of the probe and Hybond N for blotting were used according to the instructions of the manufacturer (Amersham). The temperature for hybridization was 60 °C, and the final washing of the filter was done with 0.1 × SSC at 60 °C.

Organ culture: The samples of resected tissues were observed under a dissecting microscope, removed the damaged part, and cut into a 5 × 5 × 7 mm block with a razor blade. Each block put into a petri dish (Falcon 3002) and weighed. Into several parts of a block, various concentrations of one of the following solutions was injected with a 32 gauge needle and a microsyringe (Hamilton, Reno): 16 or 8 mg / ml of antibody to Epo (R2), 0.4, 0.2 or 0.08 mg of soluble EpoR (sEpoR), 0.4 mg / ml of denatured sEpoR, 8 mg / ml of monoclonal antibody, mouse serum or saline. The petri dish was covered and incubated at 37 °C with 5 % CO_2 in air for the first 90 minutes. The second injection was done without removal of the former solution released from the block, and incubation was continued for 60 minutes under the same conditions. The process was repeated 2-4 times, and the block was removed from the petri dish, put on a metal grid (Falcon, 3014) in a well filled with α-MEM and 10 % FCS (Gibco BRL) in a multiwell dish (Falcon 3047) and incubated for 8.5 hours or longer. The overall time from the beginning of the first injection to the end of the culture on a raft was planned within 12 hours. Then the blocks were examined under a dissecting microscope and fixed in Zamboni solution.

Injection materials: Monoclonal mouse antibody to Epo (R2), a gift from the Snow Brand Milk Product CO. (Tokyo, Japan) was dissolved in saline (Ohtsuka, Tokyo, Japan). sEpoR was prepared by the method of Nagao et al. [41] and diluted with saline. sEpoR denatured by incubation at 56 °C for 1 hour, mouse monoclonal antibody against S-100 (Cosmo, Tokyo), mouse serum and saline were used as controls. To these injection materials, Evans blue dye (Merck, Darmstadt, Germany) was added to yield a final concentration of 0.025 % in each solution for coloring.

Transplantation: Hairless female mice (Balb/c, Jcl-nu) were purchased from Clea Inc. Japan, at 5 weeks of age, placed one by one in aseptic chambers and given sterilized pellets and water freely in a pathogen-free room. At 6 weeks of age or older, they were inoculated a piece of cancer specimen. For resected tumor specimens, blocks of the specimens, adenocarcinoma from uterus and ovary or cervical squamous cell carcinomas were cut into 5 × 5 × 5 mm and transplanted at the interscapular region subcutaneously. For Hela cell line, 2-4 × 10^6 cells per 0.1 ml of α-MEM medium were injected subcutaneously. The length and width of the implants were measured 3 times a week. Tumor growth was calculated according to the Battle Memorial Institute Protocol [42].

Transfection of cDNA for sEpoR: Hela cells maintained in α-MEM medium (Gibco BRL) supplemented with 10 % FCS were transfected with the expression vector for sEpoR (typically 0.67 μg for 3.5 cm dish) using LipofectAMINE plus (Life Technologies) according to the manufacturer's recommendations. After selection with 500 μg / ml G418 (Life Technologies) for 10-14 days, the resistant clones were isolated and expanded. The positive Hela cell line secreting sEpoR, epo-sepharose beads [41] were screened by adding them to the supernatant of each clone to immobilize sEpoR, incubated for 1 hr at room temperature, and washed 3 times with phosphate-buffered saline (PBS). Proteins were then eluted in loading buffer by boiling and subjected to 15 % SDS-PAGE, and processed for western blotting.

Construction of expression plasmid for a sEpoR: A cDNA coding for Ig_K signal sequence followed by 4 amino acids (A-R-V-V) after signal cleavage site was prepared synthetically with *Nhe*I site introduced at the 5' end (fragment 1). A cDNA encoding most of the extracellular region of human EpoR with *Bgl*II site introduced at the 3' end was amplified by the PCR (fragment 2). A DNA fragment coding for Histidine-tag $(His)_6$ was generated by digestion of pQE60 (Qiagen) with *Bgl*II and *Hind*III (fragment 3). These fragments were cloned in tandem into the *Nhe*I and *Hind*III site of pcDNA3.1(–) (Invitrogen). The resulting plasmid produces a soluble (secreted) form of EpoR (amino acids 3 to 226) with five additional amino acids A-R-V-V-A at the N-terminus and R-3-$(H)_6$ at the C-terminus.

Viability assay: The percent ratio of surviving areas of the xenograft transfected or not was determined using formazan, 2, 3, 5- triphenyl tetrazolium chloride (TTC, Wako Chemicals), was used. In this assay the viability of cells is based on the mitochondrial dehydrogenase activity, the development of red colour in response to the viable cells [43]. After removing from nude mice, the xenograft was cut into slices 1 mm in thickness on a mouse brain slicer (MBS-01, Aster Indust). The slices were incubated in 2 % TTC in 0.1 mM PBS at 37 °C for 10 minutes in darkness, and then fixed in 10 % formalin for 5 minutes to stabilize the red colour. In the coloured slices, red and white areas were determined.

Capillary counting: Sections of all specimens were stained with anti- FVIII antiserum. Cross- and longitudinally- sectioned capillaries were counted in 100 areas (2.85×10 mm^2) in each specimen with an eye-piece ocular micrometer or in 40 of the definite area (2.3×10^{-3} mm^2) with an image analyzer.

Results and Discussion

Role of Erythropoietin in Normal Uterine and Ovarian Tissues

In the mouse uterine endometrium Epo is expressed in an estrogen-dependent manner and involved in the angiogenesis [16]. The occurrence of similar phenomena in the human reproductive organs was confirmed by examining the expression of Epo signaling, identification of Epo responsive sites, co-existence of EpoR and estrogen receptor α (EstRα) and the vascular density in the uterus and ovary. This section shows that female reproductive organs can produce Epo, that EpoR expression sites are distributed in various tissue components and that the EpoR co-exists with EstRα. Vascular density was highest in the secreting phase of endometrium and in the theca interna of the ovary. Signal transduction of Epo appears to contribute to the cyclic changes and cellular differentiation through angiogenesis concomitant with estrogen.

Expression of Epo mRNA

Eight resected normal specimens, three cervical, two endometrial and three ovarian tissues, were examined with RT-PCR for the expression of Epo mRNA. Figure 1 shows the results of Southern analysis of the RT-PCR products. Epo mRNA was detectable in two cervical (NC-44), one endometrial (NC-39) and two ovarian (NO-34, and NO-46) tissues. Hep3B is a human hepatoma cell line that produces Epo in a hypoxia-inducible manner [44]. Epo mRNA was clearly detected in Hep3B cultured in 21 % oxygen and its level was elevated when the cells were cultured in 2 % oxygen.

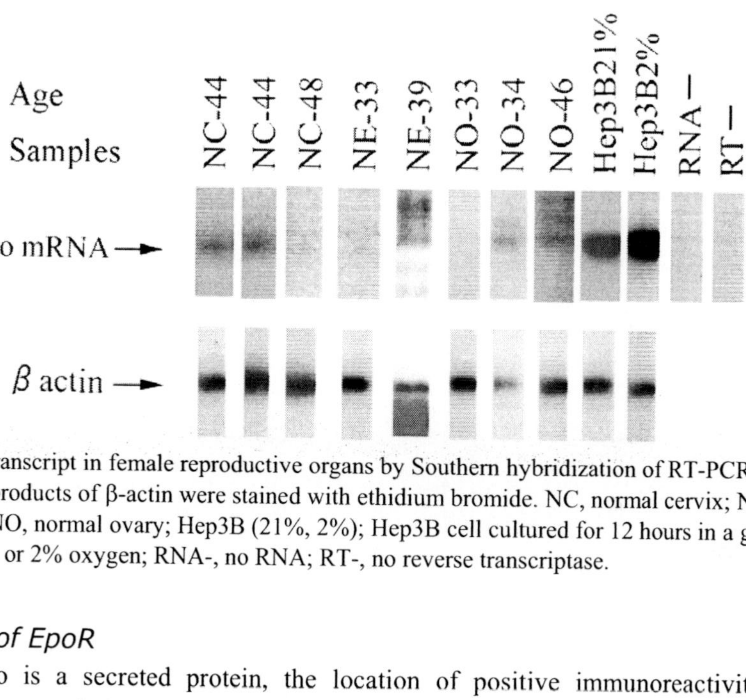

Figure 1. Epo transcript in female reproductive organs by Southern hybridization of RT-PCR products. The amplified products of β-actin were stained with ethidium bromide. NC, normal cervix; NE, normal endometrium; NO, normal ovary; Hep3B (21%, 2%); Hep3B cell cultured for 12 hours in a gas mixture containing 21% or 2% oxygen; RNA-, no RNA; RT-, no reverse transcriptase.

Expression of EpoR

Since Epo is a secreted protein, the location of positive immunoreactivity to Epo antibody does not strictly reflect the production sites of Epo. EpoR exists on the surface of the cell so that the sites of positive EpoR are more reliable to demonstrate the Epo-reactive sites. Immunoreactive EpoR was detectable both in the cytoplasm including cell surface and sometimes only in the cell surface clearly. For immunohistochemical examinations, 14 cervical, 10 endometrial, proliferative and secretory phases, and three decidual and six ovarian tissues were used. In the cervix, the surface epithelium showed positive immunoreactivity to the EpoR antibody. In the uterine endometrium, additionally glandular epithelium, decidual cells and fibroblasts showed positive EpoR reactivity (Figure 2A). The staining specificity of the EpoR was confirmed in the section of endometrium (Figure 2B). In the ovary, most cellular components, oocytes, follicular cells and theca cells showed EpoR immunoreactivity (Figure 2C). Moreover, endothelial cells of capillaries (Figure 2A), arterioles and venules reacted positively to the EpoR antibody. The expression sites of these tissues are summarized in Table 1. These EpoR expression sites expressed also EstRα protein as shown in Figure 2D, where granulosa cells and cells of the theca interna showed a characteristic distribution pattern of EstRα with many capillaries in the theca interna (Figure 2D). The co-expression of EpoR and EstRα was confirmed in the same section of ovarian tissue showing positive immunoreactivity to the EpoR and EstRα antibody (Figure 2E, F). In Table 1, co-expression sites of EpoR and EstRα in the tissues are summarized. In Figure 3, EpoR and EstRα were detected in the lysates from normal endometrial and ovarian tissues by the western blotting.

Table 1. Co- expression of erythropoietin receptor and estrogen receptor α in human female reproductive organs

Regions	Expression sites	
	Tissue components	Blood vessels
Uterine cervix	• stratified epithelial cells[a]	• capillary endothelium
Uterine endometrium	• surface and glandular epithelial cells • decidual cells • fibroblasts	• capillary endothelium
Ovary	• mesothelium • oocytes • follicular cells • granulosa cells • theca interna cells • theca lutein cells • granulosa lutein cells • fibroblasts in corpus albicans	• capillary endothelium • arteriole endothelium • venule endothelium

[a] Co-localization is detected in lower half of the epithelium

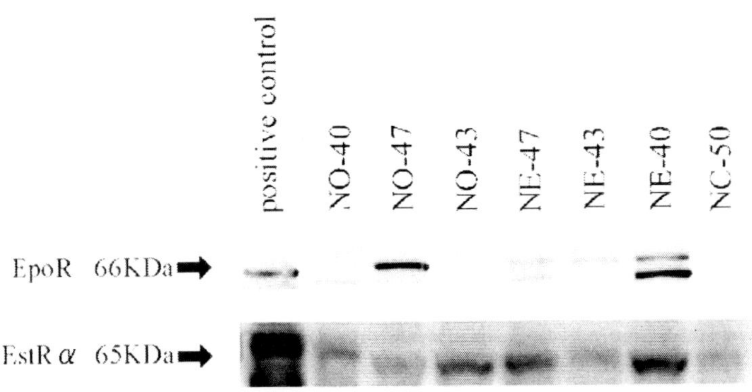

Figure 3. Western blotting of EpoR and EstRα proteins in the human uterus and ovary. NO, normal ovary; NE, normal endometrium; NC, normal cervix. Number after abbreviation shows age of patient. Positive control for EpoR using cell lysate of UT-7, and for EstRα, lysate of mouse ovary.

Demonstration of Tyrosine Phosphorylation

The expression of Epo mRNA and EpoR protein in the female reproductive organs indicate the existence of Epo signal transduction, which proceeds through tyrosine phosphorylation of JAK2 associated with the intracellular domain of EpoR [3,4]. In the hyperplastic endometrium, glandular epithelial cells, decidual cells and endothelium expressed both JAK2 and PY (data not shown). In the ovarium, follicular cells of the developing follicles showed immunoreactive EpoR, EstRα, JAK2 and PY, and the co-expression of EpoR and EstRα (Figure 2E, F), and JAK2 and PY (Figure 2G, F) were detected. The staining specificity was detected by confirming the absence of stainability in the sections incubated with rabbit serum for JAK2 antibody, and with supernatant preabsorbed with PY antigen, 4OH phenylalanine 4-phosphate (data not shown). JAK2 and PY was co-expressed in the cells positively stained for EpoR in the uterine endometrium and in the ovaries.

Demonstration of STAT5 in EpoR-expressing Sites

STAT5 is a transcriptional factor that is considered to be one of the mitogenic substrates in Epo-responsive cells. The surface and glandular epithelial cells of the decidua at the 7th week pregnancy showed positive EpoR (Figure 2I) and positive STAT5 (Figure 2J) reactivity. No immunoreactivity was discernible in adjacent sections treated with mouse IgG (data not shown). EpoR and STAT5 was co-expressed in the uterine endometrium and in the ovaries. These reactive sites corresponded to the regions expressing JAK2 and PY. To confirm the Epo signaling, Epo antagonist, sEpoR, was injected into a piece of resected samples four times in organ culture and then processed for immunostaining with anti-STAT5 and anti-PY antibody. Figure 4 shows that glandular epithelium with STAT5 (green fluorescence), PY (red fluorescence) and coalesce into a double fluorescent (overlay) in the control endometrium (Figure 4A) but not PY (middle) in the experimental block (Figure 4B). Moreover, capillary endothelium was confirmed in a section with double fluorescence of EpoR (green) and FVIII (red), and coalesce into a double fluorescent (overlay) (Figure 4C). In Figure 5, Western blotting of EpoR, JAK2, PY and STAT5 proteins showed the bands for these proteins in the same lysate from normal endometrial, cervical, and ovarian tissues. These findings indicate that Epo signal transduction exists in uterine and ovarian tissues, especially in cells undergoing cyclic changes or turn over and that angiogenesis appears to contribute to performing the cyclic changes concomitant with estrogen.

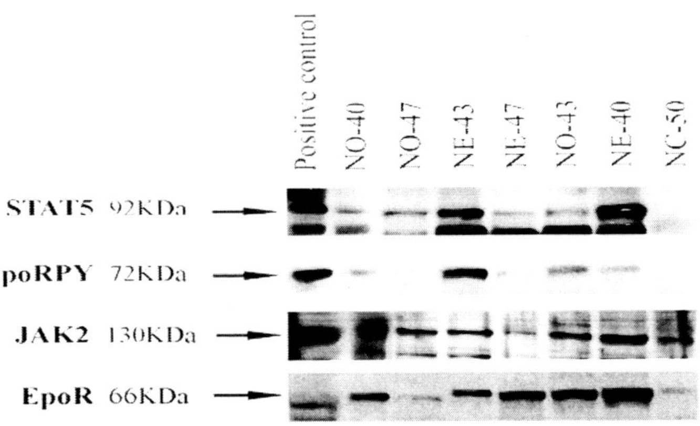

Figure 5. Western blotting of EpoR, JAK2, phosphotyrosine and STAT5 proteins in the human uterus and ovary. The lysates were from the same origin as those shown in Figure 3. Positive control for JAK2 and phosphotyrosine (PY) is cell lysates from EGF stimulated A431, and for STAT5, from human aortic endothelial cells.

Vascular Density in the Tissues

The average number of vessels in each region is shown in Figure 6. In sections of all specimens stained with anti-FVIII antibody, cross- and longitudinally- sectioned capillaries and endothelial cells of arterioles and venules were counted in 40 areas of $2.3 \times 10^{-3}mm^2$ under $10 \times$ magnification. The vascular density of the region of theca interna was highest of all regions. In the uterine endometrium, vascularity was significantly higher in the secretory phase than in the proliferative phase ($P<0.001$). The decidua showed less vascularity than the proliferative endometrium ($P<0.001$).

The plasma concentration of E_2 is peak just before the beginning of the secretory phase and gradually decreases the last half of the menstrual cycle but the level in still higher in the secretory phase than in the proliferative phase of endometrium. Theca interna cells and granulosa cells have a system to make E_2. In the former, E_2 is secreted into the circulation, and in the latter, into the follicular fluid. In the present study, vascular density was higher in the endometrium in the secretory phase than in the other two, proliferative phases or decidua, and that the highest vascularity was detectable in the theca interna of the ovary. Thus, the Epo signal appears to be involved in angiogenesis which is responsible for the normal physiology of the uterus and ovary in concomitant with E_2.

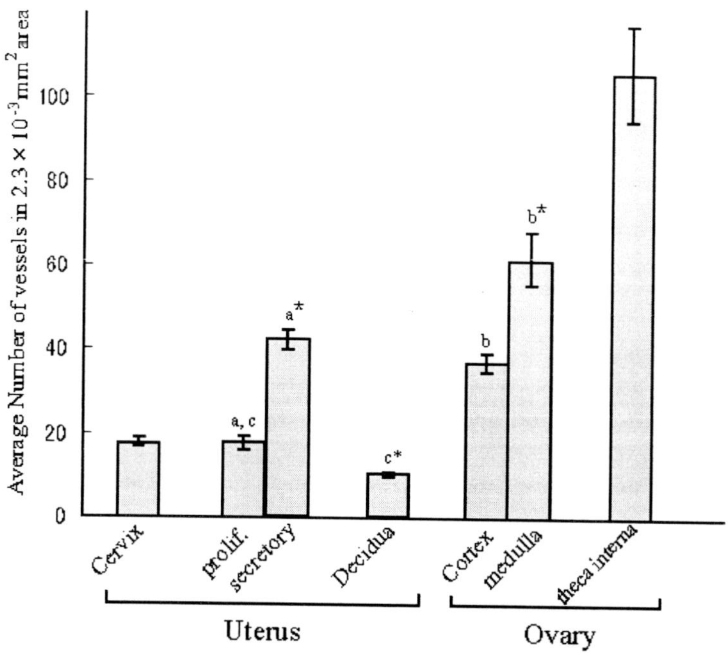

Figure 6. Average number of capillaries in a definite area in normal uterine and ovarian tissues. Cervix, uterine cervix; prolif, proliferative phase; secretory, secretory phase; Decidua, decidual tissue from 7th week of pregnancy; Cortex, cortical layer; medulla, medullary region; theca interna; theca interna cells of mature follicle. * Values with the same letter are significantly different by Student's t-test, $P<0.001$.

Blockade of Erythropoietin Signal Destroys the Vascularities in Ovarian and Uterine Cancers in Vitro

The widespread expression sites for Epo and EpoR in our body suggest that Epo signaling might be involved in the growth of tumors, but this possibility has not been studied adequately. mRNAs for Epo and EpoR are expressed in cervical squamous cell carcinoma (SCC), endometrial adenocarcinoma (ADCE), and ovarian adenocarcinoma (ADCO), and the extracts from these tissues contained more Epo protein than did those from respective normal controls. In these malignant tumors, tumor cells themselves and the capillary endothelial cells showed EpoR immunoreactivity. The dependency of the promotion of the tumor growth and angiogenesis on the Epo-EpoR pathway was clarified by blocking the signal by injection of antibody against Epo (R2) or soluble form of the EpoR (sEpoR) into blocks of resected tumor specimens, and cultured the blocks. Twelve hours after injection, these blocks were examined and compared with control blocks that were injected with saline, mouse serum or heat-denatured sEpoR. A marked decrease in capillaries and tumor cells was seen, and the reduction showed in a dose-dependent manner. Many cells showed apoptotic cell death. Moreover, co-existence of STAT5 and phospho-STAT5 (P-STAT5), which is involved in the mitogenic signaling of Epo, was detected in the control blocks, but not in the treated blocks. These results indicate that the proliferation and survival of both tumor cells and the capillary endothelial cells depend on Epo signaling in ovarian and uterine cancers.

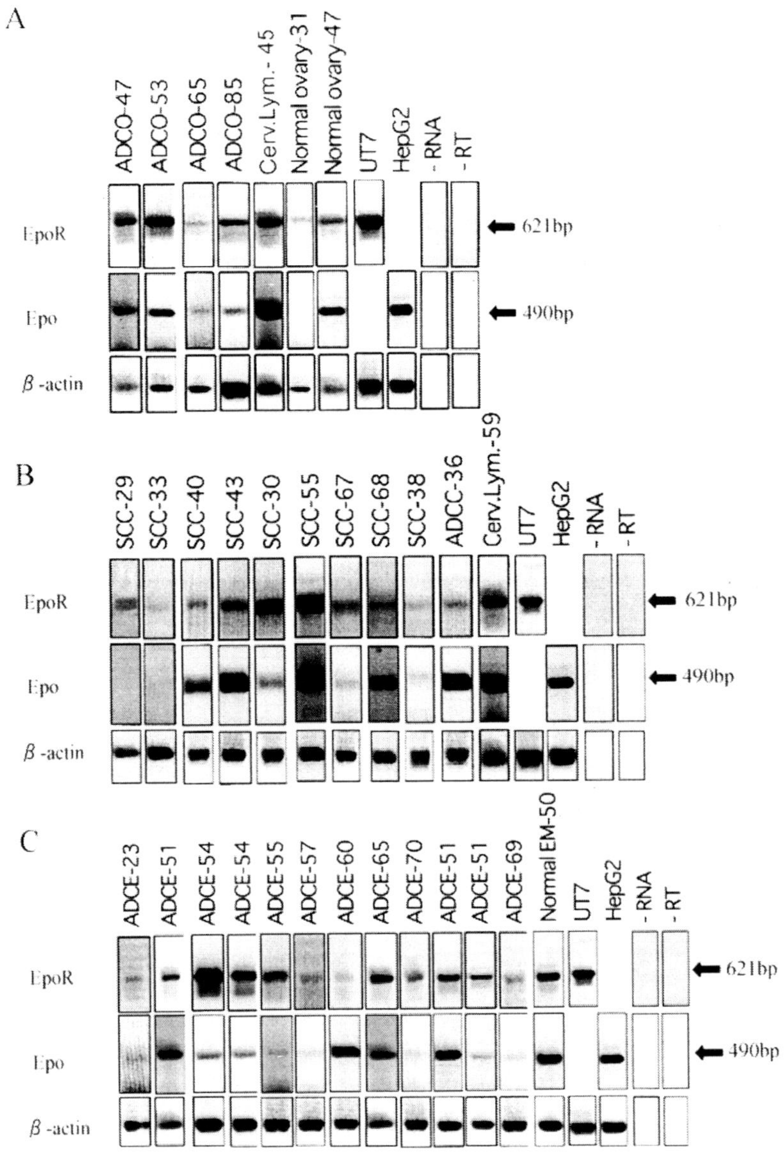

Figure 7. Expression of Epo and EpoR mRNA in malignant tumors of female reproductive organs. RT-PCR analysis of ADCO (A), SCC (B), ADCE (C), metastatic lymph nodes and control normal specimens shows mRNAs for Epo and EpoR and β-actin. RT-, no reverse transcriptase in RNA. RNA-, no RNA.

Expression of Epo and EpoR mRNA

Twenty eight tumor specimens, four ADCO, nine SCC, one ADCC, 12 ADCE, and two cervical metastatic lymph nodes and two normal ovarian, and one normal endometrial specimens were examined with RT-PCR for expression of Epo and EpoR mRNA. Figure 7 shows the results of ADCO (A), SCC (B) and ADCE (C). Ten tumor specimens and two metastatic lymph nodes showed high expression of both Epo and EpoR mRNA, and seven specimens (ADCO-65, SCC 33, SCC 38, ADCC 36, ADCE 23, ADCE 60, ADCE 69) showed weak expression of EpoR mRNA, and 10 specimens (SCC 29, SCC 33, SCC 67,

SCC 38, ADCE 23, ADCE 55, ADCE 57, ADCE 70, ADCE 51, ADCE 69) showed weak expression of Epo mRNA. UT-7, a human megakaryoblastic leukemia cell line was used as a control for EpoR mRNA [45] and HepG2, a hepatoma cell line as a control for Epo mRNA [44].

Content of Epo Protein

The content of Epo in the resected samples was determined by enzyme-linked immunoassay [46]. The average Epo protein was significantly higher in the malignant ovarian (67.75 ± 19.01; mean ± SEM, range 41.93 - 88.25) and uterine tumors (65.31 ± 19.14, 8.86 – 124.85) than in normal ovarian (28.13 ± 14.81, 6.4 – 39.09) and uterine tissues (19.14 ± 5.58, 7.01 – 30.65) ($P<0.05$, Table 2).

Table 2. Erythropoietin in extracts of ovarian and uterine cancers

Sample (number)	Epo (mU/ml) mean±SEM	Protein (mg/mg of tissue) mean±SEM	Epo (mU/g of tissue) mean±SEM
Adenocarcinoma ovary (4)	0.32 ± 0.11	0.75 ± 0.48	62.75 ± 19.01*
Normal ovary (3)	0.17 ± 0.06	0.36 ± 0.07	28.13 ± 14.81
Adenocarcinoma endometrium (5)	0.55 ± 0.15	0.65 ± 0.08	65.31 ± 19.14*
Normal endometrium (3)	0.13 ± 0.02	0.51 ± 0.11	19.14 ± 5.58
Squamous cell carcinoma cervix (4)	0.42 ± 0.19	0.55 ± 0.22	57.33 ± 28.30

*Significant difference from normal controls by Student's t-test ($P<0.05$).
(Modified and rearranged from Carcinogenesis 23: 1797-1805, 2002 with permission from Oxford University Press)

Epo-responsive Sites in Tumors

Sections stained with anti-EpoR antibody of all tumors, five ADCO, nine SCC and 12 ADCE, showed the EpoR immunoreactivity as shown in Figure 8, which shows the loci of EpoR in ADCO-55 (Figure 8A), ADCE-57 (Figure 8B) and SCC-63(Figure 8C). In these tumors, malignant cells and capillary endothelial cells reacted with the anti-EpoR antibody (Figure 8A, B and C). The staining specificity was confirmed in the adjacent sections to those shown in Figure 8A, B and C; no immunoreactivity was detectable in malignant cells and capillary endothelial cells (data not shown). Moreover, sections adjacent to that shown in Figure 8C, were stained with anti-FVIII antibody, demonstrating the capillary endothelium (Figure 8D). Figure 9 shows immunoblots of tumor tissue extracts from three SCC, two ACC, three ADCE and two ADCO. The bands for EpoR were clearly detected in all tissue lysates, indicating the presence of EpoR protein in these tumors.

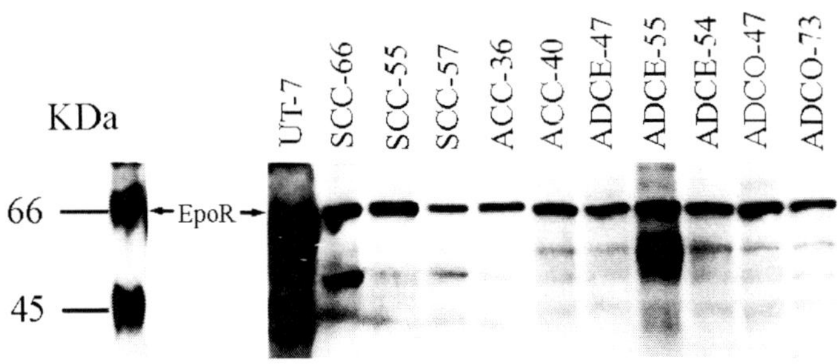

Figure 9. Western blotting of EpoR protein in malignant female reproductive tumors. SCC, squamous cell carcinoma cervix; ACC, adenocarcinoma cervix; ADCE, endometrial adenocarcinoma; ADCO, ovarian adenocarcinoma. Number after abbreviation is age of the patient. UT-7, control for EpoR protein from lysate of UT-7 cell line.

Alteration of Macroscopic Features in Tumor Blocks

Figure 10 shows one of the typical features of blocks intercepting Epo signaling. The block before injection had many capillaries and blood coagulation (Figure 10A). The saline – injected blocks retained blood vessels (Figure 10B,C and D). The block injected sEpoR once (Figure 10E) was less vascularized than the control block injected with saline (Figure 10B). There was less vascularization in the block injected with sEpoR three times (Figure 10F). Four injections resulted in pale blocks with only a few twigs of capillaries after 12 hours of injection (Figure 10G).

Alteration of Vascularization in Tumor Blocks

Figure 11 shows the histopathological characteristics, especially of vascularization of blocks of tumors in organ culture. Before culture blocks of ADCO-68 (Figure 11A, B) showed many vascular nets (Figure 11A) with canals (Figure 11B). After the injection with saline there still were many vascular nets (Figure 11C) with a rigid canal (Figure 11D) in blocks after 12 hours of injection. The treatment with 0.2 mg/ml of sEpoR destroyed the vascular nets (Figure 11E) with broken capillary walls (Figure 11F). A few apoptotic cells were seen in the control saline-injected blocks (Figure 11G), but many apoptotic nuclei were detectable in the blocks treated with sEpoR (Figure 11H) and that apoptotic death was also discerned in the nuclei of capillary endothelial cells (Figure 11H inset).

Change in Vascularization

In all experimental and control blocks, the number of cross- or longitudinally-sectioned capillaries was counted in a definite area and compared among the blocks. All experimental blocks had significantly fewer capillaries than the controls ($P<0.01$, $P<0.001$, Figure 12).

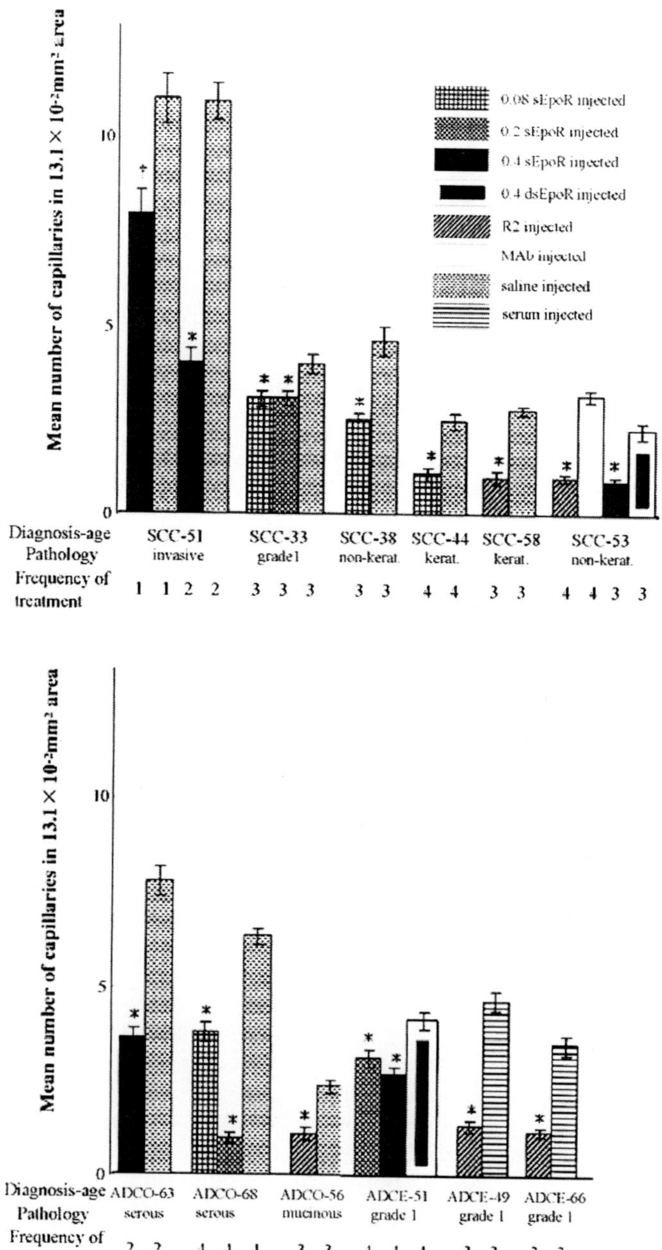

Figure 12. Average number of capillaries in a definite area in all experimental and control blocks treated in vitro. The positively stained cross- and longitudinally sectioned capillaries were counted in 100 areas ($13.1 \times 10^{-2}mm^2$) under 200- fold magnification in every third section. * Significant difference from controls by Student's t-test, † $P<0.01$, * $P<0.001$ (Modified and rearranged from Carcinogenesis 23: 1797-1805, 2002 with permission from Oxford University Press).

Abolishment of Tyrosine Phosphorylation

The expression of Epo and EpoR mRNA, the presence of EpoR and the effect of sEpoR on the tumors strongly indicate the operation of Epo signaling. The effect of injection of sEpoR or R2 on tyrosine phosphorylation in the tumor blocks was examined since Epo signal transduction proceeds through tyrosine phosphorylation of JAK2, EpoR and other substrates, including STAT5, by activated JAK2. Western blot analysis of 7 ADC and 3 SCC showed STAT5, PY and JAK2 proteins (Figure 13). In 5 ADC and 5 SCC, the loci of PY and JAK2 were detectable in tumor cells and capillary endothelial cells (data not shown). Next, the co-expression of PY and JAK2 was demonstrated by double staining with both antibodies (Figure 14A and B). The location of JAK2, PY, STAT5 and P-STAT5 was examined immunohistochemically in eight ADC and eight SCC. In all tumors, JAK2, PY (Figure 14A, B), STAT5 and P-STAT5 were present in tumor cells and capillary endothelial cells; all substances were detectable in the cytoplasm of the responsive cells, STAT5 and P-STAT5 were additionally detectable in the nucleus (data not shown). In the sections from tumor blocks treated with sEpoR, STAT5 was detectable in the tumor cells (Figure 14C), but P-STAT5 was not frequently detectable in the nuclei (Figure 14D), while in the sections from tumor blocks treated with deN-sEpoR, both STAT5 and P-STAT5 were detectable (Figure 14E and F). Moreover, western blotting analysis of STAT5 immunoprecipitates revealed a weak tyrosine phosphorylation of STAT5 in the lysates from the blocks treated with sEpoR or R2 compared with the blocks injected saline, but the expression of STAT5 was comparable (Figure 15).

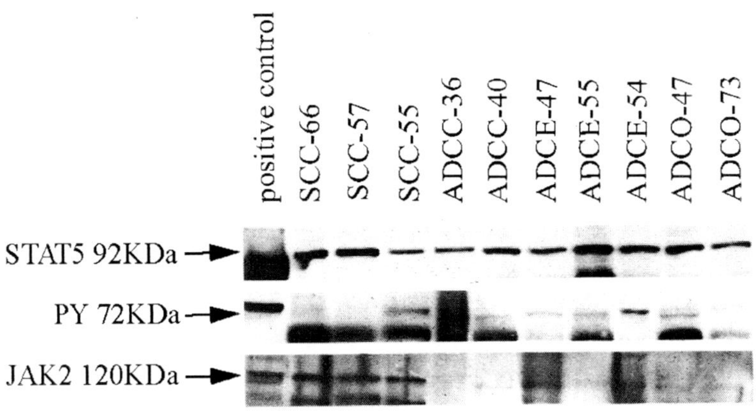

Figure 13. Western blotting of STAT5 phosphotyrosine and JAK2 in malignant female reproductive tumors. SCC, squamous cell carcinoma cervix; ADC, cervical adenocarcinoma; ADCO, ovarian adenocarcinoma number after the abbreviation means age of a patient.

The present study revealed that the malignant tumors of female reproductive organs express Epo and EpoR mRNA, the signaling pathway of which is stimulated to cause proliferation of the EpoR- expressing cells, tumor cells themselves and capillary endothelial cells. This is demonstrated by withdrawal of Epo signaling in tumors in vitro. Blockade of Epo-EpoR signal inhibited the survival of the tumor cells and the angiogenesis in tumor blocks through injection of R2 or sEpoR in vitro. The present in vitro methods are useful to see the direct effects of deprivation of Epo signal in tumor blocks on the vascular endothelial cells, but can not be used to see the effects on developing vascular nets, angiogenesis in the tumor in situ.

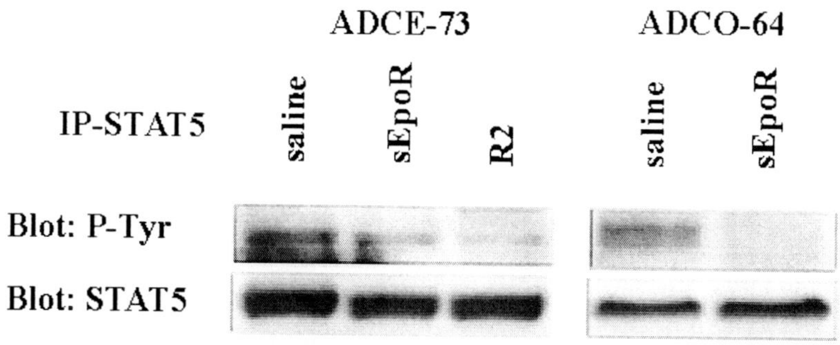

Figure 15. Tyrosine phosphorylation of STAT5 in tumor blocks treated in vitro. Cell lysates from two tumors (ADCE-73, ADCO-64) were immunoprecipitated with anti-STAT5. Western blotting with anti-phosphotyrosine shows weak or no band in lysates of tumor blocks treated with sEpoR and R2, but strong in the controls. (From Carcinogenesis 23: 1797-1805, 2002 with permission from Oxford University Press).

Deprivation of Erythropoietin Signal Destroys Xenografts of Ovarian and Uterine Cancers in Nude Mice

The previous experiments revealed that malignant tumors of female reproductive organs express the Epo and EpoR mRNAs and that the Epo signaling pathway is involved in the survival of tumor cells and their angiogenesis. Moreover, blockade of Epo signal in the resected tumor masses destroyed the tumor mass through the death of tumor cells and capillary endothelial cells in vitro. Then in this study, we explored whether deprivation of the Epo signal in the transplants of uterine and ovarian cancers induces similar phenomena in nude mice.

Thirty five transplants derived from 11 resected specimens of ovarian and uterine cancers were transplanted; a block, 5 × 5 × 5 mm was implanted one by one in the interscapular region of the nude mouse. When the tumors grew larger than three times or more their initial size, the antibody against Epo (R2) or soluble form of EpoR (sEpoR) was injected into the tumor 3 to 4 times at a 0.5 or 1- hour interval, and at 0.5 to 14 days after the injection the tumors were extirpated and examined. The tumor size was reduced to 60 to 11% of that before the injection in Epo-deprivated grafts. In contrast, the tumor size was comparable or larger than that in the control grafts.

Microscopic examinations of the experimental grafts revealed that tumor cells and the capillary endothelial cells were destroyed through their apoptotic death leading to destroyal of the grafts, while, control grafts with saline injections or needle insertion showed well-developed tumor masses as seen in control non-treated grafts. Angiogenesis was inhibited significantly in treated grafts with R2 or sEpoR in a dose-dependent manner. RT-PCR analysis of the non-treated grafts demonstrated the expression of Epo and EpoR mRNAs. Western blotting of the lysates from the grafts showed the band for EpoR protein in these transplants. These results indicate that Epo signal is involved in tumor growth and angiogenesis of the grafts in nude mice.

Expression of Epo and EpoR mRNA

Five extirpated grafts, three ADCE, one SCC and one ADCO were analyzed by RT-PCR for expression of Epo and EpoR mRNA. Figure 16A shows the results. Figure 16B shows that western blotting of EpoR in the lysates of each graft. These results indicate that Epo signaling exists through autocrine or paracrine route in the grafts of tumor masses of uterine and ovarian cancers.

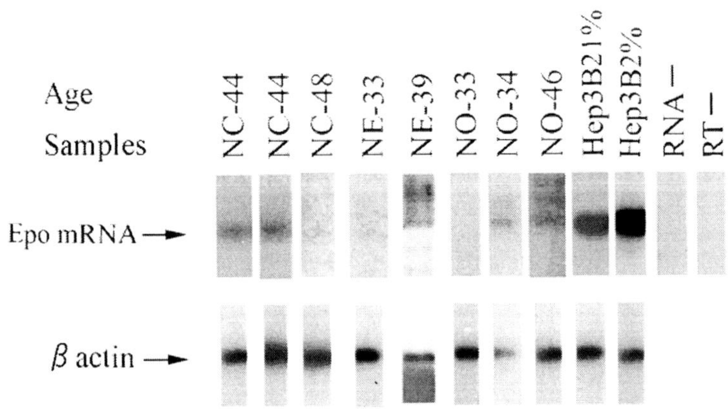

Figure 16. A. Expression of Epo and EpoR mRNA in grafts of ovarian and uterine cancer by RT-PCR analysis. ADCE, SCC, and ADCO, resected specimens of endometrial, squamous cell and ovarian cancers. The number after the abbreviation means age of a patient. RNA-: no RNA; RT-: no reverse transcriptase; UT-7: megakaryoblast cell line; HepG2; hepatoma cell line. β-actin, amplified product stained by ethidium bromide. (From Brit. J. Cancer 84: 844-850, 2001 with permission from © 2001 Cancer Research Campaign) B. Immunoblot for EpoR protein in lysates of grafts of ovarian and uterine cancer.

Tumor Growth and Treatment

Growth curves of all grafts were plotted from the beginning of the transplant till 160 to 195 days after the transplant. Most grafts grew 5 to 35 times larger than the initial size. After injection of R2 or sEpoR the degree of tumor regression was calculated from each growth curve as shown in Figure 20. The tumor size of all transplants was reduced after injection of R2 or sEpoR (Figure 20). However, the control tumors injected saline were 93 to 95 % of their original size or larger than before injection. Needle injection caused no regression. Of 16 tumors injected R2 or sEpoR locally, 2 mice showed scab formation as shown in Figure 17. The R2 injected graft enlarged and bled 7 days after of the injection and the covering skin was torn off to make a thick scab over the tumor (Figure 17).

Macroscopy of the Extirpated Xenografts

All 35 grafts, 16 tumors treated and 19 control tumors, were examined under a dissecting microscope. Typical effects of R2 (Figure 18A, B) or sEpoR (Figure 18D, E) on tumors are shown in Figure 18. Transplants at 14 days after the injection of 8 mg/ml of R2 (ADCO-78, Figure 20) had few fresh compact tumor masses and vascular twigs under the scab (Figure 18A) or a few masses (Figure 18B), while control saline injected transplant had a compact fresh tumor mass with vivid vessels (Figure 18C). Grafts at 7 days after injection of 0.2 mg/ml of sEpoR had pulverized tumor mass (Figure 18E) or few fresh tumor mass under the scab (Figure 18D), but the control grafts inserted only the needle had a vivid fresh tumor mass with vascular vessels (Figure 18C) or a pus-like material in the central region of the tumor (Figure 18F).

Microscopy of the Grafts

The sections of all grafts were immunostained with anti-EpoR, anti- FVIII and anti-mouse macrophage antibodies, and were adapted to TdT assay. Microscopic examinations of all these sections revealed that the grafts injected locally R2 or sEpoR had various destroyed foci as detected by macroscopic examinations, and the degree of the destruction correlated with the dose of R2 or sEpoR and that associated with disappearance of vasculature. Many macrophages and neutrophil leukocytes recruited to the degenerating foci containing many cells in apoptosis (data not shown). The distribution patterns of capillaries in the grafts are shown in Figure 19. The grafts injected 8 mg / ml of R2 showed the degenerative changes in tumor tissues and endothelial cells leaving amorphous masses with many dead or recruited neutrophil leukocytes (ADCE-64, Figure 19A), while the graft inserted only the needle at 7 days after transplant (ADCE-64) showed well-developed malignant tissues with abundant vasculature (Figure 19B). The grafts from ovarian cancer (ADCO-78) injected with 8 mg / ml of R2 showed large necrotic foci (Figure 19C) with or without fragmented capillaries (Figure 19D). The grafts from ovarian cancer (ADCO-78) injected with saline showed the characteristic features of adenocarcinoma (Figure 19E, F) with many small vessels (Figure 19F).

Effects on Vascularity in Grafts

In sections of all grafts stained with anti- FVIII antibody, cross- and longitudinally-sectioned capillaries were counted in 100 definite areas under 400 times magnification. The results are shown in Figure 20. The number of capillaries was comparable among the specimens before transplant and in the control grafts injected with saline or inserted only the needle (Figure 20) but, the number was significantly lower in the grafts injected R2 or sEpoR than that in controls ($P<0.001$).

Vascular formation in the grafts from human resected specimens consists of two origins, the original pre-existing vessels of the tumor tissues, vasculogenesis, and the newly-formed vessels from the host animal, angiogenesis. In the present experiment, withdrawal of Epo signaling in the grafts of ovarian and uterine cancers that expressed the Epo and EpoR mRNAs, by intra-tumor injection of R2 or sEpoR caused marked degeneration of the tumor cells and disappearance of capillaries. The present results suggested that deprivation of Epo signaling is effective to inhibit not only promotion of tumor growth but also vasculogenesis and angiogenesis of the grafts.

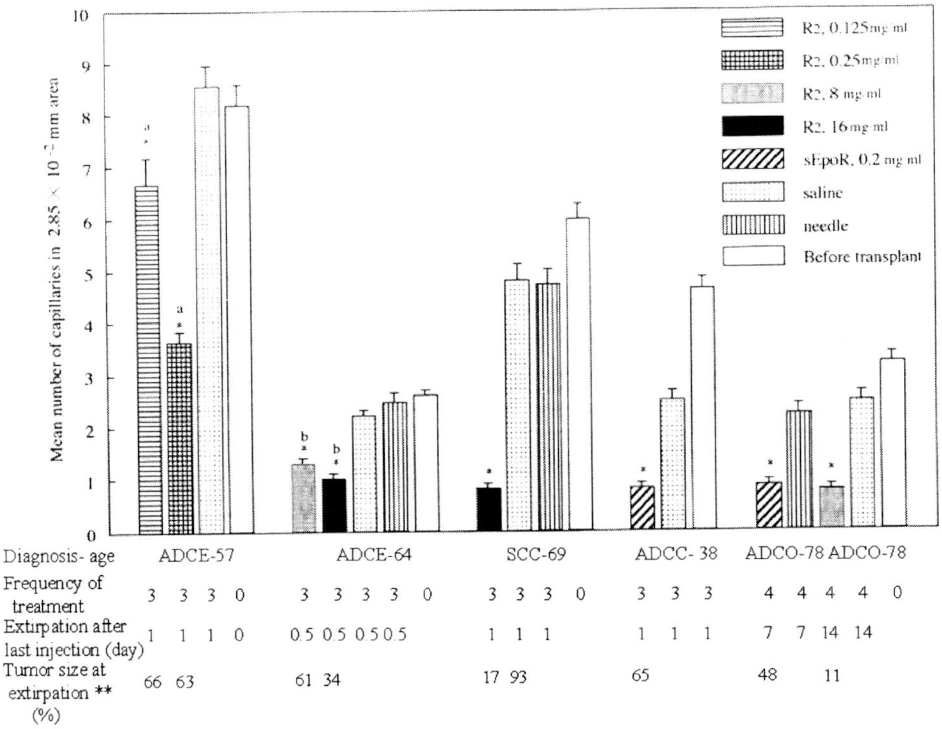

Figure 20. Average number of capillaries in a definite area of sections of xenografts and original tumors. Significant differences from controls by Student's t-test. * P<0.001. Columns with the same letter show significant differences (a, P<0.001; b, P<0.05) **, Tumor size was calculated relative to that just before the injection. (Modified data from Brit. J. Cancer 84: 844-850, 2001 with permission from © 2001 Cancer Research Campaign).

Endogenous Soluble Erythropoietin Receptor Destroys Angiogenesis in Xenografts of Hela Cell Line

The fact that withdrawal of Epo signaling through Epo antibody or soluble EpoR in the resected specimens in vitro and in the grafts of cancer specimens in mice caused marked degeneration of tumor cells and disappearance of capillaries promoted us to create such xenografts that can abolish the Epo signal endogenously. We transfected the cDNA of sEpoR into the cells of Hela cell line, and injected the transfected cells into nude mice at the interscapular region subcutaneously. Non-transfected cells were also transplanted similarly. Forty days after the injection, the xenografts were extirpated and examined: the xenografts of transfected-cells expressed significantly less Epo mRNA, showed less viable regions, and had fewer vascular nets than did those of xenografts of non-transfected cells. These results indicate that deprivation of Epo signaling interrupts the proliferation of tumor growth through induction of death of tumor cells and suppression of the angiogenesis from the host animal.

Expression of sEpoR Protein

The production of sEpoR protein was confirmed by western blotting of the lysates from the xenograft was performed. The band for sEpoR was detectable in the sEpoR-Hela, but not in the Hela (Figure 21A).

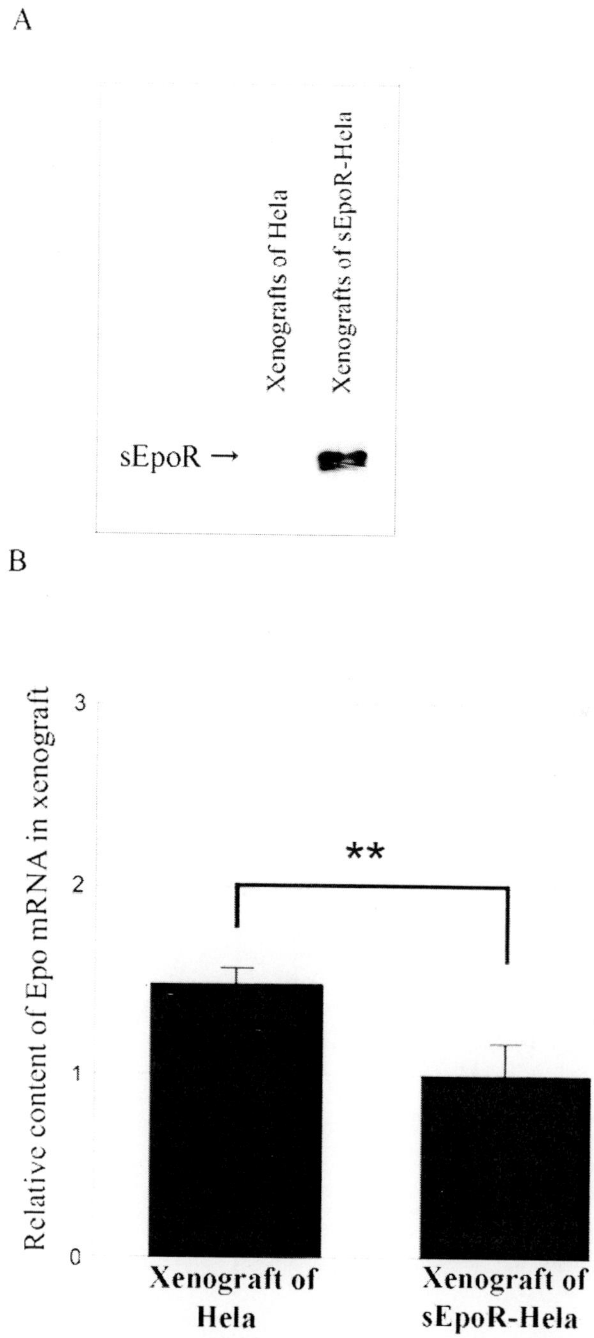

Figure 21. Western blotting of sEpoR protein in xenografts. A. sEpoR was detected in the lysates from xenografts of sEpoR-Hela, not from xenografts of Hela. B. Content of Epo mRNA in xenografts. Epo mRNA expression of xenografts of Hela cell line transfected with or without cDNA of sEpoR. The ordinate indicates the copies of Epo mRNA of xenografts. Bars represent means ± SEM (n = 9).

Expression of Epo mRNA

Epo mRNA in the xenografts of cells transfected (sEpoR-Hela), or not (Hela) was measured by the quantitative RT-PCR method. Figure 21B shows Epo mRNA content in the xenografts of sEpoR-Hela and of Hela, relative to the xenografts of sEpoR-Hela content that was defined as 1. Xenografts of Hela contained about 1.5 fold more Epo mRNA than that of sEpoR-Hela, and that the content showed significant difference (P<0.01; Figure 21B).

Macroscopy of the Xenografts

At 40 days after the cell transplantation, the tumors were detected externally and examined the tumor under the skin. The main vascular vessels were connected to the vessels from the host (Figure 22A, B). The extirpated tumors had well-developed vessels (Figure 22C, D). The tumor slices incubated with formazane, showed the red (alive) and white (dead) foci (Figure 22E, F). The slices from the xenograft of sEpoR-Hela showed larger white areas (Figure 22F) than those seen in slices from the xenograft of Hela (Figure 22E). The percent ratio of the dead and alive areas were determined in each slice of all xenografts (Figure 23). The xenograft of sEpoR-Hela showed significantly smaller viable areas (P<0.01) than those in the xenograft of Hela (Figure 23).

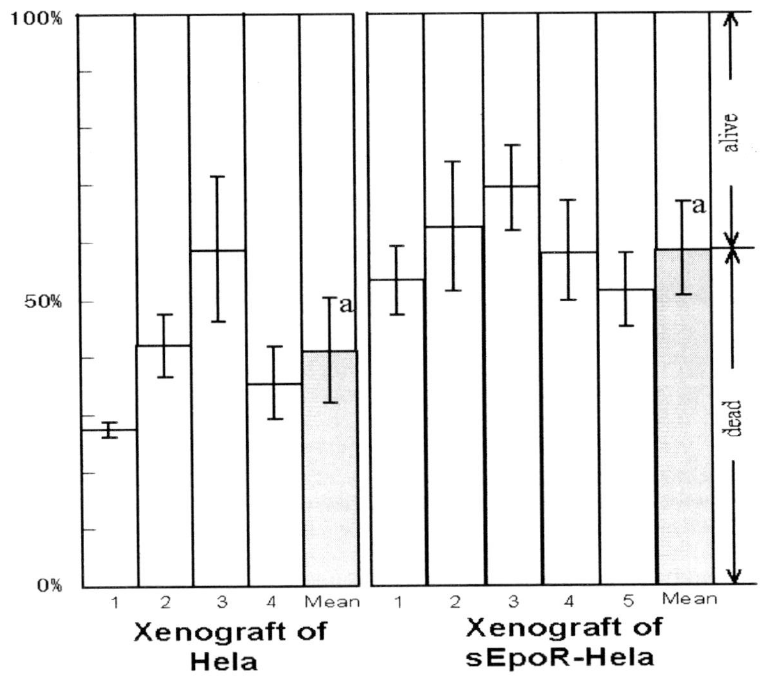

Figure 23. Destruction of xenografts of Hela cell line with or without transfection of the cDNA of sEpoR. Each column represents the mean of the viable and dead areas of a tumor. The most right column indicates the average of the all tumors. The same letter indicates significant difference between the columns by Student's t-test (p<0.01).

Microscopy of the Xenografts

All sections of xenografts with or without transfection were stained with anti- FVIII antibody, hematoxylin and eosin and processed for microscopic examinations. The tumor cells were connected with each other with endothelial linings that showed a positive reaction to anti- FVIII antibody, and fibrous tissues. The tumors consisted of a lobule-like structure containing tumor cells with thick fibrous tissues and blood vessels. In these tumors supporting fibrous tissues and blood cells are derived from the host animal. We confirmed this in the xenografts of the cells introduced green fluorescent protein (data not shown). In the xenograft of Hela, many endothelial layers and capillaries were detectable in the peripheral region of the lobule (Figure 24A, B) and they were decrease in number at the central necrotic region (Figure 24B). In the xenograft of sEpoR-Hela, a thin endothelial lining was seen in the peripheral region (Figure 24C) and a thin lining in the necrotic region (Figure 24D). Then, in sections stained with anti- FVIII antibody, the number of capillaries and endothelial layers was counted in 40 areas of a definite area in the peripheral, intermediate and central zones separately. The average numbers of capillary are summarized in Figure25. The peripheral zone of the tumor masses showed highest density among the other zones in both xenografts (Figure 25). The peripheral and the intermediate zones of the xenograft of sEpoR-Hela showed less vascularity than those of the xenografts of Hela ($P<0.01$, $P<0.05$ in Figure 25).

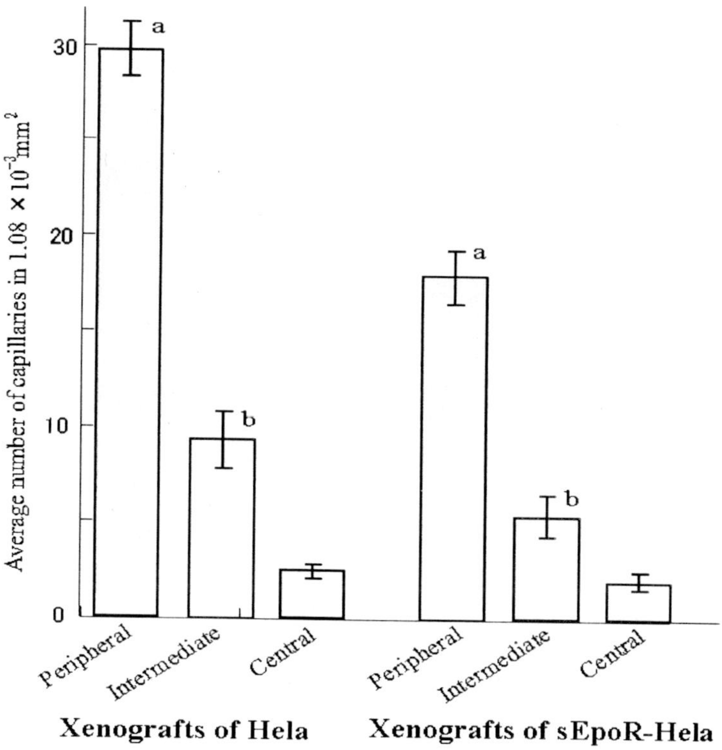

Figure 25. Average number of capillaries in a definite area of three zones, peripheral, intermediate and central. Bars, means ± SEM. The same letter means significant difference between the columns (a, $P<0.001$; b, $P<0.05$).

Thus endogenous sEpoR that is secreted from transplanted cells was effective not only to induce the cell death but also to suppress the angiogenesis from the host animal.

REFERENCES

[1] Kranz, S. B. (1991). Erythropoietin. *Blood, 77,* 419-434.

[2] Jelkmann, W. (1992). Erythropoietin: structure, control of production, and function. *Physiol. Rev, 72,* 449-489.

[3] Youssoufian, H., Longmore, G., Neumann, D., Yoshimura, A. & Lodish, H. F. (1993). Structure, function, and activation of the erythropoietin receptor. *Blood, 81,*2223-2236.

[4] Ihle, J. N. (1995). Cytokine receptor signaling. *Nature, 377,* 591-594.

[5] Anagnostou, A., Lee, E. S., Kessimian, N., Levinson, R. & Steiner, M. (1990). Erythropoietin has a mitogenic and positive chemotactic effect on endothelial cells. *Proc. Natl. Acad. Sci. USA, 87,* 5978-5982.

[6] Anagnostou, A., Liu, Z., Steiner, M., Chin, K., Lee, E. S., Kessimian, N. & Noguchi, C. T. (1994). Erythropoietin receptor mRNA expression in human endothelial cells. *Proc. Natl. Acad. Sci. USA, 91,* 3974-3978.

[7] Carlini, R. G., Reyes, A. A., & Rothstein, M. (1995). Recombinant human erythropoietin stimulates angiogenesis in vitro. *Kidney Int, 47,* 740-745.

[8] Yamaji, R., Okada, T., Moriya, M., Naito, M., Tsuruo, T., Miyatake, K. & Nakano, Y. (1996). Brain capillary endothelial cells express two forms of erythropoietin receptor mRNA. *Eur. J. Biochem., 239,* 494-500.

[9] Haller, H., Christel, C., Dannenberg, L., Thiele, P., Lindschau, C. & Luft, F. C. (1996). Signal transduction of erythropoietin in endothelial cells. *Kidney Int., 50*, 481-488.

[10] Bikfalvi, A. & Han, Z. C. (1994). Angiogenic factors are hematopoietic growth factors and vice versa. *Leukemia, 8*, 523-529.

[11] Masuda, S., Okano, M., Yamagishi, K., Nagao, M., Ueda, M. & Sasaki, R. (1993). Functional erythropoietin receptor of the cells with neural characteristics: Comparison with receptor properties of erythroid cells. *J. Biol. Chem, 268,* 11208-11216.

[12] Digicaylioglu, M., Bichet, S., Marti, H. H., Wenger, R. H., Rivas, L. A., Bauer, C. & Gassmann, M. (1995). Localization of specific erythropoietin binding sites in defined areas of the mouse brain. *Proc. Natl. Acad. Sci. USA, 92,* 3717-3720.

[13] Marti, H. H., Wenger, R. H., Rivas, L. A., Straumann, U., Digicaylioglu, M., Henn, V., Yonekawa, Y., Bauer, C. & Gassmann. (1996). Erythropoietin gene expression in human, monkey and murine brain. *Eur. J. Neurosi, 8,* 666-676.

[14] Morishita, E., Masuda, S., Nagao, M., Yasuda, Y. & Sasaki, R. (1997). Erythropoietin receptor is expressed in rat hippocampal and cerebral cortical neurons, and erythropoietin prevents in vitro glutamate-induced neuronal death. *Neuroscience, 76,* 105-116.

[15] Liu, C., Shen, K., Liu, Z. & Noguchi, C. T. (1997). Regulated human erythropoietin receptor expression in mouse brain. *J. Biol. Chem, 272*, 32395-32400.

[16] Yasuda, Y., Masuda, S., Chikuma, M., Inoue, K., Nagao, M. & Sasaki, R. (1998). Estrogen-dependent production of erythropoietin in uterus and its implication in uterine angiogenesis. *J. Biol. Chem, 273,* 25381-25387.

[17] Conrad, K. P., Benyo, D. F., Westerhausen-Larsen, A. & Miles, T. M. Expression of erythropoietin by the human placenta. *FASEB. J, 10*, 760-768.

[18] Yasuda, Y., Nagao, M., Okano, M., Masuda, S., Sasaki, R., Konishi, H. & Tanimura, T. (1993). Localization of erythropoietin and erythropoietin receptor in postimplantation mouse embryos. *Develop. Growth. Differ, 35*, 711-721.

[19] Juul, S .E., Li, Y., Anderson, D. K. & Christensen, R. D. (1998). Erythropoietin and erythropoietin receptor in the developing human central nervous system. *Pediatr. Res, 43,* 40-49.

[20] Yasuda, Y., Okano, M., Nagao, M., Masuda, S., Konishi, H., Ueda, K., Matsuo, T., Tsujiguchi, K., Tajima, S., Sasaki, R. & Tanimura, T. (1996). Erythropoietin in mouse avascular yolk sacs is increased by retinoic acid. *Dev. Dyn, 207,* 184-194.

[21] Fandrey, J. & Bunn, H. F. (1993). In vivo and in vitro regulation of erythropoietin mRNA: measurement by competitive polymerase chain reaction. *Blood, 81,* 617-623.

[22] Yasuda, Y., Musha, T., Tanaka, H., Fujita, Y., Fujita, H., Utsumi, H., Matsuo, T., Masuda, S., Nagao, M., Sasaki, R. & Nakamura, Y. (2001). Inhibition of erythropoietin signalling destroys xenografts of ovarian and uterine cancers in nude mice. *Brit. J. Cancer, 84,* 836-843.

[23] Kobayashi, T., Yanase, H., Iwanaga, T., Sasaki, R. & Nagao, M. (2002). Epididymis is a novel site of erythropoietin production in mouse reproductive organs. *Biochem. Biophys. Res. Commun, 296,* 145-151.

[24] Vogt, C., Pentz, S. & Rich, I. N. (1989). A role for the macrophage in normal hemopoiesis; III. In vivo and in vitro erythropoietin gene expression in macrophages detected by in situ hybridization. *Exp. Hematol, 17,* 391-397.

[25] Ohls, R. K., Li, Y., Trautman, M. S. & Christensen, R. D. (1994). Erythropoietin production by macrophages from preterm infants; implication regarding the cause of the anemia of prematurity. *Pediatr. Res, 35,* 169-170.

[26] Hermine, O., Beru, N., Pech, N. & Goldwasser, E. (1991). An autocrine role for erythropoietin in mouse hematopoietic cell differentiation. *Blood, 78,* 2253-2260.

[27] Kambe, T., Tada, J., Chikuma, M., Masuda, S., Nagao, M., Tsuchiya, T., Ratcliffe, P. J. & Sasaki, R. (1998). Embryonal carcinoma P19 cells produce erythropoietin constitutively but express lactate dehydrogenase in an oxygen-dependent manner. *Blood, 91,* 1185-1195.

[28] Minoni, R., Gottardello, F., Bordon, P., Montini, G. & Foresta, C. (1992). Evidence for specific binding and stimulatory effects of recombinant human erythropoietin on isolated adult rat Leydig cells. *Acta. Endocrinol, 127,* 459-465.

[29] Ohneda, O., Yanai, N. & Obinata, M. (1993). Erythropoietin as a mitogen for fetal liver stromal cells which supports erythropoiesis. *Exp. Cell. Res, 208,* 327-331.

[30] Heberlein, C., Fischer, K-D., Stoffel, M., Nowock, J., Ford, A., Tessmer, U. & Stocking, C. (1992). The gene for erythropoietin receptor is expressed in multipotential hematopoietic and embryonal stem cells: Evidence for differentiation stage-specific regulation. *Mol. Cell. Biol, 12,* 1815-1826.

[31] Liu, Z-Y., Chin, K. & Noguchi, C. T. (1994). Tissue specific expression of human erythropoietin receptor in transgenic mice. *Dev. Biol, 166,* 159-169.

[32] Benyo, D. F. & Conrad, K. P. (1999). Expression of the erythropoietin receptor by trophoblast cells in the human placenta. *Biol. Reprod, 60,* 861-870.

[33] Kusano, E., Akimoto, T., Inoue, M., Masunaga, Y., Umino, T., Ono, S., Ando, Y., Homma, S., Muto, S., Komatsu, N. & Asano, Y. (1999). Human recombinant erythropoietin inhibits interleukin-1β-stimulated nitric oxide and cyclic guanosine monophosphate production in cultured rat vascular smooth-muscle cells. *Nephrol. Dial. Transplant, 14,* 597-603.

[34] Masuda, S., Okano, M., Yamagishi, K., Nagao, M., Ueda, M. & Sasaki, R. (1994). A novel site of erythropoietin production: Oxygen-dependent production in cultured rat astrocytes. *J. Biol. Chem, 269,* 19488-19493.

[35] Sakanaka, M., Wen, T-C., Matsuda, S., Masuda, S., Morishita, E., Nagao, M. & Sasaki, R. (1998). In vivo evidence that erythropoietin protects neurons from ischemic damage. *Proc. Natl. Acad. Sci. USA, 95,* 4635-4640.

[36] Sadamoto, Y., Igase, K., Sakanaka, M., Sato, K., Otsuka, H., Sasaki, S., Masuda, S. & Sasaki, R. (1998). Erythropoietin prevents place navigation disability and cortical infarction in rats with permanent occlusion of the middle cerebral artery. *Biochem. Biophys. Res. Commun, 253,* 26-32.

[37] Chikuma, M., Masuda, S., Kobayashi, T., Nagao, M. & Sasaki, R. (2000). Tissue-specific regulation of erythropoietin production in the murine kidney, brain, and uterus. *Am. J. Physiol. Endocrinol. Metab, 279,* E1242-E1248.

[38] Trimble, M., Garo, J., Talalla, A. & Brain, M. (1991). Secondary erythrocytosis due to a cerebellar hemangioblastoma: demonstration of erythropoietin mRNA in the tumor. *Blood, 78,* 599-601.

[39] Bruneval, P., Sassy, C., Mayeux, P., Belair, M-F., Casadevall, N., Roux, F-X., Varet, B. & Lacombe, C. (1993). Erythropoietin synthesis by tumor cells in a case of meningioma associated with erythrocytosis. *Blood, 81,* 1593-1597.

[40] Matsumoto, S., Ikura, K., Ueda, M. & Sasaki, R. (1995). Characterization of a human glycoprotein (erythropoietin) production in cultured tobacco cells. *Plant. Mol. Biol, 27,* 1163-1172.

[41] Nagao, M., Masuda, S., Abe, S., Ueda, M. & Sasaki, R. (1992). Production and ligand-binding characteristics of the soluble form of murine erythropoietin receptor. *Biochem. Biophys. Res. Commun, 188,* 888-897.

[42] Ovejara, A. A., Houchens, D. P. & Barker, A. D. (1978). Chemotherapy of human tumor xenografts in genetically athymic mice. *Ann. Clin. Lab. Sci, 8,* 50-56.

[43] Ohba, N., Kiryu-Seo, S., Maeda, M., Muraoka, M., Ishii, M. & Kiyama, H. (2004). Transgenic mouse overexpressing the Akt reduced the volume of infarct area after middle cerebral artery occlusion. *Neurosci. Letter, 359,* 159-162.

[44] Goldberg, M. A., Glass, G. A., Cunningham, J. M. & Bunn, H. F. (1987). The regulated expression of erythropoietin by two human hepatoma cell lines. *Proc. Natl. Acad. Sci. USA, 84,* 7972-7976.

[45] Komatsu, N. & Fujita, H. (1993). Induced megakaryocytic maturation of the human leukemic cell line UT-7 results in down-modulation of erythropoietin receptor gene expression. *Cancer Res, 53,* 1156-1161.

[46] Okano, M., Ohneta, H. & Sasaki, R. (1992). Protein deficiency impairs erythropoiesis in rats by reducing serum erythropoietin concentration and the population size of erythroid precursor cells. *J. Nutr, 122,* 1376-1383.

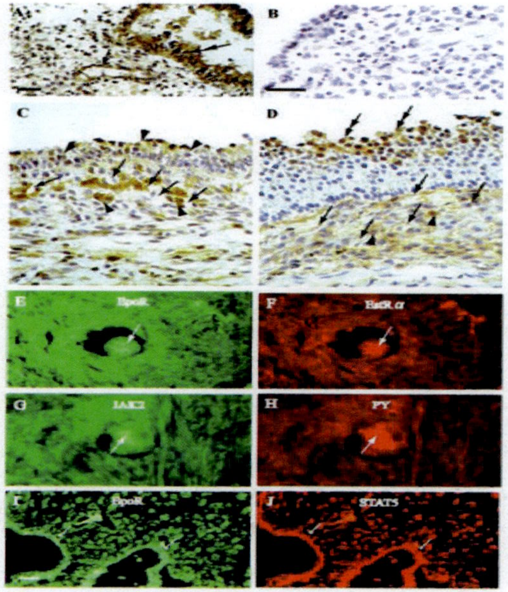

Figure 2. Detection of EpoR and co-expression of EpoR and EstRα, JAK2 and phosphotyrosine, and EpoR and STAT5 in uterus and ovary. (A) Section of endometrium in secretory phase of a 42-yr-old patient shows prominent immunoreaction to EpoR antibody in glandular epithelium (double arrows) and capillary endothelial cells (arrow). (B) Section incubated with supernatant preabsorbed with EpoR antigen. No immunoreactivity is detectable. (C) Section of a part of wall of mature follicle with granulosa cell layer and theca interna layer. Note many intervening capillaries (arrows) and strong EpoR positive cells (arrowheads). (D) Section of a similar region shown in C. Note many EstRα-positive granulosa cells (double arrows) and capillaries (arrows) in theca interna cells (arrowheads). (E, F) Section of ovarian cortex stained with anti-EpoR and EstRα antibody. Note co-expression of EpoR (E) and EstRα (F) in the follicular cells. (G, H) Section of the same specimen shown in (E, F) stained with anti-JAK2 antibody (G) and anti- phosphotyrosine (PY) (H). Note co-expression of JAK2 and PY in the follicular cells. (I, J) Section of decidua at 7th week of pregnancy stained with anti- EpoR (I) and anti- STAT5 (J) antibody. Note co-existence of EpoR (I) and STAT5 (J) in enlarged glandular epithelium (arrows). A, C and D, B, E, F, G and H, and I and J are at the same magnification. Bar = 50 μm.

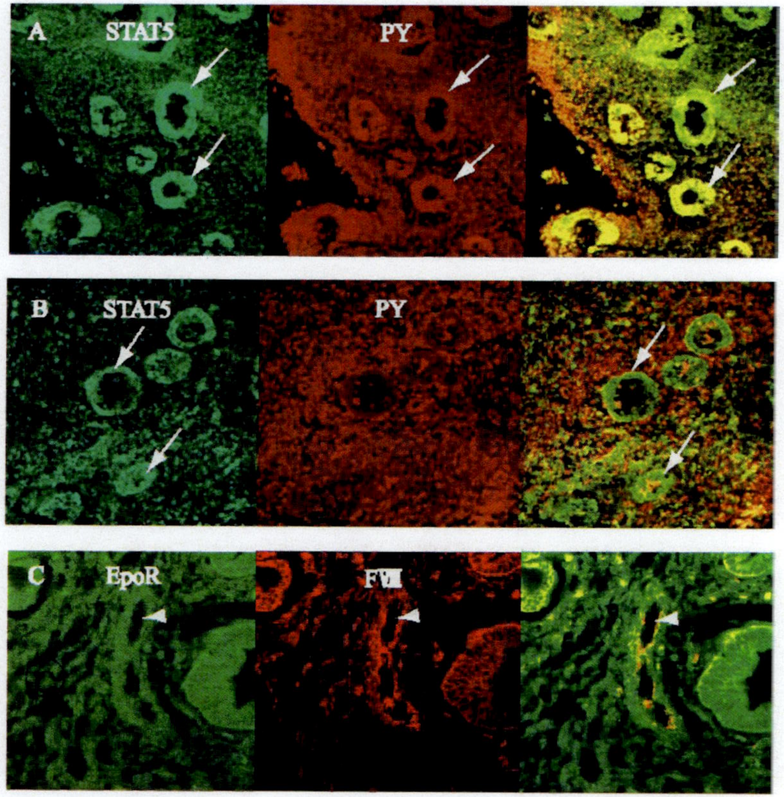

Figure 4. Confocal image of uterine endometrium. A. Shows positive immunoreactive sites of STAT5 (green), positively reacted to PY (red) and merge image of control sections. Arrows indicate glandular epithelium. B. Shows positive reaction to EpoR antibody in the glandular epithelium (green), no reactivity to PY antibody in the glandular epithelium (red) and merge image shows clearly detectable glandular epithelium only with STAT5 immunoreactivity. C. Shows positive reaction in glandular epithelium and endothelial cells to EpoR (green), positive reaction to FVIII anti- serum (red), and merge image to EpoR and FVIII antibody. Arrowhead indicates endothelium.

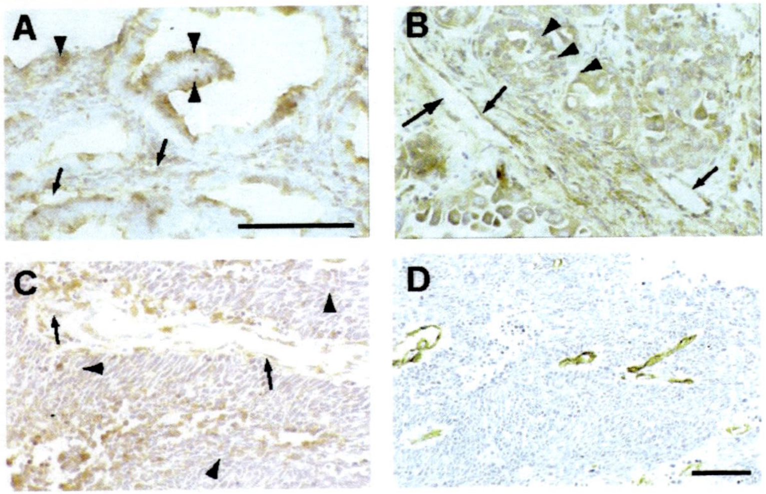

Figure 8. Expression of EpoR in malignant female reproductive tumors. A. Section of ADCO in a 55-yr-old patient shows tumor cells (arrowheads) and capillary endothelium (arrows) with EpoR immunoreactivity. B. Sections of ADCE in a 57-yr-old patient show positive EpoR immunoreactive glandular epithelium (arrowheads) and capillaries (arrows). C. Section of SCC in a 63-yr-old patient shows positive immunoreactive squamous epithelial cells (arrowhead) and intervening capillary endothelium (arrows). D. Adjacent section shown in C stained with anti- FVIII antibody. Note location of capillaries among proliferating epithelium. A-C are at the same magnification. Bar = 50 μm.

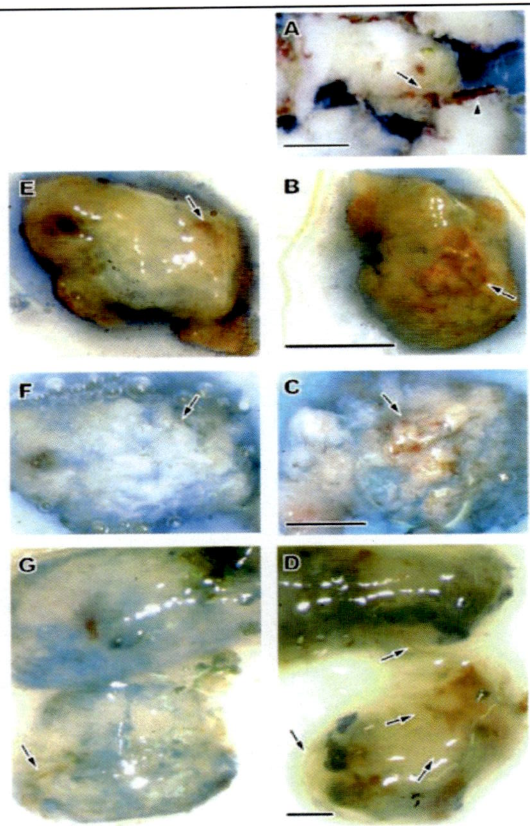

Figure 10. Macroscopy of blood vessels in tumor specimens injected with saline or a sEpoR. Panel A shows blocks in PBS; the other panels show blocks on petri dish. A, Blocks of SCC from a 44-yr-old patient (SCC-44 in Figure 12) before culture. B-D show tumor blocks injected once with saline (B), 3 times (C) and 4 times (D). E-G show tumor blocks injected 0.08 mg/ml of sEpoR once (E), 3 times (F) and 4 times (G). Arrows indicate capillaries and arrowhead, blood coagulation. Blue colouring is due to Evans blue dye for colouring of the solutions. B and E, C and F, D and G are the same magnification. Bar = 2 mm.

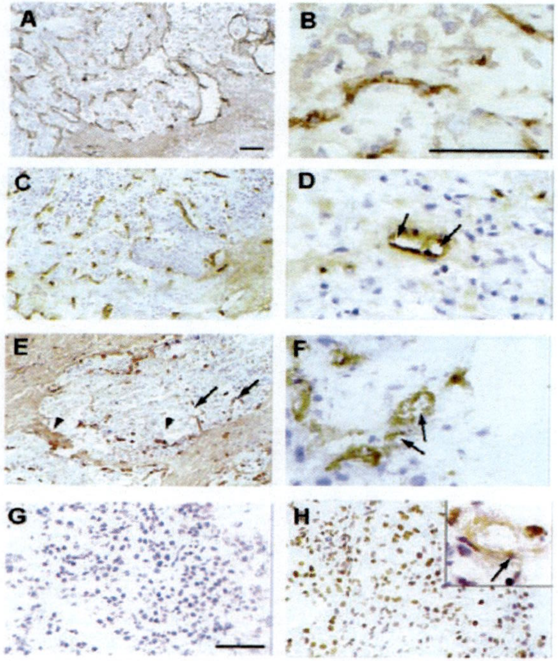

Figure 11. Destructive features of tumor specimens intercepting Epo signaling. All panels are from blocks of ADCO from a 68-yr-old patient (ADCO-68 in Figure 12). A-F, sections stained with anti- FVIII antibody; G and H, sections adapted to TdT assay. A. Section of tumor block before culture shows many capillaries with vascular nets and compact tumor masses with many nuclei. B. High power view of a part of A shows capillary lumens. C. Section of tumor block after 4 injections of saline shows many capillaries. D. High power view of a part of C shows capillary lumen (arrows). E. Section of a tumor block after 4 injections with 0.2 mg/ml of sEpoR shows fragmentation of capillaries (arrows) and many foci of defective tumor masses (arrowheads). F. High power view of a part of E shows many defective capillary walls (arrows). G. Section of tumor block after 4 injections of saline shows a few apoptotic nuclei in the tumor mass. H. Section of tumor block after 4 injections with 0.2 mg/ml of sEpoR shows many apoptotic nuclei in tumor mass. Inset shows apoptotic nuclei in capillary endothelial cell (arrow) of another section of tumor block injected 0.08 mg / ml sEpoR (SCC-44 in Figure 12). A, C and E, B, D, F and inset, and G and H are at the same magnification. Bar = 100 μm.

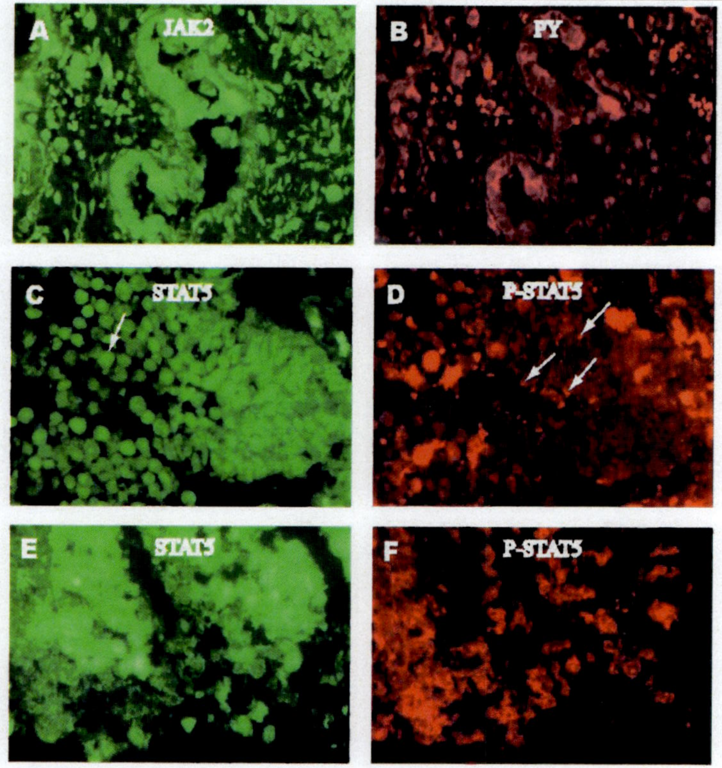

Figure 14. Co-existence of JAK2 and phosphotyrosine, and STAT5 and P-STAT5 in tumors treated with or without sEpoR. A-B, ADCE from a 72-yr-old patient. C-F, SCC from a 53-yr-old patient (SCC-53 in Figure 12). Each left and right panel shows the same section. (A) indicates JAK2 and (B) indicate PY. (C) and (E) indicate STAT5, and (D) and (F) indicate P-STAT5. (C) and (D), section from the block injected with 0.4 mg / ml of dsEpoR three times. Note cells with positive STAT5 in the cytoplasm and in the nucleus (arrow), and P-STAT5, prominently detectable in the nucleus (arrows). (E) and (F), section from the block injected with 0.4 mg/ml of sEpoR three times showing loss of P-STAT5 positive nuclei on the cytoplasm.

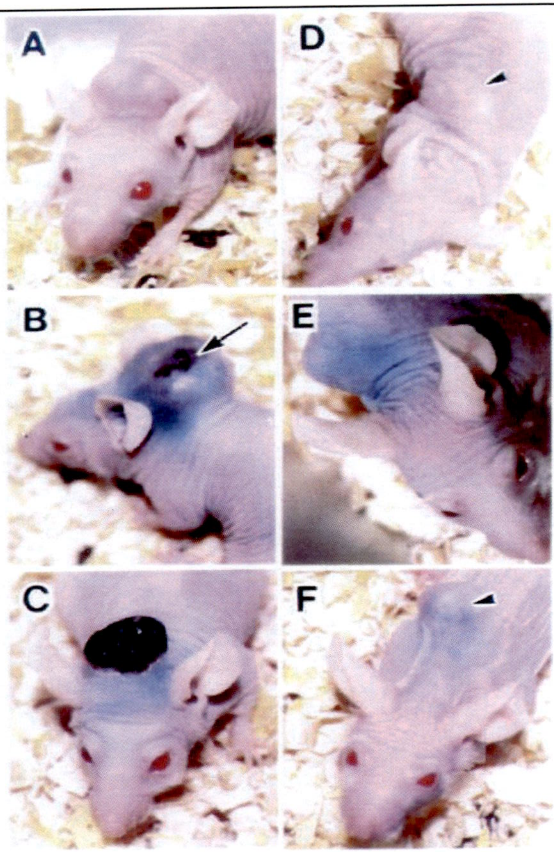

Figure 17. Nude mice with graft of primary ovarian tumor before and after treatment. The blue tint of tumor is due to Evans blue dye for coloring the injection solution. A – C. A mouse receiving a local injection of R2 (ADCO-78 in Figure 20). A, At the time of injection; B, 7 days after injection; Note dark-red exudates (arrow); C, 14 days after injection, showing shrinkage of tumor with scab at the top. D – F. A mouse receiving saline injection locally (ADCO-78 in Figure 20). Arrowhead points to tumor. D, Before injection; E, 7 days after injection; F, 14 days after injection. Note that tumor is larger than before injection.

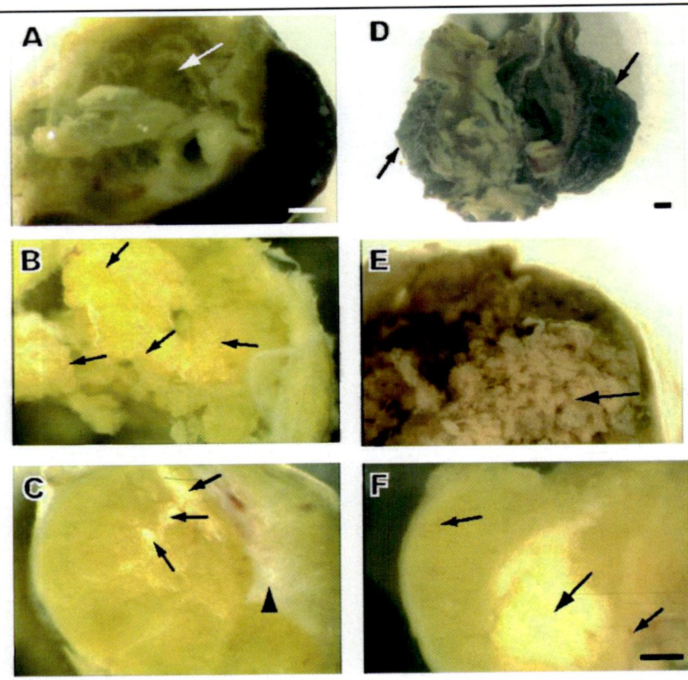

Figure 18. Interior or cut surface of resected tumors. A – C, extirpated 14 days after treatment; D – F, extirpated 7 days after treatment. A. Graft of primary ADCO treated with R2 (ADCO-78 in Figure 20). Note thick scab with large hole (arrow) and large defect of tumor masses leaving fibrous tissues with many holes. B. Another graft of primary ADCO treated with R2 (ADCO-78 in Figure 20), showing destruction of tumor masses with large holes and some tumor masses with broken capillary twigs (arrows) under capsule. C. Control xenograft of (A, B) injected with saline, showing compact tumor masses under thin capsule (arrowhead) and many capillaries and a few calcium deposits (arrows). D. Xenograft of secondary ADCO treated with sEpoR (ADCO-78 in Figure 20). Note covering scab (arrows) and interior with destroyed tumor masses leaving membranous tissues with broken capillary twigs. E. Another xenograft of secondary ADCO treated with sEpoR (ADCO-78 in Figure 20), showing large defective hole with pulverization of tumor masses (arrow). F. Control xenograft of (D, E) inserted only the needle showing compact tumor masses, central pus (arrow) and vessels (small arrows). A, B, C and E are at the same magnification. *, Scale bar = 100 μm.

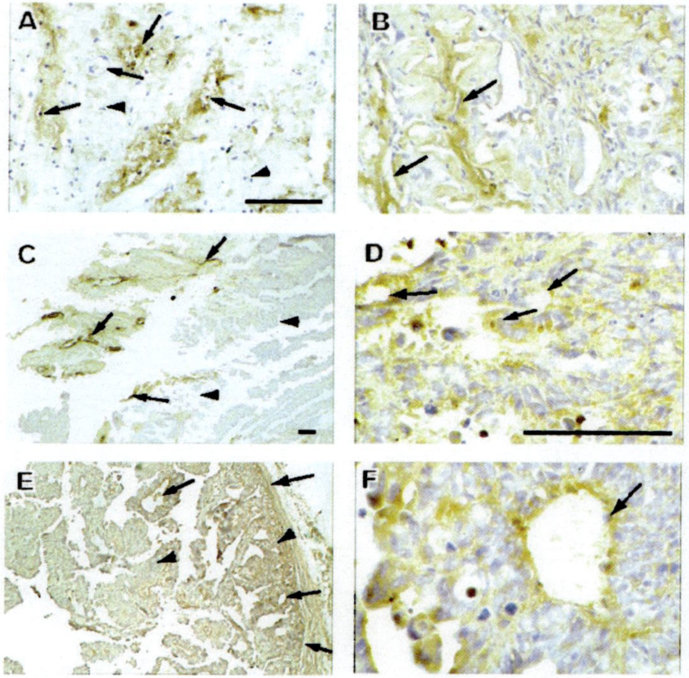

Figure 19. Destruction of angiogenesis in xenografts of ovarian and uterine tumors. A and B, C and E, and D and F are at the same magnification. All panels from sections stained with anti- FVIIIantibody. A. Section of xenograft of ADCE injected with 8 mg / ml of R2 (ADCE-64 in Figure 20), showing amorphous masses infiltrated with many neutrophil- like cells (arrowheads) and destructed endothelium (arrows). B. Control xenograft of (A) injected needle (ADCE-64 in Figure 20), showing well-developed tumor masses with many vessels (arrows). C. Section of xenograft of ADCO injected with R2 (ADCO-78 in Figure 20), showing necrotic region with remnant of vessels (arrows) and thinning tumor masses with few vessels (arrowheads). D. High power view of (C). Note absence of intact capillaries and degenerating capillaries (arrow). E. Control xenograft of ADCO injected with saline (ADCO-78 in Figure 20), showing well-developed tumor masses (arrowheads) with many capillaries (arrows). Long arrows indicate capsule. F. High power view of (E). Note centrally located vessel (arrow) containing red blood cells. Bar = 100 μm.

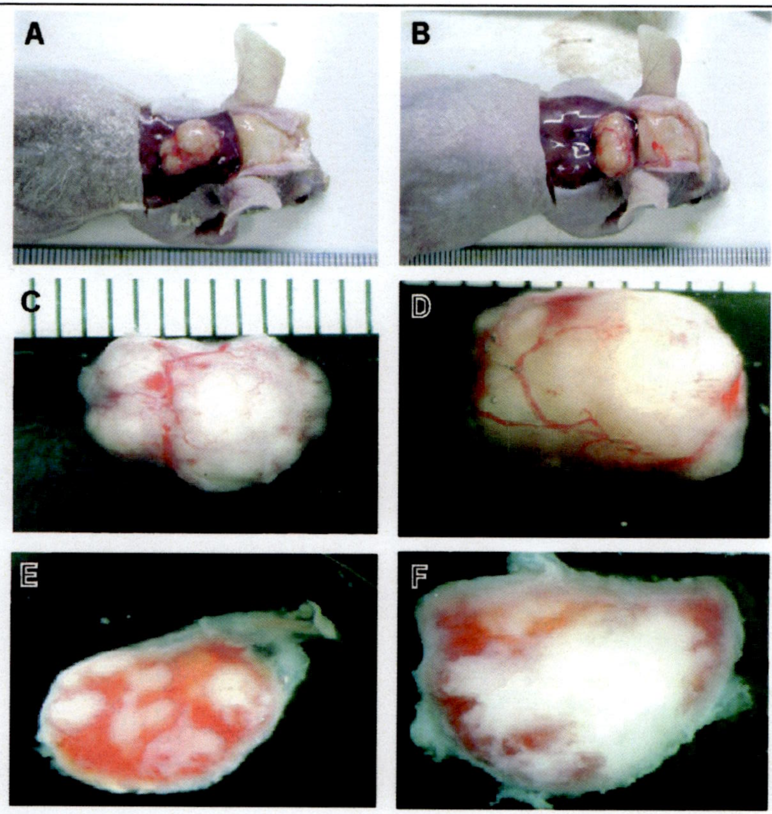

Figure 22. Xenografts of Hela cell line. A. Tumor of non-transfected cells injected in nude mouse. B. Tumor of sEpoR-transfected cells injected in nude mouse. C. Extirpated tumor (A) with well-developed vascular vessels on the dorsal surface. D. Extirpated tumor (B) with vascular nets on the dorsal surface. E. A slice of the tumor from C incubated with formazane, showing viable, (red), and dead, (white) regions. F. A slice of the tumor from D incubated with formazane, showing huge dead region. Scale = 1mm.

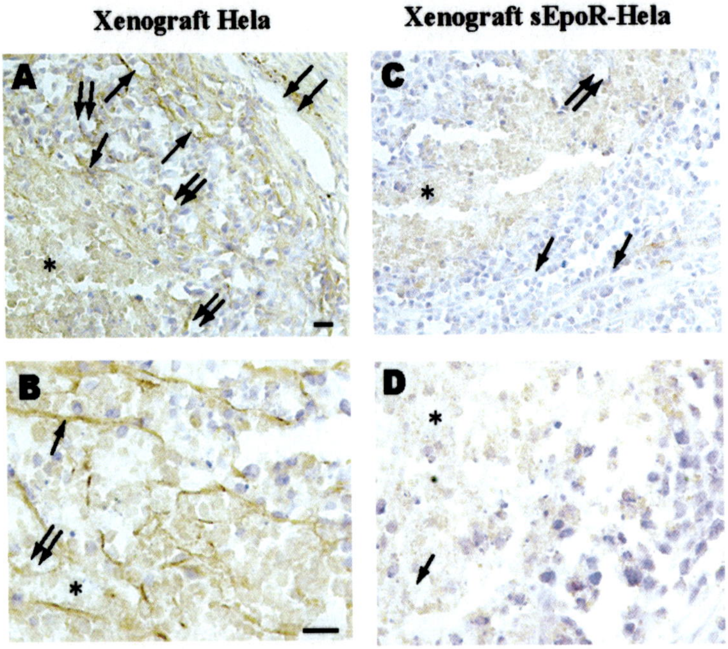

Figure 24. Angiogenesis in xenografts of Hela and sEpoR-Hela A and C, and B and D are at the same magnification. A. Peripheral region of a section of xenografts of Hela. Note many endothelial linings (arrows) and capillaries (double arrows). B. High power view of A. Note extending endothelial lining into necrotic dead area (arrow). C. Peripheral region of a section of xenograft of sEpoR-Hela. Note a thin endothelial linings (arrows) and capillaries (double arrows). D. High power view of C. Note loss of endothelial lining (arrow). Asterisk in each panel points to necrotic dead region. Bar = 10 μm.

INDEX

A

aberrant, 193
acid, 13, 25, 29, 40, 107, 126, 128, 130, 155, 156, 235
acute, 23, 24, 38, 39, 47, 77, 147, 152, 155, 184
acute myelogenous leukemia, 39
adaptation, 22, 47, 184, 199
adhesions, 14, 16, 33, 36, 135
adjuvant, 195, 196, 197, 198, 207, 208
adrenal, 137, 166
adsorption, 119
aerobic, 184
age, 11, 23, 139, 141, 142, 143, 144, 145, 147, 149, 192, 203, 215, 218, 224, 226, 228
agonist, 158, 171, 179, 198
airways, 155
alanine, 28
albumin, 9, 142
aldolase, 184
alkaline, 12, 13
allele, 52, 63, 186, 201
allergic reaction, 27
allergic reactions, 27
amino acids, 5, 6, 7, 9, 12, 15, 126, 127, 129, 135, 153, 154, 155, 156, 157, 216
anaerobic, 184
analogous, 160
anemia, 140, 235
angina, 141
angiogenic process, vii, 3, 49, 103, 104, 108, 109, 110, 113, 115, 117, 120, 195
antagonism, 164, 170, 179
anti-angiogenic agents, 20, 25, 26, 27, 28, 43, 46, 47, 48, 50
antibiotics, 106, 107, 141
antibodies, 6, 7, 14, 27, 45, 48, 49, 60, 90, 101, 194, 203, 213, 226, 229
antibody (Ab), 15, 20, 21, 32, 46, 48, 57, 58, 60, 68, 74, 81, 90, 107, 129, 133, 211, 212, 213, 214, 215, 217, 218, 219, 220, 221, 223, 227, 229, 230, 232, 237, 238, 239
anticoagulant, 58
antifungal, 107
antigens, 90, 106, 194, 214, 219, 237
anti-inflammatory, 80
aorta, 127, 130, 170
apoptosis, 2, 6, 7, 16, 17, 20, 22, 26, 27, 32, 36, 40, 41, 51, 52, 53, 61, 119, 120, 122, 125, 127, 132, 135, 137, 138, 153, 154, 159, 162, 163, 170, 173, 176, 178, 181, 184, 185, 190, 192, 193, 195, 199, 207, 229
appearance, 4, 51, 188
arginine, 12, 128
arterioles, 171, 178, 217, 220
arteries, vii, 6, 11, 33, 43, 55, 87, 99, 100, 141, 142, 149, 151, 152, 164, 179, 195, 236
ascites, 201
aseptic, 215
asymptomatic, 150
atherogenesis, 140, 147
atherosclerosis, viii, 140, 142, 143, 147, 148, 149, 150, 151, 152, 155
atherosclerotic plaque, 147
attenuated, 48, 171
Australia, 71, 81, 82
autosomal recessive, 11
axon, 34

B

basement membrane, 1, 2, 3, 5, 7, 8, 11, 12, 19, 21, 23, 30, 31, 32, 34, 44, 50, 127, 136, 137, 167, 169, 185, 186
benign, 161, 165
beta-blockers, 141
binding, 2, 3, 4, 6, 7, 9, 12, 13, 14, 15, 16, 17, 18, 20, 21, 22, 25, 27, 28, 29, 31, 32, 33, 35, 38, 40, 45, 50, 51, 54, 65, 66, 98, 116, 117, 121, 126, 127, 128, 132, 135, 154, 158, 159, 166, 168, 177, 184, 186, 188, 190, 191, 192, 202, 204, 211, 234, 235, 236
biology, 19, 26, 35, 43, 55, 56, 58, 121
biomarkers, viii, 26, 29, 183, 192
biopsy, 26, 58, 196
biosynthesis, 35, 179
bladder, 23, 24, 38, 46, 47, 59, 68
bleeding, 72, 97, 98, 100
blood, viii, 2, 3, 11, 16, 26, 28, 29, 30, 35, 44, 45, 46, 47, 50, 52, 53, 55, 58, 60, 63, 68, 76, 89, 97, 104, 105, 111, 116, 121, 141, 149, 153, 155, 156, 166, 167, 170, 171, 178, 179, 183, 184, 185, 186, 187, 194, 199, 201, 204, 224, 233, 238
blood pressure, 155, 171
blood vessels, viii, 2, 3, 11, 28, 30, 35, 44, 50, 53, 55, 58, 68, 76, 89, 97, 104, 155, 166, 183, 185, 186, 199, 224, 233, 238
BMI, 143
body weight, 104
bone marrow, 2, 19, 45, 48, 59, 191
brain tumor, 185
Brazil, 25
breast cancer, viii, 23, 30, 39, 49, 60, 82, 137, 154, 159, 161, 168, 173, 176, 177, 181, 183, 187, 188, 189, 190, 191, 194, 195, 196, 197, 198, 199, 202, 204, 205, 206, 207, 208
breast carcinoma, 23, 138, 166, 172, 176, 188, 198, 203, 205, 206, 207, 208, 209
bronchial epithelium, 175

C

C reactive protein (CRP), 139, 142, 144, 145, 147, 148, 149
calcium, 19, 22, 137, 141, 154, 157, 180, 240
calcium channel blocker, 141
calcium channel blockers, 141
cancer progression, 31
cancers, viii, 8, 10, 11, 20, 21, 23, 24, 25, 27, 28, 29, 30, 31, 33, 34, 38, 40, 41, 46, 49, 56, 58, 59, 117, 121, 153, 154, 158, 159, 160, 161, 162, 167, 172, 173, 174, 176, 178, 183, 184, 185, 186, 188, 189, 190, 194, 195, 196, 197, 198, 199, 201, 203, 207, 208, 209, 211, 215, 228, 229, 230
capillaries, 2, 7, 9, 10, 12, 41, 45, 47, 54, 57, 65, 66, 74, 79, 89, 90, 91, 92, 104, 105, 109, 120, 126, 127, 137, 169, 211, 212, 214, 219, 221, 223, 224, 226, 227, 233, 234, 237, 238, 239, 240
capsule, 240, 241
carcinoma, 7, 8, 19, 21, 23, 24, 28, 31, 38, 40, 41, 59, 68, 117, 121, 136, 154, 160, 161, 164, 168, 170, 173, 174, 175, 176, 179, 187, 191, 194, 203, 205, 207, 213, 235
cardiac, 8, 12, 155, 170, 178
cardiovascular disease, viii, 139, 140, 141, 147, 150, 151
carotid arteries, viii, 139, 142
carrier, 126
cast, 108
cell cycle, 17, 20, 40, 74, 78, 107, 111, 117, 130, 135, 190
cell death, 163, 176, 204, 221, 233
cell line, 10, 14, 18, 19, 20, 21, 28, 82, 125, 127, 129, 130, 132, 133, 135, 154, 159, 160, 161, 162, 163, 164, 165, 168, 172, 175, 177, 179, 189, 198, 212, 213, 214, 215, 217, 223, 224, 228, 230, 231, 232, 236, 241
cell surface, 2, 3, 4, 5, 6, 8, 9, 13, 14, 15, 16, 19, 21, 27, 29, 49, 51, 65, 87, 97, 104, 132, 140, 164, 217
cells, 2, 3, 5, 6, 7, 8, 10, 11, 12, 13, 16, 17, 18, 21, 27, 28, 30, 32, 36, 37, 38, 40, 44, 45, 47, 48, 49, 50, 51, 52, 53, 54, 55, 59, 62, 64, 65, 68, 72, 73, 74, 76, 78, 79, 80, 81, 82, 83, 84, 86, 87, 88, 91, 95, 99, 102, 104, 105, 106, 107, 109, 110, 111, 113, 115, 116, 117, 118, 120, 121, 123, 125, 126, 127, 128, 129, 130, 131, 132, 133, 134, 135, 136, 137, 138, 140, 153, 154, 156, 157, 159, 160, 161, 163, 164, 165, 166, 167, 168, 169, 170, 172, 173, 175, 176, 179, 180, 181, 182, 184, 185, 186, 187, 188, 189, 190, 192, 193, 196, 199, 201, 203, 204, 205, 211, 212, 213, 215, 216, 217, 218, 219, 220, 221, 223, 224, 226, 227, 229, 230, 232, 233, 234, 235, 236, 237, 239, 241
central nervous system (CNS), 169, 235
cervical, 46, 59, 200, 215, 217, 219, 221, 222, 226
cervical cancer, 46, 59, 200
cervix, 179, 217, 218, 221, 224, 226

chemokines, 165, 167, 185
chemotaxis, 65, 164, 181
chemotherapeutic, 45, 48, 171
chemotherapeutic agents, 45, 48, 171
chemotherapy, 10, 25, 27, 28, 39, 40, 48, 57, 171, 183, 196, 198, 199, 208
chi, 142
China, 125, 127
cholesterol, 142, 143, 144, 145, 146
chromosome, 23, 202
chronic, viii, 47, 117, 139, 140, 142, 143, 144, 145, 146, 147, 148, 149, 150, 151, 155, 183
chronic renal failure, viii, 139, 140, 143, 144, 145, 146, 149, 150, 151, 155
chronically, 184
cleavage, 9, 11, 28, 216
clinical trials, 1, 2, 8, 10, 23, 27, 29, 157, 158, 162, 171, 172, 173, 199
clone, 90, 191, 216
cloning, 174
cluster of differentiation (CD), 121, 200
coagulation, 4, 224, 238
collagen, 1, 2, 3, 5, 6, 7, 8, 9, 10, 11, 12, 13, 18, 21, 23, 29, 31, 32, 34, 35, 38, 39, 41, 105, 107, 109, 110, 111, 115, 117, 120, 125, 126, 127, 129, 135, 136, 137, 138, 169
collateral, vii, 43, 55
colon, 2, 20, 38
colon cancer, 20, 38
colorectal cancer, 41, 45, 179
combination therapy, 57
complementary DNA (cDNA), 13, 81, 82, 84, 88, 127, 129, 133, 174, 212, 213, 214, 215, 216, 230, 231, 232
complications, 46, 148, 152
concentration, 18, 19, 22, 25, 54, 81, 85, 86, 93, 108, 111, 113, 117, 118, 128, 129, 132, 160, 165, 166, 184, 187, 188, 189, 190, 192, 193, 194, 197, 215, 220, 236
congestive heart failure, 155
conservation, 12
contraceptive, 72, 189
control, vii, 3, 9, 23, 24, 25, 29, 43, 49, 81, 82, 83, 84, 85, 86, 91, 93, 94, 96, 111, 112, 113, 118, 123, 125, 126, 127, 129, 132, 134, 136, 141, 143, 144, 145, 151, 155, 156, 171, 172, 173, 185, 192, 193, 195, 218, 219, 220, 221, 222, 223, 224, 225, 227, 228, 229, 234, 237
controlled study, 66
cornea, 57, 91, 97, 98, 167
corneal, 19, 126, 137, 188
coronary arteries, 97, 99, 147
correlation coefficient, 145, 146
cortex, 237
cortical neurons, 234
corticosteroids, 141
creatinine, 141, 148
crystals, 34
cultured, 36, 44, 45, 47, 48, 50, 51, 52, 53, 54, 59, 66, 80, 87, 106, 120, 129, 155, 162, 166, 170, 177, 178, 217, 221, 236
cultures, 11, 45, 47, 57, 86, 87, 88, 98, 104, 106, 107, 108, 110, 111, 120, 126, 128, 133, 134, 137, 161, 164, 213, 215, 219, 224, 238, 239
cycling, 81, 214
cyclophosphamide, 60, 198, 208
cystitis, 46, 58
cytokines, vii, 25, 36, 48, 49, 52, 69, 97, 103, 104, 139, 154, 155, 163, 164, 165, 166, 167, 169, 177, 181
cytoplasm, 109, 188, 217, 226, 239
cytotoxic, 25, 26, 28, 37, 45, 113, 117, 141, 199, 209

D

death, 23, 24, 32, 51, 52, 53, 61, 147, 151, 163, 170, 199, 212, 213, 224, 227, 230, 234
degenerate, 12
deletion, 11, 12, 51, 52, 53
denaturation, 214
dendritic cell (DC), 31, 226
dephosphorylation, 18, 22
dermis, 80, 88
diabetes, viii, 140, 141, 143, 144, 183
diabetes mellitus, 141, 143, 144
diabetic, 46, 58, 117, 141, 145
diabetic nephropathy, 141
diabetic patients, 145
diabetic retinopathy, 46, 58, 117
diacylglycerol, 180
diagnosis, 41, 56, 208
dialysis, 149, 150, 151, 152
diastolic blood pressure, 143
differentiation, 5, 50, 53, 61, 63, 68, 118, 120, 121, 126, 154, 155, 162, 169, 185, 212, 216, 235
diffusion, 2, 185
digestion, 44, 216
disability, 236
distal, 142, 208

DNA, 45, 74, 81, 83, 100, 122, 127, 130, 163, 184, 214, 215, 216
DNase, 81, 82, 83
dorsal, 241
dosage, 141
Down syndrome, 38
down-regulation, 37, 62, 84, 85, 88
duplication, 17
dyslipidemia, 140

E

ectoderm, 167
edema, 46, 98
efficacy, 23, 28, 39, 40, 47, 48, 117, 171, 172, 196, 208
elastin, 126
elderly, 204
electrophoresis, 81, 214
emboli, 55, 66
embolization, 55, 66
embryo, 50, 51, 52, 53, 60, 98, 126, 167, 213
endocrine, 183, 194, 197, 199
endogenous, vii, 1, 2, 4, 9, 15, 25, 27, 28, 29, 33, 34, 45, 54, 57, 137, 187, 189, 190, 196, 207, 212, 233
endometrial hyperplasia, 41
endometriosis, 100
endothelial cells, vii, 2, 3, 4, 7, 10, 12, 14, 16, 17, 18, 19, 20, 21, 22, 27, 28, 29, 31, 32, 36, 37, 40, 41, 44, 45, 46, 48, 49, 50, 51, 52, 53, 54, 55, 56, 57, 59, 61, 62, 64, 65, 66, 67, 68, 71, 72, 73, 74, 76, 78, 79, 80, 82, 83, 84, 87, 88, 90, 91, 93, 97, 98, 99, 100, 101, 103, 104, 120, 121, 122, 126, 128, 130, 131, 135, 137, 138, 139, 140, 153, 154, 155, 157, 159, 160, 161, 165, 166, 167, 169, 170, 173, 177, 178, 179, 181, 182, 185, 186, 188, 194, 196, 199, 201, 202, 203, 211, 212, 213, 214, 217, 220, 221, 223, 224, 226, 227, 229, 234, 237
endothelium, 11, 33, 46, 56, 74, 76, 77, 78, 97, 99, 174, 177, 186, 200, 202, 204, 212, 219, 223, 237, 238, 241
end-stage renal disease, 148, 149
energy, 47, 184
enzyme-linked immunoassay, 106, 223
enzyme-linked immunosorbent assay (ELISA), 142
enzymes, 3, 16, 55, 106, 121, 153, 155, 163, 164, 174, 175, 185, 191, 192, 198, 223
epididymis, 213
epithelial cells, 21, 38, 99, 127, 155, 157, 162, 188, 190, 199, 219, 238
epithelial ovarian cancer, 38, 41
epithelium, 11, 187, 217, 219, 237, 238
erythrocytosis, 236
erythroid cells, 212, 234
erythropoietin, vi, viii, 52, 62, 141, 178, 211, 212, 216, 218, 221, 227, 230, 234, 235, 236
estrogen, vii, viii, 71, 72, 73, 75, 76, 78, 79, 82, 83, 84, 87, 88, 91, 93, 94, 97, 98, 99, 101, 183, 188, 189, 190, 191, 193, 198, 204, 211, 213, 214, 216, 218, 219
ethanol, 82, 86, 107
eukaryotic cell, 136
evolution, 174
excision, 196
excretion, 155
exercise, 12
exogenous, 8, 27
extracellulaar matrix (ECM), viii, 2, 3, 8, 9, 104, 105, 108, 110, 111, 115, 116, 117, 123, 125, 126, 127
extracellular, vii, viii, 1, 2, 3, 9, 13, 16, 18, 19, 28, 29, 30, 45, 49, 51, 103, 104, 120, 122, 125, 126, 136, 137, 157, 164, 186, 202, 211, 216
extracellular matrix (ECM), vii, viii, 1, 2, 3, 8, 9, 13, 16, 28, 29, 30, 103, 104, 108, 110, 111, 115, 116, 117, 122, 123, 125, 126, 127, 136, 137, 164, 202
extracellular matrix (protein) (ECM), viii, 2, 3, 8, 9, 104, 105, 108, 110, 111, 115, 116, 117, 123, 125, 126, 127

F

factor i, 88, 104, 169, 178, 179, 199, 203
fasting, 141
fat, 187
feedback, 19, 45, 166
fetal growth, 63
fetus, 212
fibers, 36, 135
fibrin, 105, 109, 110, 111, 115, 117, 120
fibrinogen, 9, 107, 143, 144, 148
fibroadenoma, 161
fibroblast growth factor, 3, 30, 35, 39, 41, 45, 57, 60, 65, 67, 77, 100, 104, 121, 125, 126, 127, 137, 154, 178
fibroblasts, vii, 13, 19, 51, 103, 104, 153, 154, 164, 181, 212, 217
fibrosarcoma, 171, 179

flu, 190
fluorescence, 108, 132, 219
follicles, 219, 221, 237
follow-up, 176, 195

G

gastric, 19
gastrointestinal, 33
gender, 142, 144, 145
gene, 5, 6, 11, 17, 19, 21, 22, 23, 25, 27, 28, 29, 37, 38, 44, 50, 52, 53, 55, 62, 63, 64, 71, 83, 84, 85, 86, 87, 88, 93, 94, 95, 96, 99, 127, 128, 129, 132, 136, 155, 159, 163, 174, 175, 177, 178, 182, 184, 185, 186, 188, 193, 201, 202, 204, 206, 234, 235, 236
gene expression, 6, 11, 17, 19, 21, 22, 23, 28, 29, 37, 62, 71, 83, 84, 85, 86, 87, 88, 93, 94, 95, 99, 163, 177, 178, 206, 234, 235, 236
gene therapy, 27, 28
genetic factors, 194
genome, 20
Germany, 103, 106, 107, 108, 119, 215
gland, 17, 102, 187, 203, 204
glatiramer acetate (GA), 31, 32, 120, 174, 202
glioma, 10, 33
glomerulonephritis, 141
glucose, 26, 47, 184
glycerol, 214
glycoprotein, viii, 9, 19, 186, 211, 212, 236
granules, 91
growth factors, vii, 3, 14, 17, 30, 31, 35, 37, 38, 39, 41, 44, 47, 48, 49, 50, 51, 52, 53, 56, 57, 58, 59, 60, 61, 62, 63, 65, 66, 68, 71, 77, 78, 79, 86, 97, 98, 99, 100, 101, 103, 104, 109, 111, 121, 126, 130, 137, 138, 159, 160, 161, 162, 164, 168, 175, 176, 177, 179, 184, 185, 186, 188, 200, 201, 202, 203, 204, 205, 206, 207, 208, 234
guidelines, 141, 197, 213

H

headache, 46
heart attack, 151, 184
heart failure, 172
heat shock protein, 36
hemangioma, 213
hematopoietic stem cells, 50
hemodialysis, viii, 139, 140, 149, 150, 151, 152
hemorrhage, 46, 51
heparin, 9, 12, 13, 15, 27, 29, 32, 35, 82, 86, 106, 116, 126
hepatic, 9, 24, 195
hepatocellular carcinoma, 23, 24, 39, 41, 55, 66, 200
hepatocyte, 31, 49, 68
hepatoma, 125, 127, 129, 132, 133, 217, 223, 228, 236
heterogeneity, 12, 87
histidine, 12
histone, 104, 107, 117, 121, 122
HLA, 164
homeostasis, 56, 63, 64, 154, 156, 184
homologous, 125, 127, 135
homozygous, 50, 51, 52
hormones, viii, 57, 72, 76, 78, 82, 86, 87, 88, 94, 99, 156, 172, 179, 183, 188, 189, 190, 191, 192, 195, 197, 199, 205, 208
host, 2, 118, 208, 229, 230, 232, 233
human leukocyte antigen (HLA), 164
human neutrophil elastase, 90, 102
human neutrophils, 98, 164
hybrid, 9, 54
hyperplasia, 187
hypertension, 140, 141, 155, 157, 172
hypertrophy, 155
hypoglycemia, 177, 185
hypothermia, 199
hypothesis, 4, 23, 76, 89, 147, 149, 188, 189, 190, 197, 198, 204
hypoxia, viii, 22, 26, 27, 44, 47, 48, 52, 56, 59, 62, 66, 104, 110, 111, 116, 120, 121, 153, 154, 155, 159, 160, 165, 166, 168, 176, 177, 178, 181, 182, 183, 184, 185, 187, 188, 189, 195, 198, 199, 200, 201, 203, 204, 206, 213, 217
hypoxia-inducible factor (HIF), 153, 183, 184
hysterectomy, 80

I

identification, vii, 1, 3, 13, 17, 21, 29, 55, 65, 76, 109, 110, 123, 126, 194, 196, 202, 216
immune reaction, 199
immunodeficiency, 60
immunogenicity, 27
immunoglobulin (Ig), 140
immunohistochemistry, 77, 82, 148, 187, 192, 213
immunoprecipitation, 16
immunoreactivity, 217, 218, 219, 221, 223, 237, 238
immunostaining, 76, 89, 90, 213, 219

in situ hybridization, 235
in vitro, v, viii, 5, 6, 7, 8, 10, 11, 12, 13, 15, 17, 18, 20, 21, 27, 28, 29, 32, 37, 40, 41, 45, 57, 58, 71, 73, 78, 79, 80, 82, 84, 87, 88, 93, 103, 104, 105, 107, 108, 109, 110, 111, 113, 114, 115, 116, 117, 118, 119, 120, 121, 122, 123, 125, 126, 127, 130, 135, 136, 152, 158, 160, 162, 164, 169, 172, 176, 189, 203, 211, 212, 213, 221, 225, 226, 227, 230, 234, 235
in vivo, vii, viii, 2, 3, 4, 5, 6, 7, 9, 11, 13, 17, 19, 20, 21, 22, 26, 28, 29, 31, 32, 33, 37, 38, 40, 44, 45, 47, 57, 58, 65, 88, 103, 104, 105, 115, 116, 117, 119, 121, 125, 127, 132, 136, 152, 158, 162, 163, 166, 167, 169, 172, 176, 177, 178, 179, 185, 188, 200, 203, 212, 213
inducer, 186
infarction, 236
inflammation, 19, 93, 104, 117, 140, 144, 147, 148, 149, 150, 151, 152, 154
inflammatory, 91, 93, 95, 140, 148, 150, 152, 154, 155, 160, 165, 176, 181, 185
inflammatory cells, 155, 185
inflammatory response, 140, 148, 150, 152
inhibitor, 4, 17, 28, 30, 31, 32, 33, 34, 35, 36, 39, 40, 76, 77, 78, 87, 99, 104, 107, 111, 117, 121, 125, 126, 127, 136, 137, 161, 166, 168, 170, 188, 199, 207
innate immunity, 64
inositol, 19, 180
insertion, 227
insulin, 47, 162, 165
integrin, 3, 4, 5, 6, 7, 8, 9, 14, 15, 17, 22, 27, 29, 31, 32, 33, 38, 40, 48, 122, 126, 135, 137, 138
interactions, vii, 4, 5, 6, 9, 15, 16, 35, 61, 97, 103, 104, 120, 163
intercellular, vii, 103, 104, 115, 120, 139, 151
intercellular adhesion molecule (ICAM), viii, 139, 140, 142, 143, 145, 146, 147, 148, 149, 150, 151, 152
interleukin (IL), 96, 151, 158, 160, 164, 165, 169, 170, 177, 178, 236
interleukin-8, 178
interstitial, 2, 44, 45, 46, 50, 137, 167, 185
intestine, 155
intima, 139, 140, 144, 146, 149, 150, 152
intracellular, 4, 9, 17, 18, 19, 20, 22, 36, 37, 49, 54, 109, 154, 157, 170, 174, 180, 189, 212, 219
intravascular, 73, 97, 98
intravenous (IV), v, viii, 2, 3, 5, 6, 7, 8, 9, 24, 25, 27, 29, 31, 32, 38, 39, 103, 135, 171
intravenously, 155
ischemia, 46, 200, 213
ischemic, vii, 43, 45, 46, 236
isolation, 3, 4, 29, 83, 106, 164, 214

K

kidneys, 32, 137, 155, 212, 236
kinase activity, 22, 54, 64, 65, 77

L

lactate dehydrogenase, 184, 235
lactation, 187
laminar, 122
lateral, 5
lesions, 148, 149, 185, 188, 190, 195, 203, 204
leukemia, 38, 39, 223
leukocytes, 19, 97, 140, 229
life cycle, 187, 203
lipid, 14, 15, 22, 36, 152
lipoproteins, 152
liver, 40, 41, 202, 207, 212, 213, 235
liver metastases, 41, 207
lumen, 44, 49, 76, 89, 109, 115, 123, 142, 147, 239
lung cancer, 24, 38, 39, 47, 159, 175
lymph, 161, 192, 194, 196, 206, 222
lymph nodes, 161, 192, 194, 196, 222
lymphocytes, 90, 148, 164
lymphoma, 23, 24, 38
lysine, 25
lysis, 214

M

macrophages, vii, 90, 103, 104, 148, 154, 155, 161, 163, 164, 167, 170, 173, 174, 176, 179, 181, 200, 212, 213, 229, 235
magnetic resonance imaging (MRI), 26
malignancy, 26, 31, 63, 194, 195
malignant, vi, vii, viii, 2, 23, 43, 47, 48, 55, 58, 154, 162, 187, 195, 203, 211, 212, 213, 221, 222, 223, 224, 226, 227, 229, 238
malnutrition, 151
mammals, 126
mast cells, 90
mat, 23, 139, 141, 142, 147, 149, 171, 192

matrix, 1, 2, 3, 7, 11, 31, 32, 33, 36, 38, 88, 104, 105, 109, 115, 120, 125, 126, 135, 137, 160, 164, 170, 186, 202
matrix metalloproteinase (MMP), 7, 8, 9, 10, 16, 21, 31, 32, 33, 36, 38, 120, 159, 160, 161, 163, 164, 167, 170, 173, 181
matrix metalloproteinase (MMP)-2, 8, 9, 10, 16, 36, 120, 163, 167, 173
matrix metalloproteinases (MMP), 3, 7, 8, 9, 10, 16, 21, 31, 32, 33, 159, 160, 161, 163, 164, 167, 173, 181
maturation, 51, 236
MCP-1, 87, 100, 152
mean, viii, 24, 86, 94, 110, 114, 128, 131, 141, 143, 147, 154, 171, 223, 232
mean arterial pressure, 171
median, 8, 83, 192, 193
medulla, 137, 221
melanoma, 5, 7, 10, 16, 25, 30, 32, 40, 162, 163, 168, 172, 173, 176, 179
men, 32
meningioma, 213, 236
menopause, 188
menstruation, 2
mesoderm, 63
messenger ribonucleic acid, 204
messenger RNA (mRNA), 17, 22, 76, 78, 80, 82, 83, 87, 88, 89, 94, 96, 101, 161, 163, 168, 169, 174, 178, 184, 185, 186, 189, 195, 204, 213, 214, 217, 219, 222, 226, 228, 230, 231, 232, 234, 235, 236
metabolism, 26, 47, 184, 185
metalloproteinase, 33
metastases, 4, 10, 16, 23, 24, 31, 41, 58, 161, 167, 176, 181, 191, 195, 196, 200, 207
metastasis, vii, 1, 2, 9, 30, 31, 40, 44, 56, 117, 121, 136, 137, 164, 173, 183, 194, 195, 196, 198, 201, 203, 206
metastatic, 10, 25, 27, 41, 44, 45, 160, 162, 163, 191, 194, 196, 197, 203, 205, 206, 222
metastatic cancer, 25, 162
metastatic disease, 27, 162
mg, 25, 74, 77, 86, 107, 128, 131, 136, 142, 143, 144, 145, 147, 191, 192, 193, 197, 215, 224, 228, 229, 238, 239, 241
mg/dl, 143
microarray technology, 20
micrometer, 216
microscope, 108, 128, 215, 228
migration, 2, 3, 4, 5, 6, 9, 11, 12, 13, 14, 18, 19, 21, 29, 31, 34, 35, 36, 37, 40, 41, 44, 45, 53, 60, 64, 66, 68, 115, 120, 126, 128, 130, 131, 135, 140, 159, 160, 163, 166, 169, 179, 182, 185, 186
mild, 25, 162
mitogen, 50, 51, 61, 62, 63, 121, 162, 166, 170, 186, 201, 235
mitosis, 212
MMP-9, 8, 21, 32
mode, 18, 152
modelling, 25
moderate, 25
molecule, viii, 4, 7, 8, 10, 11, 12, 15, 25, 28, 29, 45, 49, 50, 51, 53, 54, 68, 97, 99, 100, 139, 140, 142, 145, 147, 148, 149, 154, 158, 163, 172, 173
monoclonal antibody (mAb), 3, 45, 60, 215
monocyte chemoattractant protein (MCP), 87, 100, 152
monolayer, 113, 114, 118
morphogenesis, 5, 21, 38, 45, 54, 57, 63, 65, 109, 115, 117, 120, 126, 166, 167
morphology, 45, 109, 115, 126, 133
mortality, viii, 23, 139, 140, 148, 149, 151, 208
mortality rate, viii, 139, 140
mRNA, 17, 22, 76, 78, 80, 82, 83, 87, 88, 89, 94, 96, 101, 161, 163, 168, 169, 174, 178, 184, 185, 186, 189, 195, 204, 213, 214, 217, 219, 222, 226, 228, 230, 231, 232, 234, 235, 236
mucosa, 46
multifactorial, 140, 148, 199
multiple myeloma, 25, 39, 41
multiple sclerosis (MS), 31, 33, 40, 41, 120, 121, 177, 207, 208
mutant, 25, 28, 40, 50, 51, 52, 53, 65, 206
mutation, 13, 25, 206
mutations, 11, 185, 200
myocardial infarction, 141
myocardium, 51
myopathy, 35, 137
myopia, 11

N

natural killer cell (NK), 90
nausea, 46
necrosis, 165, 172, 188
neoangiogenesis, 184, 189
nephrectomy, 23
nephritis, 32, 141
nervous system, 11, 212
neuroblastoma, 37, 173, 179
neurons, 213, 236

neutrophils, 71, 90, 91, 97, 98, 100, 102
ng/ml, 24, 106, 107, 110, 128, 129, 131, 142, 145, 146, 147
nitrates, 141
NK cells, 90
nodes, 23, 24, 161, 181, 194, 196, 197, 198, 204, 205, 206, 207, 208, 222
nodules, 6, 168
norepinephrine (NE), 217, 218
nuclear receptors, 97
nucleotide, 50, 69
nucleus, 182, 185, 188, 226, 239
nutrients, 2, 170
nutrition, 136

O

occipital, 11
occlusion, vii, 43, 195, 236
occult, 185
oedema, 75, 76
oncogenes, 47, 188
organ, 3, 11, 179, 213, 219, 224
organism, 184
ovarian cancer, 28, 154, 159, 160, 164, 175, 227, 228, 229
ovarian tumor, 240
ovaries, 154, 159, 167, 212, 213, 215, 216, 217, 218, 219, 220, 237
oxidative stress, 62, 140, 148, 151

P

p53, 122, 190, 192, 193, 206
paclitaxel, 173
pain, 162
parenchyma, 188
pathogen, 215
pathogenesis, viii, 58, 100, 148, 183
pathogenic, 7
pathologic, 60, 117, 184, 185
pathologist, 187
pathology, 60, 97
pathophysiology, 29, 56, 58, 104, 120, 208
peptide, 7, 15, 16, 29, 32, 33, 36, 54, 135, 155, 156, 158, 159, 166, 172, 174, 178
peptides, viii, 3, 7, 8, 15, 29, 40, 153, 154, 155, 174, 179
perfusion, 46, 74, 171
peripheral vascular disease, 141, 150
peritoneum, 191
pertussis, 164
pH, 4, 11, 12, 107, 128, 129, 185, 214
pharmacokinetics, 25
phenotype, 2, 11, 12, 14, 17, 46, 51, 105, 113, 114, 116, 118, 161, 164, 177, 178, 183, 185, 186, 187, 188, 189, 193, 203, 205
phenylalanine, 219
phosphate, 12, 19, 216, 219
phosphorylation, 7, 16, 17, 18, 20, 22, 51, 52, 53, 54, 61, 63, 64, 65, 163, 212, 219, 226, 227
physiology, 120, 220
placenta, 6, 30, 51, 52, 53, 60, 61, 100, 186, 202, 234, 235
plasma, 4, 9, 15, 23, 28, 33, 38, 41, 50, 51, 54, 132, 166, 190, 202, 220
plasma levels, 190
plasma membrane, 50, 51, 54, 132
plasma proteins, 4
plasmid, 127, 128, 132, 136, 214, 216
plasmin, 64
plasminogen, 1, 4, 36, 40, 60, 87, 107, 121, 128, 130, 188
platelet, 30, 49, 53, 59, 60, 77, 162, 184, 186, 206
platelets, 202
plexus, 89, 90, 91, 92
point mutation, 28
polycystic kidney disease, 141
polymerase, 80, 81, 127, 235
polymerase chain reaction, 235
polymerase chain reaction (PCR), 80, 81, 82, 83, 87, 127, 129, 132, 133, 174, 189, 214, 216, 217, 222, 227, 228, 232, 235
polymorphism, 39, 152
polypeptide, 10
polysaccharides, 3
population, viii, 23, 25, 38, 104, 106, 140, 147, 148, 149, 150, 164, 236
precursor cells, 45, 50, 56, 212, 236
pregnancy, 78, 187, 219, 221, 237
prematurity, 235
preterm infants, 235
prevention, 38, 58, 198
primary tumor, 40, 117, 190, 195, 196, 198, 208
primate, 97, 99, 204
probe, 9, 12, 80, 82, 86, 132, 142, 215
proctitis, 58

progesterone, vii, 71, 72, 73, 74, 75, 78, 79, 80, 81, 82, 83, 84, 86, 87, 88, 89, 93, 94, 95, 96, 97, 98, 99, 100, 189, 190, 191
progestin, 72, 97, 189
progestins, 72, 189, 204
prognosis, viii, 23, 24, 25, 28, 38, 154, 190, 193, 194, 195, 198, 206
prognostic, 23, 194, 196, 197, 198, 201, 206, 207
progression, 10, 27, 37, 38, 59, 109, 111, 117, 140, 147, 148, 149, 161, 168, 172, 173, 179, 187, 189, 190, 191, 193, 194, 195, 197, 199, 200
prolactin, 4, 31
proliferation, viii, 2, 3, 4, 6, 7, 9, 10, 12, 18, 22, 26, 29, 32, 41, 44, 45, 50, 58, 61, 62, 63, 68, 71, 72, 73, 74, 76, 77, 78, 86, 89, 91, 93, 97, 98, 101, 111, 116, 117, 118, 125, 126, 127, 128, 130, 131, 133, 135, 138, 140, 159, 162, 163, 164, 166, 167, 168, 172, 173, 176, 179, 182, 183, 185, 186, 187, 192, 193, 194, 195, 199, 205, 207, 208, 212, 221, 226, 230
promoter, 9, 17, 72, 93, 129, 166, 169, 177, 182, 183, 184, 188, 193
prostaglandin, 176
prostate, 154, 158, 159, 162, 165, 172, 175, 177, 179
prostate cancer, 154, 158, 159, 162, 165, 172, 175, 177, 179
prostate gland, 162
protease, 5, 10, 11, 12, 16, 104, 107, 111, 117, 166
protease inhibitor, 104, 107, 111, 117
protease inhibitors, 104
protein synthesis, 5, 6, 7, 15, 32, 188
proteinase, 11, 175
proteins, vii, 1, 2, 3, 4, 5, 7, 8, 9, 13, 16, 19, 20, 28, 29, 33, 34, 45, 47, 48, 49, 50, 51, 54, 60, 97, 104, 105, 117, 126, 127, 129, 132, 136, 148, 163, 184, 186, 190, 192, 201, 212, 218, 219, 220, 226
proteolysis, 2, 28, 32, 56, 120
proteolytic enzyme, 105
proteolytic enzymes, 105
proteomics, 16
prothrombin, 41
proto-oncogene, 64
proximal, 7, 32, 166, 177
psoriasis, viii, 183
pulmonary, 6, 7, 16, 59, 99, 155, 158, 164, 179, 184
pulmonary arteries, 158
pulmonary hypertension, 155, 158, 184
pus, 229, 240

Q

quality of life, 179

R

RA, 34, 151, 153, 154, 155, 156, 157, 158, 159, 160, 161, 162, 163, 164, 165, 166, 167, 168, 169, 170, 171, 172, 173, 180, 181, 182
radiation, 40, 46, 57, 58, 191, 196, 201, 205, 208
radiation cystitis, 46, 58
radiation therapy, 191, 205
radiotherapy, 28, 47, 171, 196, 201, 208
rapidly progressive glomerulonephritis, 7
reagents, 81
receptor, viii, 5, 6, 14, 18, 25, 29, 32, 44, 45, 47, 49, 50, 51, 53, 54, 56, 57, 60, 61, 63, 65, 66, 68, 69, 73, 76, 79, 80, 81, 82, 83, 88, 89, 97, 98, 99, 100, 101, 117, 121, 135, 137, 141, 155, 157, 158, 159, 161, 162, 163, 164, 165, 166, 168, 170, 171, 172, 173, 174, 175, 176, 178, 179, 180, 183, 185, 186, 188, 189, 191, 193, 198, 201, 202, 203, 204, 211, 212, 214, 216, 218, 230, 234, 235, 236
rectal, 46, 58
recurrence, 24, 194, 195, 196, 198, 206
red blood cell, 212, 241
red blood cells, 241
regression, vii, 10, 11, 43, 46, 47, 48, 57, 97, 109, 142, 145, 198, 228
regulators, vii, 1, 20, 31, 60, 72
remission, 196
Remodeling, 79, 155
remodelling, 79, 155
renal, viii, 8, 12, 21, 23, 24, 38, 55, 66, 139, 140, 141, 147, 148, 150, 151, 158, 172
renal cell carcinoma, 12, 21, 23, 24, 38, 55, 66
renal failure, 8, 148, 151
renal replacement therapy, viii, 139, 140, 141, 147, 148, 150
repressor, 62
resection, 23
residual disease, 27, 195
response, 6, 8, 12, 17, 19, 20, 23, 25, 27, 33, 37, 44, 48, 53, 55, 57, 59, 78, 84, 87, 93, 94, 96, 98, 99, 100, 116, 117, 118, 119, 139, 148, 152, 155, 160, 163, 165, 166, 168, 169, 171, 172, 184, 188, 193, 194, 196, 199, 200, 201, 204, 208, 216
retinal detachment, 11
reverse transcriptase, 81, 214, 217, 222, 228

rheumatoid arthritis, viii, 183
risk, viii, 8, 23, 24, 25, 27, 46, 140, 143, 144, 147, 148, 150, 151, 190, 194, 196, 197, 198
risk factor, 140, 143, 144, 148, 150, 151
risk factors, 140, 143, 144, 148, 150, 151
RNA, 80, 81, 82, 83, 93, 94, 127, 129, 132, 202, 213, 214, 217, 222, 228
rodents, 46, 47, 48
RS, 39

S

secrete, 49, 100, 160, 164, 166, 169, 201
secretion, 2, 16, 64, 99, 105, 129, 132, 133, 160, 163, 164, 165, 168, 177, 203
sensitivity, 19, 64, 88, 104, 142, 196
serum, 8, 9, 23, 25, 28, 38, 39, 41, 52, 62, 77, 86, 129, 139, 140, 143, 144, 145, 146, 147, 148, 149, 150, 151, 152, 161, 170, 178, 190, 194, 202, 204, 214, 215, 219, 221, 236, 237
serum albumin, 143
serum erythropoietin, 236
severe, 47, 52, 53, 60, 212
sex hormones, 187
shock, 48
side effects, 60, 172
side-effects, 162
sign, 149
signal peptide, 128, 130, 136
signalling pathways, 8, 15, 17, 19, 21, 27, 29, 154, 157, 161, 180, 182
silica, 107
skeletal muscle, 12, 127
skin, 8, 25, 26, 60, 129, 134, 228, 232
smoking, 143, 144
smooth muscle, vii, 2, 31, 44, 72, 79, 97, 99, 103, 104, 106, 140, 157, 165, 169, 178, 186, 213
smooth muscle cells, vii, 2, 31, 44, 72, 79, 97, 99, 103, 104, 157, 165, 169, 178, 186, 213
solution, 9, 107, 108, 122, 128, 213, 214, 215, 240
Southern blot, 80, 81, 83
species, 73, 119, 166, 184, 202
specificity, 17, 165, 171, 217, 219, 223
spindle, 130
spleen, 213
squamous, 215, 221, 224, 226, 228, 238
squamous cell, 215, 221, 224, 226, 228
squamous cell carcinoma, 215, 221, 224, 226
standard deviation, 108, 114
stenosis, 151
sterile, 81, 149, 152
steroids, vii, 71, 72, 73, 75, 76, 78, 79, 87, 100, 101, 189, 191, 193, 194, 204, 207
stimulus, 20, 87, 88, 93, 97, 126, 189
stroke, 141, 184
stroma, 72, 76, 78, 99, 102, 154, 160, 163, 167, 169, 173, 187, 203
stromal cells, 74, 88, 126, 163, 186, 199, 213, 235
subcutaneous, 8, 27, 40, 132, 136
subcutaneous (SC), 8, 27, 40, 132, 136, 203
subcutaneous injection, 40, 132
superficial bladder cancer, 59
superior, 29
surgical resection, 23
survival, vii, 18, 19, 23, 28, 43, 45, 49, 51, 52, 63, 66, 163, 170, 172, 178, 184, 190, 194, 197, 198, 199, 206, 208, 212, 221, 226, 227
survival rate, 45
syndrome, 7, 10, 11, 23, 24, 29, 31, 32, 34, 38, 53, 185
synergistic, 20, 28, 37, 116, 119, 121
systolic blood pressure, 139

T

therapeutic interventions, viii, 140, 150
threshold, 109
thrombin, 22, 202
thrombomodulin, 87, 100
thyroid, 58
tissue inhibitor of MMP (TIMP), 33, 161, 170
tissue inhibitors of metalloproteinase (TIMP), 33, 161, 170
tissue plasminogen activator, 19
tissues, viii, 12, 16, 20, 44, 45, 46, 48, 50, 58, 74, 77, 87, 101, 104, 106, 118, 122, 127, 137, 153, 154, 155, 157, 167, 171, 179, 184, 188, 193, 200, 211, 213, 215, 216, 217, 219, 220, 221, 223, 229, 233, 240
TNF-alpha, 177
TNF-α, 22
total cholesterol, 142, 144
toxic effect, 46
toxic effects, 46
toxicity, 25, 27, 28, 29, 48
toxin, 164
transcription, 22, 55, 62, 66, 87, 88, 97, 99, 129, 132, 133, 153, 154, 160, 165, 166, 168, 180, 184, 193, 206
transcription factors, 55, 180, 184

transducer, 187
transduction, v, 17, 19, 37, 43, 44, 48, 49, 54, 55, 56, 61, 62, 65, 67, 179, 180, 202, 203, 212, 214, 216, 219, 226, 234
transfection, 18, 19, 54, 87, 129, 133, 138, 214, 232
transformation, 162, 165
transforming growth factor, 10, 47, 121, 186, 188, 196
transforming growth factor (TGF), 10, 47, 49, 121, 160, 165, 169, 170, 177, 186, 188, 196
transitional cell carcinoma (TCC), 23, 24, 38, 68
translation, 8, 96
translocation, 14, 15, 22, 44, 180
transplantation, 232
treatment, viii, 10, 13, 14, 25, 26, 27, 28, 31, 37, 38, 40, 41, 46, 48, 53, 55, 57, 58, 66, 72, 73, 74, 75, 76, 77, 78, 82, 83, 94, 109, 117, 129, 130, 131, 132, 135, 139, 140, 142, 147, 148, 149, 150, 154, 157, 158, 161, 162, 163, 168, 171, 172, 173, 175, 178, 189, 194, 195, 197, 198, 208, 224, 228, 240
triglycerides, 142, 143, 144
trimolecular complex (TMC), 14
trisomy, 23
trypsin, 128
tumor cells, 32, 37, 44, 46, 47, 49, 50, 55, 68, 104, 136, 183, 185, 189, 196, 199, 202, 203, 207, 211, 221, 226, 227, 229, 230, 233, 236, 238
tumor growth, vii, 30, 31, 32, 33, 34, 35, 40, 41, 43, 46, 47, 48, 59, 60, 98, 126, 134, 136, 137, 138, 174, 176, 183, 184, 191, 193, 195, 201, 207, 212, 213, 221, 227, 229, 230
tumor invasion, 31
tumor metastasis, 195
tumor necrosis factor, 196
tumor necrosis factor (TNF), 22, 94, 95, 151, 160, 164, 165, 169, 170, 177, 196
tumor progression, 30, 40, 45, 49, 59, 185, 187, 194, 195, 197, 198, 199, 200
tumors, vii, 30, 38, 39, 41, 43, 46, 47, 48, 55, 57, 58, 59, 60, 72, 117, 125, 127, 129, 132, 134, 136, 174, 176, 185, 187, 188, 189, 190, 191, 193, 194, 195, 197, 198, 199, 200, 203, 213, 221, 222, 223, 224, 226, 227, 228, 230, 232, 233, 238, 239, 240, 241
tumour growth, vii, 1, 2, 8, 9, 28, 160, 161, 163, 164, 169, 172, 173, 179, 199
tumour necrosis factor, 179
tyrosine, 17, 22, 28, 36, 44, 45, 48, 50, 51, 53, 54, 61, 63, 64, 65, 66, 68, 69, 168, 169, 170, 178, 180, 186, 188, 201, 202, 203, 212, 219, 226

U

ultrasonography, viii, 139, 142, 147, 152
ultrasound, 107, 176
umbilical, 5, 54, 80, 88, 166
urokinase, 60, 107, 120, 121
uterine, viii, 46, 72, 73, 74, 75, 79, 89, 97, 98, 99, 100, 204, 211, 212, 213, 216, 217, 219, 220, 221, 223, 227, 228, 229, 234, 235, 237, 241
uterine cancer, 211, 221, 223, 227, 228, 229, 235
uterus, 81, 98, 99, 212, 215, 216, 218, 220, 234, 236, 237

V

variance, 108
vascular, viii, 2, 3, 28, 30, 32, 37, 38, 39, 40, 41, 46, 49, 50, 51, 52, 53, 56, 57, 58, 59, 60, 61, 62, 63, 64, 65, 66, 69, 71, 72, 73, 74, 75, 76, 78, 79, 91, 97, 98, 99, 100, 101, 104, 120, 121, 126, 127, 137, 138, 139, 140, 141, 142, 144, 147, 148, 149, 151, 152, 153, 154, 157, 166, 167, 171, 175, 176, 177, 178, 179, 183, 184, 185, 186, 188, 191, 194, 195, 196, 198, 199, 200, 201, 202, 203, 204, 205, 206, 207, 208, 211, 213, 216, 220, 224, 226, 228, 230, 232, 236, 239, 241
vascular cell adhesion molecule (VCAM), viii, 88, 100, 139, 140, 142, 143, 145, 146, 147, 148, 149, 151, 152
vascular endothelial growth factor (VEGF), 3, 57, 72, 73, 76, 153, 154, 183, 184, 191, 202, 204, 205
vasculature, 2, 4, 6, 11, 17, 27, 41, 46, 50, 51, 57, 72, 73, 80, 93, 153, 165, 166, 168, 170, 171, 172, 184, 185, 187, 196, 201, 229
vasoactive intestinal peptide, 178
vasoconstriction, 157, 158, 172
vasodilation, 76
vasodilator, 99, 171, 174
vasopressor, 166
vector, 10, 55, 67, 127, 129, 215
VEGF expression, 89, 97, 153, 160, 161, 163, 165, 166, 167, 168, 172, 185, 188, 189, 192, 193, 198
VEGF protein, 168, 189
veins, 5, 37, 54, 80, 87, 88, 141, 166
venous, 61
ventilation, 184
ventral, 17
venules, 217, 220

vertebrate, 184
vessel, 2, 16, 26, 29, 30, 44, 45, 50, 51, 57, 63, 71, 73, 75, 76, 91, 97, 111, 116, 121, 167, 186, 194, 201, 206, 241
vessels, 2, 44, 45, 46, 47, 50, 51, 53, 55, 68, 72, 73, 76, 79, 80, 87, 89, 90, 91, 92, 104, 126, 147, 155, 160, 163, 167, 168, 172, 185, 194, 196, 199, 200, 220, 228, 229, 232, 240, 241
viral, 28
virus, 55, 67, 186, 201, 214
vision, 34
vital, vii, 1, 2, 16, 19, 108, 123
vitreous, 11
vomiting, 46
Vomiting, 46

W

western blot, 129, 132, 133, 214, 216, 218, 226, 228, 231
wild type, 8, 50, 53
women, 72, 89, 98, 99, 100, 190, 197, 204, 205
wound healing, viii, 2, 8, 9, 26, 33, 104, 113, 118, 169, 183, 195

X

xenografts, 6, 7, 10, 28, 57, 163, 172, 173, 200, 211, 212, 213, 214, 227, 228, 230, 231, 232, 235, 236, 241, 242

Y

yeast, 9, 54

Z

Zinc, 12, 35